Two week

loans return

J. Ring   H. Behrendt (Eds.)

New Trends in Allergy V

Springer

Berlin
Heidelberg
New York
Hong Kong
London
Milan
Paris
Tokyo

J. Ring   H. Behrendt (Eds.)

New Trends in Allergy V

With 60 Figures and 56 Tables

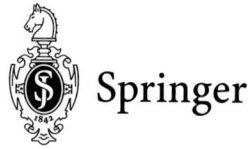 Springer

Johannes Ring, Prof. Dr. Dr.
Klinik und Poliklinik für Dermatologie
und Allergologie am Biederstein
Klinikum Rechts der Isar
Technische Universität München
Biedersteiner Straße 29
80802 München, Germany

Heidrun Behrendt, Prof. Dr.
ZAUM – Zentrum für Allergie und Umwelt
Klin. Kooperationsgruppe Umweltdermatologie
und Allergologie GSF
Technische Universität München
Biedersteiner Straße 29
80802 München, Germany

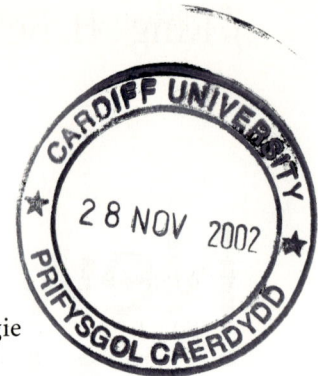

ISBN 3-540-43082-2 Springer-Verlag Berlin Heidelberg New York

Library of Congress Cataloging-in-Publication Data.
New trends in allergy V / [Johannes Ring, Heidrun Behrendt (eds.)]. p. ; cm.
Includes bibliographical references and index.
ISBN 3540430822 (alk. paper)
1. Allergy–Congresses. I. Title: New trends in allergy 5. II. Title: New trends in allergy five.
III: Ring, Johannes, 1945- IV. Behrendt, H. (Heidrun), 1945-
[DNLM: 1. Hypersensitivity–Congresses. 2. Dermatitis, Atopic–Congresses. 3. Environmen-
tal Illness–Congresses. 4. Environmental Pollutants–immunology–Congresses. 5. Hypersen-
sitivity–genetics–Congresses. 6. Hypersensitivity–therapy–Congresses. WD 300 N5324 2003]
RC584.N484 2003 616.97--dc21

Springer-Verlag Berlin Heidelberg New York
a member of BertelsmannSpringer Science+Business Media GmbH

http://www.springer.de/medizin

© Springer-Verlag Berlin Heidelberg 2002
Printed in Germany

The use of general descriptive names, registered names, trademarks, etc. in this publication
does not imply, even in the absence of a specific statement, that such names are exempt from
the relevant protective laws and regulations and therefore free for general use.

Product liability: The publishers cannot guarantee the accuracy of any information about
dosage and application contained in this book. In every individual case the user must check
such information by consulting the relevant literature.

Cover design: *design & production* GmbH, Heidelberg
Typesetting: Goldener Schnitt, Sinzheim
SPIN: 10857920   24/3130   5 4 3 2 1 0 – Printed on acid-free paper

Contents

Atopic Eczema and Allergic Skin Diseases

Food Allergy and Anaphylaxis

Occupational and Environmental Aspects

List of Chairpersons (not listed as First Authors)

W. Aberer, Graz

P. Arenberger, Praha

J. Bienenstock, Hamilton

K. Blaser, Davos

O. Braun-Falco, München

O. Herbarth, Leipzig

K. Nekam, Budapest

U. Müller, Bern

T. Platts-Mills, Charlottesville

E. Richter, München

J. Ring, München

M. Schlaak, Borstel

G. Schultze-Werninghaus, Bochum

K. Thesdrup-Pedersen, Aarhus

Ch. Virchow, Freiburg

J. Wenning, Villingen-Schwenningen

List of First Authors

Akdis M., MD
Schweizerisches Institut für Allergie und Asthmaforschung,
Obere Strasse 22, 7270 Davos, Switzerland

Becker W.-M., Dr. rer. nat.
Forschungsinstitut Borstel, Parkallee 35, 23845 Borstel, Germany

Behrendt H., Prof. Dr. med.
ZAUM – Zentrum Allergie und Umwelt, Klin. Kooperationsgruppe
Umweltdermatologie und Allergologie GSF/TU München,
Biedersteinerstraße 29, 80802 München, Germany

Braun A., Dr. med.
Klinikum der Phillips-Universität Marburg, Abteilung für
Klinische Chemie und Molekulare Diagnostik, Marburg,
Germany

Breuer K., Dr.
Fraunhofer Institut für Bauphysik, Postfach 1182, 83601 Holzkirchen,
Germany

Breuer K., Dr.
Hautklinik Linden, Medizinische Hochschule Hannover,
Germany

Ciprandi G., Dr.
Clinica de Malattie dell'Apparato Respiratorio E Allergologia,
Universitá de Genova, Largo Rosanna Benzi 10, 16132 Genova, Italy

Darsow U., Priv. Doz. Dr.
Klinik und Poliklinik für Dermatologie und Allergologie am
Biederstein, TU München, Biedersteinerstraße 29, 80802 München,
Germany

Dubakiene R., Prof. Dr.
Allergy Centre Vilnius University, Zemynos 17–10, Vilnius 2022,
Lithuania

EBERLEIN-KÖNIG B., Priv. Doz. Dr.
Klinik und Poliklinik für Dermatologie und Allergologie am
Biederstein, TU München, Biedersteinerstraße 29, 80802 München,
Germany

GAUGER, A., Dr.
Klinik und Poliklinik für Dermatologie und Allergologie am
Biederstein, TU München, Biedersteinerstraße 29, 80802 München,
Germany

JAKOB T., Dr.
Klin. Kooperationsgruppe Umweltdermatologie & Allergologie
GSF/TU München, Klinik und Poliklinik für Dermatologie und
Allergologie am Biederstein, TU München, Biedersteinerstraße 29,
80802 München, Germany

KAPP A., Prof. Dr.
Klinik und Poliklinik für Dermatologie und Venerologie der
Medizinischen Hochschule, Ricklinger Straße 5, 30449 Hannover,
Germany

KEMENY M., Prof. Dr.
Department of Immunology, Rayne Institute, 123 Coldharbour Lane,
London SE5 9NU, UK

KRÄMER U., Dr.
Medizinisches Institut für Umwelthygiene an der Heinrich-
Heine-Universität Düsseldorf, Auf'm Hennekamp 4,
40225 Düsseldorf, Germany

KRIEG A.M., Ass. Prof. MD
Department of Internal Medicine, University of Iowa, 54 EMRB,
Iowa City, IA 52242, USA

KREUTNER W., MD
Schering Plough Research Institute, 2000 Galloping Hill Road,
Kenilworth, NJ 07033-1300, USA

KOWALSKI M., Prof. Dr.
Department of Clinical Immunology, University School of
Medicine Lodz, 11 Mazowiecka Street, 93315 Lodz, Poland

KUREK M., Prof. Dr.
Department of Dermatology, Medical University of Gdansk,
Ul. Debinki 7, 80211 Gdansk, Poland

LEVI-SCHAFFER F., Prof. Dr.
Department of Pharmacology, Hadassah Medical School,
P.O. Box 12065, Jerusalem, Israel

LORBER R., MD
Schering Plough Research Institute, 2000 Galloping Hill Road,
Kenilworth, NJ 07033-1300, USA

LØWENSTEIN H., Prof. Dr.
13166 ALK A/S, Boge Allee 10–12, 2970 Horsholm, Denmark

MARINKOVICH V.A., MD
Hitachi Chemical Diagnostics Inc., 630 Clyde Court,
Mountain View, CA 94043, USA

MÉCHERI S., Dr.
Unité d'Immuno-Allergie, Institut Pasteur, 28 rue Dr. Roux,
75724 Paris, Cedex 15, France

VAN NEERVEN J., Dr.
Kruislaan 318, 1321 BW Amsterdam, The Netherlands

OROPEZA-WEKERLE R.-L., Dr.
Klin. Kooperationsgruppe an der Klinik und Poliklinik für
Dermatologie und Allergologie am Biederstein, TU München,
Biedersteinerstraße 29, 80802 München, Germany

PAWANKAR R., Prof. Dr.
Department of Otolaryngology, Nippon Medical School,
113-8603 Tokyo, Japan

PODDA M., Dr.
Zentrum der Dermatologie und Venerologie (ZDV),
Klinikum der Johann Wolfgang Goethe-Universität Frankfurt,
Theodor-Stern-Kai 7, 60590 Frankfurt, Germany

PRZYBILLA B., Prof. Dr.
Dermatologische Klinik und Poliklinik, Klinikum
Innenstadt der Ludwig Maximillians-Universität München,
Frauenlobstraße 9-11, 80337 München, Germany

SALOGA J., Priv. Doz. Dr.
Universitäts-Hautklinik Mainz, Langenbeckstraße 1, 55131 Mainz,
Germany
SIMON H.-U., Prof. Dr.

Pharmakologisches Institut der Universität Bern,
Friedbühlstrasse 49, 3010 Bern, Switzerland

SOLOMON, A., Priv.-Doz. Dr.
Department of Pharmacology, Hadassah Medical School,
P.O. Box 12065, Jerusalem, Israel

TURJANMAA K., Prof. Dr.
Department of Dermatology, Tampere University Hospital,
PO Box 2000, 33521 Tampere, Finland

VIELUF I., Dr.
Zentrum für Dermatologie, Allergologie, Pädiatrie und
Umweltmedizin, Fachklinikum Borkum, Jann-Berghaus-Straße 49,
26757 Borkum, Germany

VOCKS E., Prof. Dr.
Deutsche Klinik für Dermatologie und Allergie,
Alexanderhausklinik, Tobelmühlestrasse 2,
7270 Davos-Platz, Switzerland

DE WECK A.L., Prof. Dr.
Research Laboratory, 14 Grand Places, 1700 Fribourg,
Switzerland

WOLLENBERG A., Priv.-Doz. Dr.
Dermatologische Klinik und Poliklinik,
der Ludwig Maximillians-Universität München,
Frauenlobstraße 9-11, 80337 München, Germany

WOHLRAB W., Prof. Dr.
Universitätsklinik und Poliklinik für Dermatologie
und Venerologie, Medizinische Klinik der Universität
Halle-Wittenberg, Ernst-Kromayer-Straße 5-6,
06112 Halle, Germany

ZOLLNER T.M., Priv.-Doz. Dr.
Zentrum der Dermatologie und Venerologie (ZDV),
Klinikum der Johann Wolfgang Goethe-Universität Frankfurt,
Theodor-Stern-Kai 7, 60590 Frankfurt, Germany

Preface

Allergy is one of the major health problems of most modern societies. Allergic diseases have increased in prevalence during the last decades; the reasons for this increase are unknown, there are only hypothetical concepts for explanation.

The series *New Trends in Allergy* now covers five volumes originating from special international symposia, started in 1980 and held every 5 years, which highlight specific areas of progress in allergy research and practice. The idea behind the 5-year interval between these symposia is that real new developments do not occur very often and certainly not every year.

The contents of this book focus on specific areas where progress in allergy research has shown fascinating developments, such as:

- Elucidation of the complex genetic basis of atopy
- The influence of environmental pollutants as well as natural biological environmental factors on allergy
- Gene-environment interactions in the development of allergy
- Psycho-neuro-immunological aspects of allergic sensitisation and disease
- The nature and function of dendritic cells in skin and mucous membranes
- Interactions between lymphocytes and effector cells, such as mast cells, eosinophils and neutrophils
- Allergen carriers, allergen release and bioavailability, allergen structure
- Atopic eczema
- Asthma and rhinoconjunctivitis
- Food allergy and anaphylaxis
- Pharmacotherapy
- Unspecific (e.g. anti-IgE) and allergen-specific immunotherapy

While there has been a remarkable advancement in the understanding of complex mechanisms involved in allergic sensitisation and disease, there is still a large gap between theoretical knowledge and practical benefit to patients, as shown in this volume.

The editors would like to thank the participants, invited speakers, poster presenters, chair persons and all those involved in the organisation of the symposium in Davos, especially Mrs. Nora Enderlein and Dr. Ulf Darsow and co-workers both from the Department of Dermatology and Allergy Biederstein at the Technical University in Munich and the „Deutsche Klinik für Dermatologie und Allergie Alexanderhaus- Klinik" in Davos. Thanks also to Mrs. Wenger from Davos Tourism.

The scientific part of the symposium was enriched by the musical „The Odyssey of Allergy"performed by co-workers of the Munich Department, which allowed a humorous look at our human and scientific endeavours in allergology.

We hope that this book contributes to the better understanding of allergy for the benefit of the increasing number of patients worldwide.

Munich, March 2002   JOHANNES RING
                                                          HEIDRUN BEHRENDT

Epidemiology, Genetic and Environmental Factors

1 Pollen Grains Contain and Release Not Only Allergens, but Also Eicosanoid-Like Substances with Neutrophil Chemotactic Activity: A New Step in the Initiation of Allergic Sensitization?

H. Behrendt, A. Kasche, C. Traidl, S. Plötz, J. Huss-Marp, U. risse, C. Ebner von Eschenbach, J. Ring

Summary

Pollen grains as allergen carriers are the elicitors of the most common allergic diseases, namely seasonal allergic rhinoconjunctivitis („hay fever"), extrinsic bronchial asthma and other immediate-type allergic diseases.

All of them have increased in prevalence dramatically during the last decades. It is common belief that pollen themselves are inert and act by release of protein allergens in humid conditions on the mucosal surface, where the process of sensitization starts through the recognition of the allergen by an antigen-presenting cell. All studies dealing with the mechanism of this early phase of sensitization have used isolated allergens (from extracts or recombinant technology) as stimulus. However, under natural exposure conditions, the bioavailability of allergen depends upon allergen liberation from internal binding sites within the allergen carrier, here the pollen grain. It is not the soluble allergen, but rather the pollen grain as a particle which comes into contact with the body's surface on the skin or the mucosa. We have shown earlier that the release of allergen from pollen grains can be modulated by external factors such as gaseous or particulate air pollutants.

We now have found that pollen grains from different plants (Timothy grass = *Phleum pratense*, birch = *Betula alba*) secrete significant amounts of eicosanoid-like substances in protein-free buffer solution in a pH, time and temperature-dependent fashion. When pure pollen grains were incubated together with suspensions of human polymorphonuclear leucocytes (PMN), these cells assembled around the pollen grains and showed signs of activation and mediator release leading to destruction of the pollen grain. Leukotriene B4-like activity secreted differed between pollen species with highest values for grass and birch pollen and significantly lower values for pine pollen (*Pinus silvestris*). Furthermore there was a significant modulatory effect from traffic-related pollutants, e.g. volatile organic compounds (VOCs) leading to a significant increase in secretion of LTB4-like activity from pollen grains.

This finding opens a new dimension in understanding the early events in allergic sensitization indicating that pro-inflammatory effects of the allergen carrier itself (the pollen grain) induce activation of cellular constituents of the host. We propose to call this phase the „initiation" of allergic sensitization. The differences in allergenic „potency" of various allergens may be explained by these new findings independent of allergen release from pollen. It also may be helpful in understanding so far unexplained differences in allergy prevalence associated with automobile exhaust exposure.

New Trends in Allergy V
J. Ring, H. Behrendt (Eds)
© Springer-Verlag Berlin, Heidelberg 2002

Introduction

Allergic diseases (namely allergic rhinoconjunctivitis, bronchial asthma, atopic eczema) have increased in prevalence during the last decades world-wide; the causes for this increase are not known. Among hypothetical concepts under discussion, lack of adequate stimulation of the immune system, improved hygiene, socio-economic factors („life style") as well as influence of environmental pollutants have gained substantial public and scientific attention [1, 3, 6, 10, 11, 14, 16, 18, 22–25].

Allergies are among those few diseases in which environmental factors of both natural and anthropogenic origin have been identified as causal in the disease both in the development of sensitization as well as in the elicitation and aggravation of disease symptoms. We have shown earlier that outdoor air pollution differs strikingly in quality – not only in quantity – between former Eastern and Western European countries, whereby the modern type air pollution – characterized by organic compounds, nitrogen oxides, fine particles and ozone – was associated in multivariate regression analyses with increased prevalence of IgE-mediated sensitization and atopic disease [3, 10, 18]. Pollen grains collected from industrial regions with high polycyclic aromatic hydrocarbon load in West Germany, not in East Germany were shown to be agglomerated with fine airborne particles leading to morphological changes of the pollen surface and altered allergen release [1, 2]. Thus the bioavailability of pollen allergens may be influenced by interaction between pollen and air pollutants in the atmosphere [4]. It is common belief that allergic sensitization starts with the contact between the allergen and the surface of the antigen-presenting cell at the level of the mucosa or the skin. Most studies dealing with this aspect have used allergen extracts as stimulus. Under natural exposure conditions, however, the bioavailability of allergen depends on allergen liberation from internal binding sites within the allergen carrier (e.g. pollen grains) [4, 7, 13, 21]. Here we report the surprising finding that pollen grains themselves liberate substances with pro-inflammatory activity under humid conditions.

Allergen Liberation from Pollen Grains

Pollen grains are multicellular male gametothytes of both angiosperms and gymnosperms. Anemophilous pollen from gymnosperms (wind-transported) like grass pollen are sealed in a double-layered wall with an outer layer (exine) (containing the lipophilic sporopollenin) and a softer inner layer (intine) enclosing the cytoplasm with subcellular organelles, starch granules and polysaccharide particles [21]. Pollen allergens are bound within the pollen grain around organelles, P-particles and starch granules, some in the cytoplasmic matrix. The liberation of allergens from intracellular binding sites is the prerequisite for allergic sensitization in a pre-disposed individual. The most important stimulus for allergen liberation is humidity [4, 7, 8, 20, 21]; under humid conditions, allergens are rapidly released from pollen grains in pH and temperature-dependent fashion through small caniculi connecting the inner surface of the intine with the outer pollen surface.

Allergen liberation from pollen grains can occur in two different compartments:

- On the surface of the mucosa of the upper respiratory tract
- Outside the individual organism in the ambient air [1, 2]

Allergenic activity has been detected in air samples and fractions below 1 μm in diameter [19, 20].

Influence of Air Pollutants on Allergen Bioavailability

Pollen collected in polluted atmospheres over West German cities have been found to show particle agglomeration onto the pollen surface (see Fig. 1) as well as signs of local preactivation [1]. Pollen collected at road sides with heavy traffic showed significantly reduced allergen release compared to pollen collected from rural

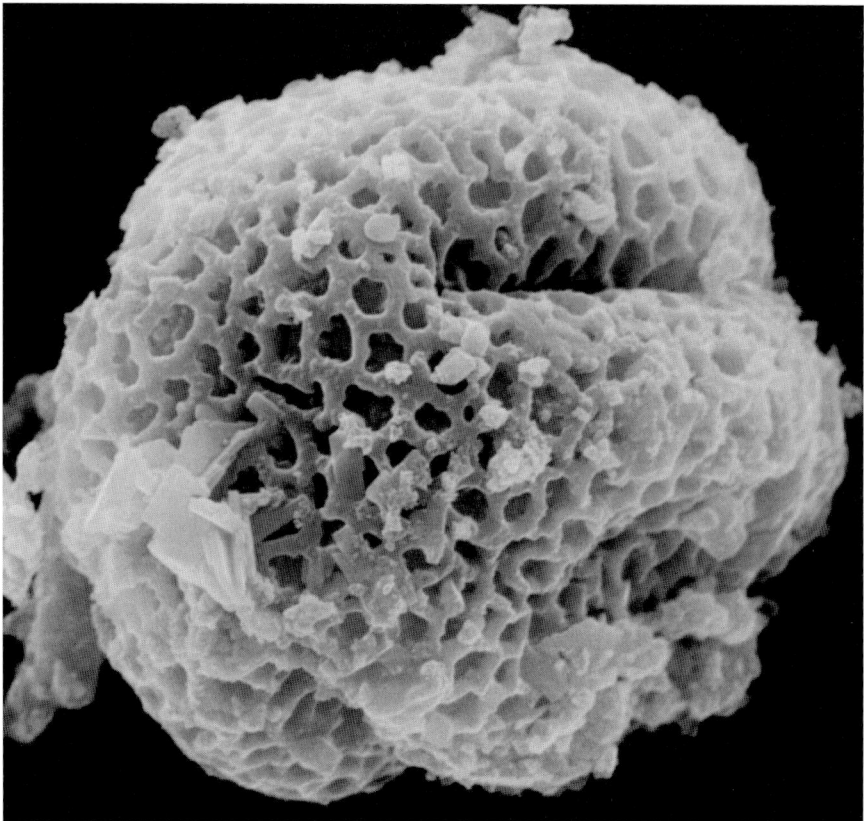

Fig. 1. Scanning electron micrograph of a pollen grain from an urban collection site showing particle agglomeration onto pollen surface.

meadows [4]. Since traffic exposure has been found to be associated with high prevalence rates of allergic sensitization and disease [10, 23], this finding might indicate a continuous release of allergen from pollen and binding of free allergen to airborne particles (e.g. diesel exhaust particles).

Using a specially constructed fluidized bed reactor, the influence of both gaseous and particulate air pollutants upon allergen release from pollen has been studied in a dose, time and humidity-dependent fashion [2, 4, 15]. Exposure of pollen to high concentrations of SO_2 did not affect allergen release [15]. This observation could help to explain the well-known paradoxic finding of lower asthma and hay fever prevalence rates in children from heavily polluted areas in former East Germany (SO_2) compared with children from West Germany (type II air pollution) [3, 12] (see below).

These findings led to the hypothesis that allergen-containing aerosols are generated through pollen-particle interaction in a moist atmosphere.

Release of Eicosanoid-Like Proinflammatory Mediators from Pollen Grains

Pollen grains incubated in phosphate-buffered saline secreted significant amounts of eicosanoid-like substances as measured by enzyme-immuno assay for leukotriene B4 (30 min at 37°C, pH 6, 7.4 and 9.0).

There were significant differences in total amounts of eicosanoid-like substance released between different pollen species: The highest values were found from birch pollen, grass and mugwort pollen, whereas pine pollen showed only little LTB4-like immunoreactivity [5].

When pollen grains were brought into contact with human neutrophil granulocytes, neutrophils were attracted and bound firmly to the pollen surface showing signs of activation and release of neutrophil mediators (C. Traidl, in prep.).

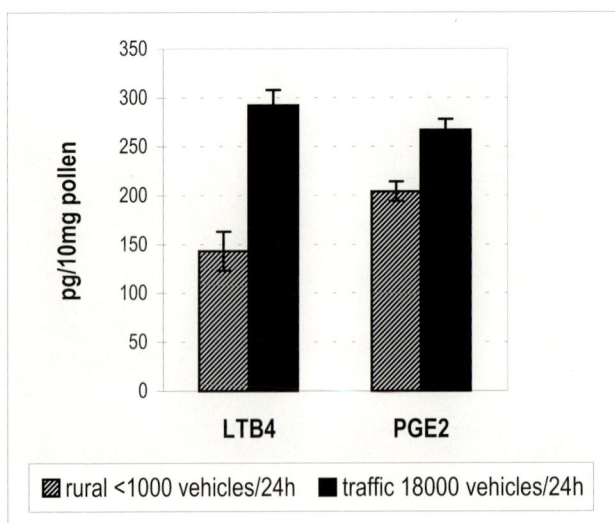

Fig. 2. Enhanced release of eicosanoid-like substances from *P. pratense* pollen freshly collected from traffic-exposed area compared to a rural meadow [5]

Similar findings were observed for the interaction between pollen grains and eosinophil granulocytes (S. Plötz, in prep.).

There were significant differences between various pollen grain sources: Pollen freshly collected from pollinating *Phleum pratense* (Timothy grass) growing on a rural meadow in upper Bavaria with a car traffic below 1,000 vehicles/24 hours showed a significantly reduced release of pro-inflammatory eicosanoid-like substances compared to pollen freshly collected and growing on the roadside of a high-traffic road in Southern Munich (car traffic more 18,000 vehicles/24 hours) (Fig. 2).

In the fluidized bed reactor, pollen grains were exposed to different types of air pollutants under various degrees of relative humidity. There was a marked enhancement of proinflammatory LTB_4-like substances by exposure to volatile organic compounds (characteristic for type II air pollution) [15].

Conclusions

These findings which have to be further studied in detail have wide implications; they open a new dimension in the understanding of the early events in allergic sensitization indicating that pro-inflammatory effects produced by the allergen carrier itself (namely the pollen grain) contribute to the activation of cellular constituents of the host, as e.g. neutrophil granulocytes or eosinophils. It is especially remarkable that pollen grains from plants with high allergenicity (birch grass, mugwort) produce significantly higher amounts of these pro-inflammatory substances than pine pollen with a much less pronounced allergenicity. Thus, the term „allergenic potency" might have to be re-defined; it should not only be considered at the molecular level of the protein structure of the allergen, but maybe also include the characteristics of allergen release and bioavailability from its carrier. The process of initiation of sensitization precedes the contact between allergen and antigen-presenting cell and may be the very first step in atopic sensitization, later followed by T-cell activation, antibody production and development of immunological memory as well as recruitment of amplificatory cells.

The aspect of allergen bioavailability should be considered more thoroughly in the future. Unfortunately, until today, only little data are available regarding a quantitative dose-response relationship for outdoor allergen exposure and allergic sensitization or disease.

Acknowledgements. This work was partly supported by a Federal grant (BMBF) „Klinische Forschergruppe Molecular and Applied Allergotoxicology" and a grant from the Bavarian Minister for Environment and Land Development (BStLU).

References

1. Behrendt H, Friedrichs K, Kainka-Staenicke E, Darsow U, Becker WM, Tomingas R: Allergens and pollutants in the air – A complex interaction; in Ring J, Przybilla B (eds): New Trends in Allergy III. Berlin, Springer, 1991, pp 467–478

2. Behrendt H, Becker WM, Friedrich KH, Darsow U, Tomingas R: Interaction between aero-allergens and airborne particulate matter: Int Arch Allergy Immunol 1992;99:425–428

3. Behrendt H, Friedrichs KH, Krämer U, Hitzfeld B, Becker WM, Ring J: The role of indoor and outdoor air pollution in allergic diseases. Prog Allergy Clin Immunol 1995;3:83–89

4. Behrendt H, Becker WM: Localization, release and bioavailability of pollen allergens: the influence of environmental factors. Curr. Opinion Immunol 2001;13:709–715

5. Behrendt H, Tomczok J, Sliwa-Tomczok W, Kasche A, Ebner von Eschenbach C, Becker WM, Ring J: Timothy grass (*Phleum pratense* L.) pollen as allergen carriers and initiators of an allergic response. Int Arch Allergy Immunol 1999;118:414–418

6. Burney PGJ, Luczynska C, Chinn S, Jarvis D: The European Community Respiratory Health Survey. Eur Respir J 1994;7:954–960

7. Grote M, Vrtala S, Niederberger V, Valenta R, Reichelt R: Expulsion of allergen-containing materials from hydrated rye grass (*Lolium perenne*) pollen revealed by using immunogold field emission scanning and transmission electron microscopy. J Allergy Clin Immunol 2000;105:1140–1145

8. Knox RB: Grass pollen, thunderstorms and asthma. Clin Allergy 1993;23:354–359

9. Kowalski ML, Grzegorczyk J, Sliwinska-Kowalska M, Wojciechowska B, Rozniecka M, Rozniecka J: Neutrophil Chemotactic activity (NCA) nasal secretions from atopic and nonatopic subjects. Allergy 1993;48:409–414

10. Krämer U, Koch T, Ranft U, Ring J, Behrendt H: Traffic-related air pollution is associated with atopy in children living in urban areas. Epidemiology 2000;11:64–70

11. Miyamoto T, Takafuji S: Environment and allergy; in Ring J, Przybilla B (eds): New Trends in Allergy III. Berlin, Springer, 1991, pp 459–468

12. Mutius E, von Weiland SK, Fritzsch C, Duhme H, Keil U: Increasing prevalence of hay fever and atopy among children in Leipzig, East Germany. Lancet 1998;351:862–866

13. Rantio-Lehtimäki A: Aerobiology of pollen and pollen allergens. In: Bioaerosols Handbook. Edited by Cox CS, Wathes CM. Boca Raton: Lewis, 1995:387–406

14. Ring J: Allergy and modern society: Does „western life style" promote the development of allergies? Int Arch Allerg Immunol 1997;113:7–10

15. Risse U, Tomczok J, Huss-Marp J, Darsow U, Behrendt H: Health-relevant interaction between airborne particulate matter and aeroallergens (pollen). J Aerosol Sci 2000;31, Suppl 1:27–28

16. Rusnak C: The impact of pollution on allergic disease. Allergy 1994;49:21–27

17. Sass-Kuhn SP, Moqbel R, Mackay JA, Cromwell O, Kay AB: Human granulocyte/pollen-binding protein: Recognition and identification as transferrin. J Clin Invest 1984;73:202–210

18. Schäfer T, Vieluf D, Behrendt H, Krämer U, Ring J: Atopic eczema and other manifestations of atopy: Results of an East-West-German comparison. Allergy 1996;51:532–539

19. Schäppi GF, Monn C, Wüthrich B, Wanner HU: Direct determination of allergens in ambient aerosols: Methodological aspects. Int Arch Allergy Immunol 1996;110:364–370

20. Spieksma F, Kramps JA, van der Linden AC, Nikkels BH, Plomp A, Koerten HK, Dijkman JH: Evidence of grass pollen allergenic activity in the smaller micronic atmospheric fraction. Clin Exp Allergy 1990;20:273–280

21. Stanley RG, Linskens HF (eds): Pollen. Biology – Biochemistry – Management. Berlin, Springer, 1974

22. The International Study of Asthma and Allergies in Childhood (ISAAC) Steering Committee: Worldwide variation in prevalence of symptoms of asthma, allergic rhinoconjunctivitis, and atopic eczema: ISAAC. Lancet 1998;351:1225–1232

23. Weiland SK, Mundt KA, Rückmann A, Keil U: Self-reported wheezing and allergic rhinitis in children and traffic density on street of residence. Ann Epidemiol 1994;4:243–247

24. Wichmann H: Environment, life-style and allergy: The German answer. Allergo J 1995;6:315–316

25. Wüthrich B: Epidemiology of the allergic diseases; are they really on the increase? Int Arch Allerg Appl Immunol 1989;90:3–10

2 House Dust Mites in Stuffed Toys as a Cause of Allergy in Lithuania

R. Dubakiene, A. Dautartiene

Introduction

The house dust mites as a cause of allergy were studied from 1980 in Lithuania. In our previous studies, it was proved that the mite *Dermatophagoides pteronyssinus* is the main house dust allergen in Lithuania [1]. The sensitization to *D. pteronyssinus* (Dpt) among patients with asthma reached more than 90% of cases [1]. It was established that the main source of Dpt allergen is the inherited pillows and quilts from native village houses in Lithuania [1, 2]. The changes in social-economic life reflect on ecological conditions in the country. So, the aim of recent study was to compare the possible changes in house dust mite acarofauna and to investigate new sources of mite Dpt as a cause of allergy in Lithuania.

Methods

The house dust mite samples were collected by vacuum cleaner with special filters from mattresses, stuffed toys and carpets. Dust samples for detecting the mites were poured into Petri dishes and examined by light microscopy. All living mites and a part of the dead individuals were picked out. Further, the flotation method was used [3]. The mites were isolated from the upper fraction of the flotation solution and examined under the microscope. In addition, the „Acarex" test was used to detect the presence of mite guanin (feces). House dust samples were mixed with reagents, and by color change the existence of mite allergen was detected. The house dust samples were collected four times a year in Vilnius pre-schools, taking 14 samples at each institution per day.

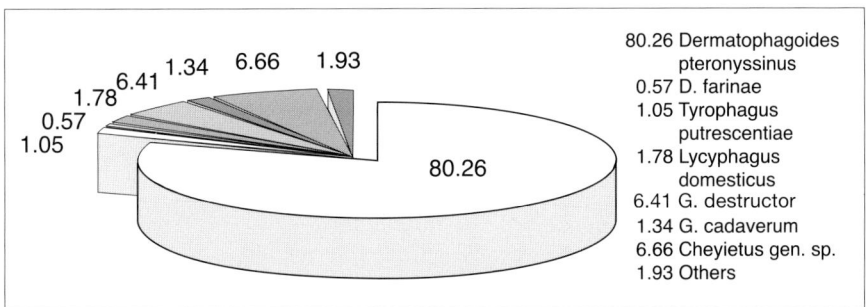

Fig. 1. The house dust mite fauna in Lithuania (%)

Results

The data on house dust mite fauna are presented in Figure 1. The figure shows that the main mite is *D. pteronyssinus* – 80.21% of all species. Glycyphagidae and Cheyletidae form more than 62% of acarofauna. The rest of the species are in fewer amounts. The comparative data in a 20-year period are presented in Table 1. The great changes in acarofauna had happened after 20 years in Lithuania. the lower amounts of *D. pteronyssinus*, 66±20 instead of 399±170 ($p<0.001$), the more *D. farinae* than *D. pteronyssinus* per 1 g of dust and the higher the rate of occurrence: 20.68% instead of 5.71% detected 20 years ago ($p<0.001$). Similar findings are presented by another mite species.

Table 1. The house dust acarofauna in a 20-year period in Lithuania

| Species | Rate of occurrence (%) | | Mite number per 1 g of dust | | | |
| | | | Limits | | In average | |
	1	2	1	2	1	2
Family Pyroglyphidae						
Dermatophagoides pteronyssinus	82.86	74.14	1–4,600	1–2,000	399±170	66±120
D. farinae	5.71	20.68	2–66	2–1,000	34±22	68±37
Hirstia chelidonis	8.57	2.59	1–65	5–57	24±16	27±16
D. evansi	–	6.89	–	7–100	–	25±10
Eurolyphus maynei	8.57	2.86	3–35	5–14	14±8	10±2
Family Acaridae						
Acarus stro	2.86	6.89	16	3–50	16	14±5
Tyrophagus putrescentiae	11.43	–	8–80	–	38±13	–
Truopeauia nova	5.71	0.86	3–20	167	10±7	167
Aleuroglyphus sp.	2.86	–	3	–	3	–
Acaroldea sp.	11.43	–	5–12	–	5±2	–
Family Glycyphagidae						
Glycyphagus domesticus	22.86	0.86	10–63	7	32±6	7
G. destructor	14.28	–	4–880	–	185±155	–
G. cadaverum	20	–	1–90	–	27±10	–
Gohieria fusca	8.57	2.86	4–40	2–14	16±9	8±6
Chortoglyphus arcuatus	2.86	0.86	19	100	19	100
Group Oribatci gen. sp.	14.28	13.79	1–5	2–50	3±1	15±5
Family Cheyletidae gen. sp.	48.57	3.45	3–420	25–100	56±24	62±67
Gamasina gen. sp.	–	0.86	–	10	–	10
Hirstionyssus sp.	2.86	–	10	–	10	–
Hypoaspis sp.	2.86	–	10	–	10	–
Macrochelis sp.	2.86	–	4	–	4	–
Proctolaelaps domestica	–	0.86	–	4	–	4

1, Species found in 1988; 2, species found in 2000.

In total, 24 species of house dust mites are recently described in Lithuania. 224 samples of house dust were collected from four randomly selected Vilnius pre-schools (2 where children stay 5 working days, and 2 where children stay 12 working hours a day).By microscope, house dust mites were detected in 109 samples; by „Acarex" test additionally in 21 samples. The mites were found in a week-stay pre-school 82 (70.7%) and day-stay 48 (44.4%) in house dust samples. The largest amounts of house dust mites were found in pre-schools where children stay for the whole week. In these pre-schools, children spend 5 days a week, sleeping after mid-day meals and at night. Both examined pre-schools were more than 20 years old. The mattresses, stuffed toys and carpets had never been changed. In the pre-schools of 12 working hours a day, mites were found more rarely because of no night sleep. The distribution of mites in different objects is

Table 2. The rates of occurrence of house dust mites in various objects

Pre-school	Mattresses Examined samples	Samples with dust mites abs (%)	Stuffed toys Examined samples	Samples with dust mites abs (%)	Carpets Examined samples	Samples with dust mites abs (%)
Week stay	88	52 (59.1)	14	11 (78.9)	12	6 (50)
Day stay	80	33 (41.3)	14	5 (35.7)	14	3 (21.4)

Table 3. Mite species found in Vilnius pre-schools

Species	Rate of occurrence (%)	Mite number per 1 g of dust Limits	Average
Order Actinotrichida (Acariformes)			
Suborder Sarcoptiformes			
Group Acaridae (Astigmata)			
Family Pyroglyphidae			
Dermatophagoides pteronyssinus	67.88	1–2,000	66±20
D. farinae	22.02	2–1,000	68±37
D. evansi	7.33	7–100	25±10
D. chelidonis	2.75	5–57	27±16
D. sp.	10.09	4–100	27±10
Euroglyphus maynei	1.83	5–14	10±2
Family Acaridae			
Acarus siro	7.33	3–50	14±5
Family Thyroglyphidae			
Thyroglyphus arcuatus	0.91	4	4
Family Glycyphagidae			
Glycyphagus sp.	1.82	7–10	8±2
Gohieria fusca	1.83	2–14	8±6
Suborder Trombidiformes			
Family Cheyletidae			
Cheyletus eruditus	0.91	33	33
Cheyletus sp.	3.66	25–100	62±18

represented in Table 2. Surprisingly high numbers of house dust mites were found in dust collected from stuffed toys from week pre-schools. During our study, it was noticed that stuffed toys had never been cleaned or washed and children were sleeping with them. It indicated that these toys could be a source of mite allergens and could perform sensitization.

Twelve mite species were determined in all examined dust samples in Vilnius pre-schools (from 24 known in Lithuania). The majority of them belong to the Pyroglyphidae family (6 species). Mite species having no influence to allergies were not included in Table 3.

Discussion

The presented data on mite acarofauna in Lithuania show after 20 years big differences in the amounts and proportion of various species. Formerly low occurrences of *D. farinae* have risen four-fold after 20 years ($p<0.05$). The Cheyletidae family nowadays is very rarely detected: 3.45% compared to 48.57% in the past ($p<0.001$) [1, 2, 4]. Similar differences occur with other species. However, *D. pteronyssinus* remains the main species in Lithuania, but with lower amounts of mites per 1 g of dust.

The studied acarofauna of pre-schools in Lithuania reveal this problem as very important, especially in stuffed toys. There are very few works on this topic [5, 6]. The contamination of soft toys with mites in Lithuania of more than 70%, may indicate new sources of house dust mite distribution. It is confirmed in a recent study. Also, by questionnaires, we found that 77% of children in Lithuania are sleeping with stuffed toys. Changing pillows, quilts, mattresses, and vacuuming did not solve the problem because the stuffed toys were not changed.

Stuffed toys are the main source of house dust mite in Lithuanian towns.

References

1. Vaicekauskaite R. Mite component in atopic bronchial asthma in Lithuania. 1983. 20 pp. Doctoral thesis (in Russian)
2. Kanchurin A, Vaicekauskaite R. Allergy to mites. 1988. Mosklas. Vilnius, 118 pp (in Russian)
3. Dubinina HV, Pletnev BD. Methods of revealing and identification of allergen house dust mites. 1977. Nauka. Leningrad. 50 pp (in Russian)
4. Dautartiene A. House dust mite studies in Lithuania. 1999. Ekologija. Vilnius 4.34–38 (in Lithuanian, English abstract)
5. Dubakiene R, Dautartiene A, Jurkuvenaite A. An acarological house dust research of Vilnius pre-schools. 2000. Environmental health. 1.13–15 (in Lithuanian)
6. Vobrazkova E, Samsinak K, Spicak V. The Possibility of a sensitization to inhalatory allergens in nursery schools. 1985. Zoologischer Anzeiger 215.3–4.195–200

3 Pharmacogenetics of β2-Adrenoceptor and Asthmatic Phenotypes

M.L. KOWALSKI, G. WOSZCZEK

Heredity has been considered an important factor in hay fever and asthma since the nineteenth century, however, more recently it has been realized, that the heredity of atopy and asthma is multifactorial and involves several levels of genetic control. One such potential area of genetic control of bronchial asthma seems to be associated with different clinical phenotypes of asthma which may be distinguished based on disease severity and response to treatment. In the last few years several „candidate genes" associated with asthma phenotypes have been identified [1]. In order to be considered as a „candidate gene" several criteria must be accomplished by the gene. The protein product of the gene must be involved in the pathomechanism of a disease and the gene itself should contain functionally relevant mutations or polymorphisms within the coding or promoter regions. Such mutations should also demonstrate association or linkage with a particular disease phenotype.

Among several identified genetic loci, that fulfil the above criteria with regard to asthmatic phenotypes is the beta-2 adrenergic receptor (β2-ADR) gene. Since the first polymorphisms of β2-ADR gene have been described a large amount of data emerged showing a significant influence of the gene on manifestation of allergic diseases. β2-ADR is widely distributed in human body, and during physiological reactions seems to respond mainly to endogenously produced hormones like epinephrine and norepinephrine. The receptor is involved in regulation of several physiologically important processes of the body homeostasis, and its genetic variants, if functionally different from the „wild type", may be potentially related to pathomechanisms leading to common disorders. In fact, several studies have shown that β2-ADR polymorphisms might be associated not only with asthma, but also with other diseases e.g. hypertension, obesity, dyslipoproteinaemia and congestive heart failure [2–6] (Table 1).

Table 1. Association of β2-ADR polymorphisms with non-atopic diseases

Disease	β2-ADR polymorphism	Citation
Essential hypertension	16 Arg/Gly	[2, 3]
Congestive heart failure	164 Thr/Ile	[4]
Obesity	16 Arg/Gly; 27 Gln/Glu	[5]
Dyslipoproteinaemia	27 Gln/Glu	[6]

New Trends in Allergy V
J. Ring, H. Behrendt (Eds.)
© Springer-Verlag Berlin, Heidelberg 2002

Structure and Functions of b2-ADR

The properties of β2-ADR include bronchodilation, inhibition of microvascular leakage and cholinergic transmission, inhibition of inflammatory mediators release and modulation of mucus production in the airways.

β2-ADR belongs to a superfamily of G protein-coupled receptors with typical structure of 7 transmembrane domains, which take a form of alfa-helix [7]. The function of β2-ADR depends on coupling to G protein, which in turn stimulates adenyl cyclase, leading to increased levels of cAMP and smooth muscle relaxation. Another possible pathway of β2-ADR action is opening large-conductance, calcium activated potassium channels, via cAMP or directly through G protein. After binding of β2-agonists the receptor exhibits a period of reduced sensitivity to further stimulation („desensitisation") which is a natural process, common for many other receptors. In the case of β2-ADR several mechanisms of desensitisation have been described. A very fast process of desensitisation (which takes seconds) is associated with uncoupling β2-ADR from protein G, through phosphorylation of specific residues. The second process called „sequestration" requires several minutes of exposure to beta agonists. In that case β2-ADR protein is functional but it is transported into intracellular compartment, where it can be digested or circulated again to the cell surface. The third mechanism of desensitisation, called down-regulation requires continuous beta agonist exposure for several hours. It involves internalisation of receptor, proteolytic digestion as well as decreased stability of mRNA for β2-ADR. In these situations the number of functional receptors on cell surface decreases and the following drug exposure may cause less physiological and clinical effects.

Genetics of β2-ADR

Very exciting data are related to the genetic polymorphisms of β2-ADR and associated with alternation of its function. The gene for β2-ADR is localized close to the IL-4 gene cluster on chromosome 5q. The group of S. Liggett [8] from Cincinnati in series of studies demonstrated that nine point mutations exist within the coding region, and that those at nucleic acid positions 46, 79, 100, 491 resulted in changes in the amino acids at positions 16, 27, 34 and 164 respectively (Fig. 1). In site-directed mutagenesis/recombinant expression studies they showed, that the changes in the amino acid sequence of the extra cellular aminoterminus of the receptor resulted in significant changes in the function of the receptor. The presence of glycine at position 16 (Gly16) is associated with enhanced down-regulation of the receptor in the response to agonist as compared to arginine at this position (Arg16), and substitution of Glu for Gln at position 27 resulted in a decreased down-regulation of the receptor, suggesting that these polymorphisms may affect bronchial smooth muscle function in vivo.

Population study, demonstrated similar frequency of Gly/Arg 16 and Glu/Gln27 polymorphisms in asthmatic atopic and normal subjects, indicating that these polymorphisms are not a major cause of asthma or atopy [9,10]. However, it has been shown, that different genetic variants of the receptor may influence the asth-

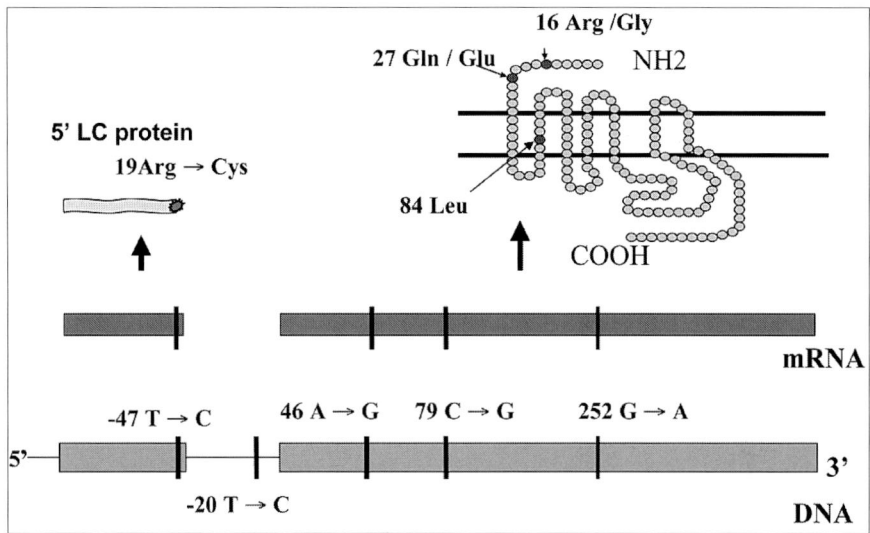

Fig. 1. Gene and protein structure of β2-adrenoceptor

matic phenotype. The study of the Gln/Glu 27 polymorphism and airway reactivity in a group of patients with mild to moderate asthma revealed that Gln27 homozygotes had a four-fold higher bronchial hyperresponsiveness to methacholin (lower threshold dose), than patients who were homozygous for the Glu 27 form of the receptor, while heterozygotes had an intermediate hyperreactivity [10]. The association of polymorphism in position 27 with bronchial hyperreactivity was also reported in our study involving patients suspected of bronchial asthma, but having negative bronchial reversibility test [11]. Furthermore, it has been shown, that the Gly 16 allele was significantly more frequent in patients with nocturnal asthma as compared to the non-nocturnal group, and the odds ratio of having nocturnal asthma and the Gly16 polymorphism was 3.8 [12] A series of other studies confirmed that β2-ADR polymorphisms may be related to the asthmatic phenotype including bronchial hyperreactivity and severity of the disease [13].

β2-ADR Polymorphism and Response to β2 Agonists Treatment

The study of Martinez et al. [14] showed that in a general population of children (which included patients with diagnosed asthma) the homozygotic form of β2-ADR with Arg in position 16 was associated with a 5 fold increase in positive response to albuterol and that in children with heterozygotic form of β2-ADR a positive response to albuterol was 2 times more frequent than in children with homozygotic Gly in position 16. This association was recently confirmed in asthmatics and in atopic patients with seasonal asthma and/or rhinitis [15, 16]. Thus, in general populations (independently of presence of asthma) there are persons responding to beta agonists with airway reversibility and groups of people in whom such a response is not observed, and that this difference may be genetically determined. This observation may help to clarify problems with airway reversibility test interpretation often encountered in clinical routine.

Tachyphylaxis of β2-ADR following chronic treatment with beta-2 mimetics has been a matter of concern for the last three decades, since it was associated with increase in asthma mortality. New data suggesting potential relation of β2-ADR polymorphism to this process were presented by Hancox et al. [17] who re-evaluated clinical data of patients treated for 6 months with regular beta-2 agonist (fenoterol) or placebo. In this study deterioration of asthma and increased death rate were significantly more frequent in fenoterol treated patients than in placebo group. Retrospective analysis of clinical data with respect to the β2-ADR polymorphism demonstrated association of treatment-induced increased non-specific bronchial hyperreactivity with Arg16. Moreover, homozygotic patients with Gln27 had higher evening PEF measurements in comparison to patients with 27 Glu in homozygotic and heterozygotic forms. Recently, Israel et al. [18] reported that among asthmatics on betamimetics, homozygotic patients 16Arg/Arg using salbutamol regularly had significantly lower morning peak expiratory flow than asthmatics who used the drug on as needed basis. In another study [19] exacerbation rate during 6 months of regular salbutamol treatment was significantly higher (in fact was doubled) in Arg 16 homozygous patients as compared to homozygous for Gly16 and heterozygous. These studies point to the conclusion that Arg 16 patients are susceptible to clinically important increases in asthma exacerbation during chronic treatment with short acting beta-agonists and strongly suggest important role of β2-ADR polymorphisms in response to regular β2-agonist treatment. If these observations are further confirmed, identification of such patients at risk by β2-ADR polymorphism typing may be justified in the future.

Long acting β2-agonists, salmeterol and formoterol, have become a valuable tool in asthma pharmacotherapy. However, regular treatment with these drugs without concomitant use of inhaled steroids may lead to decrease in their protective activity against provocation with methacholin, allergens and exercise [20]. Study by Tan et al. [21] demonstrated that decreased response to short acting β2-agonists after 4 weeks of formoterol was associated with β2-ADR genotypes, however, this observation was not confirmed by others [22]. Further studies are required to assess bronchodilator and bronchoprotective effects of long lasting β2 agonists in patients with different β2AR polymorphisms and their potential significance in different patients populations.

β2-AR and Control of IgE Production

Total IgE levels are elevated in serum of patients with atopic diseases and bronchial asthma, and an association between total serum IgE levels and nonspecific bronchial responsiveness and asthma severity has been demonstrated in epidemiological studies. Thus, serum total IgE may be considered as an important component of atopic and asthmatic phenotypes. Epidemiological studies indicate, that IgE levels have heritability in the range of 50–70%, although the mode of inher-

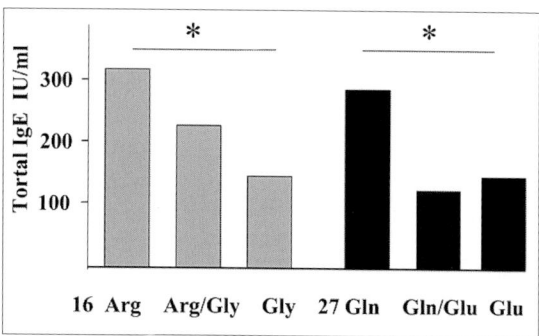

Fig. 2. Polymorphisms of β2-adrenoceptor and total serum IgE levels in atopic patients. Patients homozygotic for Arg16 and for Gln27 have significantly higher mean total serum IgE as compared to patients homozygotic for Gly16 and Glu27, respectively. *$p<0.05$ [16]

itance of high IgE levels has not been definitely established. Both single dominant and polygenic recessive mode of inheritance were concluded from different studies. In recent years the synthesis of IgE has been shown to be regulated by a cytokine network and genetic association has been reported between total IgE levels and several polymorphic genes and their receptors β2-adrenergic receptors are present on several immunological cells including T cell and B cells and their stimulation may potentially affect synthesis of regulatory cytokines and IgE production. A study by J. Dewar at al. [23] in families multiplex for asthma demonstrated that β2-adrenoceptor polymorphism (Gln27 genotype) was associated with variability in total IgE. We have recently studied an association of β2-adrenoceptor polymorphism with serum total IgE level in a group of patients with seasonal asthma and/ or allergic rhinitis [12]. We found that patients homozygous for Arg16 or Gln27 had significantly higher mean log IgE levels as compared to homozygotes for Gly16 ($p<0.05$) or Glu27 ($p<0.03$) respectively (Fig. 2). These data allow to speculate that genetic polymorphism of β2AR may play a role in regulation of IgE production in atopic patients probably by influencing cell responsiveness to endogenous catecholamines which in turn may potentially be involved in modulation of cytokine production. In fact β2AR is a predominant adrenergic receptor on PBMC (mono, T and B cells), β2-agonists (salbutamol,

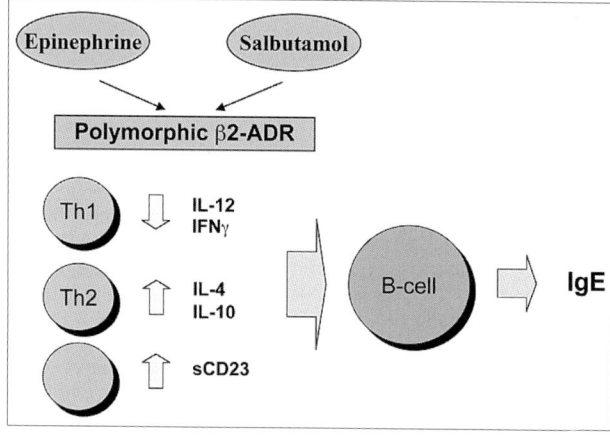

Fig. 3. Schematic diagram to illustrate a putative regulation of IgE production by polymorphisms in the β2-adrenoceptor

fenoterol) in vitro potentiate IL-4-induced IgE production and sCD23 release [24] and modulate human Th1/Th2 cytokine balance by increasing IL-4 and IL-10 release [25] and decreasing IL-12 and IFN-γ production [26]. Figure 3 summarizes possible interaction between β2 receptor stimulation and IgE production.

New β2-ADR Polymorphisms

In recent studies apart from β2-ADR polymorphism in positions 16 and 27, new polymorphic loci, which potentially can influence an expression and function of β2-ADR, have been identified. McGraw et al. [27] identified a new polymorphism in a promoter region of β2-ADR and showed that exchange of Arg for Cys in position 19 of 5' cistron leader peptide causes increased surface expression of β2-ADR. In addition, this polymorphism is in strong linkage disequilibrium with polymorphic loci 16 and 27, suggesting that it can significantly influence functions of β2-ADR (Fig. 1). The picture of β2-ADR polymorphism has become even more complicated by data from the study of Scott et al. [28] and Timmermann et al. [29] who found additional polymorphisms in 5' region of β2-ADR gene in position −20, −47, −367, −468, −654, −1023, −1343, −1429. In several studies it has been shown [9, 30], that most of these polymorphic loci are in strong linkage with polymorphisms in coding part of β2-ADR gene what implies its potential significance in regulation of β2-ADR expression and functions. Recently, Drysdale et al. [31] suggested that an individual β2-ADR polymorphism may have poor predictive power as pharmacogenetic locus and that it is the unique interaction of multiple polymorphisms within a haplotype that affects biologic and therapeutic phenotypes. Very similar data come from D'Amato et al. [32] who observed association of bronchial hyperresponsiveness with a particular β2-ADR haplotype, but not with single polymorphisms.

In conclusion, β2AR polymorphisms seem to play an important role in the modulation of asthmatic phenotype, although future studies are needed to reveal potential clinical usefulness of β2AR genotyping in asthmatic patients. It seems that earlier studies analysing associations of β2-ADR polymorphisms with asthmatic phenotypes should be re-evaluated with respect to new polymorphisms and haplotypic distribution.

References

1. Los H, Koppelman GH, Postma DS. The importance of genetic influences in asthma. Eur Respir J 1999; 14:1210–1227
2. Gratze G, Fortin J, Labugger R, et al. β2-Adrenergic receptor variants affect resting blood pressure and agonist-induced vasodilation in young adult Caucasians. Hypertension 1999; 33:1425–1430
3. Kotanko P, Binder A, Tasker J, et al. Essential hypertension in African Caribbeans associates with a variant of the β2-adrenoceptor. Hypertension 1997; 30:773–776
4. Liggett SB, Wagoner LE, Craft LL, et al. The Ile164 β2-adrenergic receptor polymorphism adversely affects the outcome of congestive heart failure. J Clin Invest 1998; 102:1534–1539
5. Large V, Hellstrom L, Reynisdottir S, et al. Human β2-adrenoceptor gene polymorphisms are highly frequent in obesity and associated with altered adipocyte β2 adrenoceptor function. J Clin Invest 1997; 100:3005–3013

6. Ehrenborg E, Skogsberg J, Ruotolo G, et al. The Q/E27 polymorphism in the β2-adrenoceptor gene is associated with increased body weight and dyslipoproteinaemia involving triglyceride-rich lipoproteins. J Intern Med 2000; 247:651–656

7. Dixon RA, Kobilka BK, Strader DJ, et al. Cloning of the gene and cDNA for mammalian β2-adrenergic receptor and homology with rhodopsin. Nature 1986; 321:75–79

8. Reihsaus E, Innis M, MacIntyre N, Liggett SB. Mutations in the gene encoding for the β2-adrenergic receptor in normal and asthmatic subjects. Am J Respir Cell Mol Biol 1993; 8:334–339

9. Borowiec M, Woszczek G, Kowalski ML. Distibution of new polymorphic loci of β2-adrenoceptor gene in atopic nad non-atopic subjects. Eur Respir J 1999; 14:117

10. Hall IP, Wheatley A, Wilding P, Liggett SB. Association of Glu 27 β2-adrenoceptor polymorphism with lower airway reactivity in asthmatic subjects. Lancet 1995; 345:1213–1214

11. Woszczek G, Borowiec M, Kosinski S, Kowalski ML. Association of bronchial hyperresponsiveness with 27 Gln/ Glu β2-adrenoceptor polymorphism. Eur Respir J 2000; 16; suppl 31, 183s

12. Turki J, Pak J, Green SA, Martin RJ, Liggett SB. Genetic polymorphisms of the β2-adrenergic receptor in nocturnal and nonnocturnal asthma. Evidence that Gly16 correlates with the nocturnal phenotype. J Clin Invest 1995; 95:1635–1641

13. Lipwworth BJ. Editorial. β2-adrenoceptor resposiveness and asthma activity. Clin Exp Allergy 1998; 28:257–260

14. Martinez FD, Graves PE, Baldini M, Solomon S, Erickson R. Association between genetic polymorphisms of the β2-adrenoceptor and response to albuterol in children with and without a history of wheezing. J Clin Invest 1997; 100:3184–3188

15. Lima JJ, Pharm D, Thomason DB et al. Impact of genetic polymorphisms of the β2-adrenergic receptor on albuterol bronchodialtor pharmacodynamics. Clin Pharmacol Ther 1999; 65:519–525

16. Kowalski ML, Woszczek G, Borowiec M. Polymorphisms of β2–adrenoceptor are associated with bronchodilator response to salbutamol and high IgE levels in patients with pollen allergy. J Allergy Clin Immunol 2000; 105:S371

17. Hancox RJ, Sears MR, Taylor DR. Polymorphism of the β2-adrenoceptor and the response to long-term β2-agonist therapy in asthma. Eur Respir J 1998; 11:589–593

18. Israel E, Drazen JM, Liggett SB, et al. The effect of polymorphisms of the β2-adrenergic receptor on the response to regular use of albuterol in asthma. Am J Respir Crit Care Med 2000; 162:75–80

19. Taylor RD, Draze JF, Herbison PG et al. Asthma exacerbations during long term b agonist use: influence of β2-adrenoceptor polymorphism. Thorax 2000; 55:762–767

20. Milot J, Boulet LP, Laviolette M, et al. Tolerance to the salmeterol protective effects on methacholine-induced bronchoconstriction and influence of inhaled corticosteroids. Am J Respir Crit Care Med 1996; 158:804

21. Tan S, Hall IP, Dewar J, Dow E, Lipworth B. Association between β2-adrenoceptor polymorphism and susceptibility to bronchodilator desensitisation in moderately severe stable asthmatics. Lancet 1997; 350:995–999

22. Lipworth BJ, Hall IP, Aziz I, Tan KS Wheatley A. β2-adrenoceptor polymorphism and bronchoprotective sensitivity with regular short- and long-acting β2-adonist therapy. Clin Science 1999; 96: 253–59

23. Dewar JC, Wilkinson J, Wheatley AP et al.. The glutamine 27 β2- adrenoceptor polymorpism is associated with elevated IgE levels in asthmatic families. J Allergy Clin Immunol 1997:100:261–5

24. Coqueret O, Duga B, Mencia-Huerta JM, Braquet P. Regulation of IgE production from human mononuclear cells by β2-adrenoceptoragonists. Clin exp Allergy 1995;25:304–11

25. Agrawal KS, Marshall GD. B-adrenergic modulation of human type-1/type-2 cytokine balance. J Allergy Clin Immunol 1999:104:91–98

26. β2-Agonists prevent Th1 developement by selective inhibition of interleukin 12. Panina-Borginion P. et al. J Clin Invest 1997: 100: 1513–1519

27. McGraw DW, Forbes SL, Kramer LA, Liggett SB. Polymorphisms of the 5' leader cistron of the human β2-adrenergic receptor regulate receptor expression. J Clin Invest 1998; 102:1927–1932

28. Scott MG, Swan C, Wheatley AP, Hall IP. Identification of novel polymorphisms within the promoter region of the human β2-adrenergic receptor gene. Br J Pharmacol 1999; 126:841–844

29. Timmermann B, Li GH, Luft FC, Lund-Johansen P, Skrabal F, Hoehe MR. Novel DNA sequence differences in the β2-adrenergic receptor gene promoter region. Hum Mutat 1998; 11:343–344
30. McGraw DW, Forbes SL, Kramer LA, Liggett SB. Polymorphisms of the 5' leader cistron of the human β2-adrenergic receptor regulate receptor expression. J Clin Invest 1998; 102:1927–1932
31. Drysdale CM, McGraw DW, Stack CB, et al. Complex promoter and coding region β2-adrenergic receptor haplotypes alter receptor expression and predict in vivo responsiveness. Proc Natl Acad Sci USA 2000; 97:10483–10488
32. D'Amato M, Vitiani LR, Petrelli G, et al. Association of persistent bronchial hyperresponsiveness with β2-adrenoceptor (ADR b-2) haplotypes. A population study. Am J Respir Crit Care Med 1998; 158:1968–1973

4   Pertussis Vaccination Is Not Associated with a Higher Prevalence of Allergies in Six-Year-Old Children from West Germany

U. KRÄMER, H. BEHRENDT, U. RANFT, T. SCHÄFER, J. RING

The association between pertussis vaccination and allergies as seen in epidemiological studies is unclear. Studies in the U.S. and in New Zealand, where vaccination coverage was nearly complete, found fewer allergies in the very small group of non-vaccinated children [1, 2]. Two studies in Great Britain found more asthma in the vaccinated than in the not vaccinated group [3, 4]. Two cohort studies found no association with wheezing, asthma or sensitisation in children up to 3 years [5, 6]. Contrary to that the evidence concerning pertussis itself is less conflicting. Studies dealing with the impact of early childhood respiratory infections on allergy in later life all found more asthma and allergies in children having had pertussis [7–10]. From 1974 to 1991 pertussis vaccination was not recommended in West Germany because of alarming reports on the side effects of the vaccine. Therefore the group of children receiving a diphteria and tetanus vaccination (DT) but no diphteria, pertussis and tetanus vaccination (DPT) is fairly big and we are able to compare these both groups with the group of children receiving neither DT nor DPT (NO) vaccination. If pertussis vaccination causes allergies then the prevalence of allergies should be highest in the DPT vaccinated group. Children in the DT or NO group should have comparable prevalences. This was investigated. We use data from our study on school beginners in West Germany where vaccinations, diagnoses of pertussis, allergies and symptoms of allergies have been recorded, atopic eczema has been diagnosed and sensitisation has been measured.

Methods

Study Population

All children on admission to first grade from predefined areas of the West German cities Duisburg, Essen, Cologne, and the small town Borken participated every third year (1991, 1994 and 1997) and children from Augsburg in 1996 in a questionnaire study with identical design. 7923 participated (response 76%). 1991, 1994 and 1997 a subgroup of these children in the same places were asked to give blood for the measurement of total and specific IgE and to undergo a dermatological investigation. The studies took place immediately after the school entrance examination compulsory for all school beginners. They were conducted between February and May of the pertinent years.

The study was approved by the ethical committee of the Medical Association of Saxony Anhalt and Bavaria.

New Trends in Allergy V
J. Ring, H. Behrendt (Eds.)
© Springer-Verlag Berlin, Heidelberg 2002

Questionnaire

A questionnaire was sent to the parents along with a letter of invitation from the local health departments. It was to be completed at home and checked by a physician on the day of the investigation. Whether the child ever had received vaccinations against diphteria, tetanus, pertussis, measles, rubella, mumps, and BCG was checked with the vaccination certificate (95% had the certificate available). Parents reported whether a physician ever had diagnosed pertussis, bronchial asthma, hay fever and eczema in the child. We used German translations of ISAAC questions to assess the symptoms of allergies wheezing ever, wheezing in the last 12 months, sneezing with reddened eyes in the last 12 months, itchy skin rash ever and itchy skin rash in the last 12 months. Wheezing in the last 12 months and itchy skin rash were included into the questionnaire in the year 1994.

Information about the following variables was taken from the questionnaire and included in the analysis as potentially confounding: Education of the parents (years of schooling, highest level of the parents was chosen to characterise the family), nationality of the parents (German for at least one of the parents/not German), gender, allergy in father or mother, bedroom sharing, damp flat, smoking of mother in pregnancy and smoking in the child's home.

Vaccination

The DPT vaccination was not recommended but the DT vaccination only [11]. A DPT vaccination was indicated for specially endangered children: those in day care centres or public homes, those living in poor socio-economic conditions and over-crowd homes and those with a tendency to bronchial illnesses. Basic immunisation was in the 3th, 4th and 5th months of life; a repetition took place after 1 year. Contraindications were illnesses of the central nervous system. 50IE Diphteriatoxoid, 50IE Tetanustoxoid and 4IE killed *Bordetella pertussis* germs were administered. Aluminiumhydroxide and Aluminiumphosphate were used as adjuvants. Preservation was Sodiumtimerfonate.

Atopic Eczema

Trained physicians from the Department of Dermatology and Allergology, Technical University Munich diagnosed atopic eczema according to standardised criteria on the day of the basic examination. In total, 3927 children from West Germany (response: 93%) participated in this investigation.

Determination of Atopic Sensitisation

The concentrations of specific IgE antibodies against birch pollen, grass pollen, mugwort pollen and house dust mites and total IgE were determined in 3411 children (response: 68% of those with a questionnaire). 1991, 1994 and 1996 this test was done by the CAP-RAST-FEIA system (Pharmacia, Uppsala Sweden) and 1996 and 1997 by ALASTAT (DPC Biermann, Los Angeles, USA). 581 analysis in 1996 were done by CAP-RAST as well as by ALASTAT. The comparability between the determination methods was very good (Kappa 0.85). A sensitisation was defined as positive, if the concentration of specific IgE antibodies was >= 0.35 kU/l. Total serum IgE concentrations above the 95th percentile for the children from Borken (180 kU/l) were considered elevated.

Statistical Analysis

The aim of the study was to find out the effect of pertussis vaccination on allergies and sensitisation. We used logistic regression analysis. The predefined covariates were included into models for all outcome variables. Parameter estimates of the model were transformed to odds ratios (OR) with 95% confidence intervals (95% CI). Only the 7338 children with complete information on pertussis and pertussis vaccination were included in the analysis.

Results

Information about all covariates and pertussis and pertussis vaccination was available in 84.8% of all children. No time trends could be detected in the percentage of missing values. Children giving blood for the analysis of specific IgE or participating in the dermatological investigation had slightly better educated parents(38.8% with more than 10 years of schooling compared to 33.0% in then non-participating group). Children in the participating group had more physician diagnosed eczema (about 2% more) than in the non-participating group in East as well as in West Germany. Other differences in covariates or health outcome variables between these both groups could not be detected.

Of all the children, 40.4% got a pertussis vaccination. If this vaccination was given, it was combined with the diphteria and tetanus vaccination (DPT); 55.8% got a diphteria and tetanus vaccination only (DT), 3.9% had neither DPT nor DT vaccination. More than 20% of the children had a physician-diagnosed pertussis. Pertussis was three times more often in non-vaccinated than in vaccinated children.

We differentiated three vaccination types: DT,DPT,NO. As Table 1 demonstrates those in the first group (DT) have parents best educated and with the least percentage of non-German children. With the exception of hay fever all allergies and allergic symptoms were most frequent in this group. Those in the third group have parents least well educated. Nearly 50% of them are non-German. Most symptoms of allergies had the lowest prevalence. Sensitisation against pollen is very uncommon in this group compared with the other groups and total IgE is fairly high in this group. As can be seen in Table 2 the differences in prevalence of allergies, allergic symptoms and sensitisation between the third group (NO) and the second group (DPT) can be largely explained by nationality and education of parents. These factors do explain the differences between the second(DPT)

Table 1. Social characteristics, allergies, symptoms and sensitisation in groups defined by different vaccination strategies in West Germany[a]

	Vaccination against diphteria and tetanus without pertussis (DT)	Vaccination against diphteria, tetanus and pertussis (DPT)	Neither vaccination against diphteria, tetanus nor pertussis (NO)
Education of parents			
<10 years schooling	22.4 (3784)	27.9 (2690)	45.9 (246)
=10 years schooling	37.7	38.6	34.2
<10 years schooling	39.9	33.5	19.9
Nationality of parents not German	17.6 (3784)	21.6 (2690)	45.9 (246)
Diagnosed:			
Bronchial asthma	2.7 (3738)	2.1 (2676)	2.5 (244)
Hay fever	3.0 (3745)	3.3 (2679)	2.5 (245)
Eczema	12.2 (3724)	10.2 (2659)	3.7 (246)
Symptoms:			
Wheezing ever	18.6 (2190)	15.8 (1855)	12.5 (112)
Wheezing l. 12 m.	6.2 (1603)	5.2 (1412)	5.0 (60)
Sneezing/ red eyes l. 12 m.	4.9 (3759)	3.9 (2668)	2.9 (242)
Itchy skin rash ever	9.7 (1635)	7.8 (1467)	4.9 (61)
Itchy skin rash l. 12 m	4.9 (1629)	4.0 (1461)	3.3 (61)
Atopic eczema at day of investigation	7.8 (1736)	5.7 (1594)	5.9 (85)
Sensitisation against:			
Birch pollen	7.2 (1624)	7.6 (1284)	**3.2 (79)**
Grass pollen	12.8 (1624)	14.1 (1290)	3.8 (79)
Mugwort pollen	3.5 (1612)	3.9 (1273)	1.3 (79)
House dust mite	12.8 (1612)	14.5 (1275)	12.8 (78)
Total IgE >180 kU/l	10.4 (1611)	12.3 (1289)	17.5 (80)

[a]Percentages, numbers in parentheses; children with information on all covariates.

and the first group (DT) to a much lesser extent. The differences between these both groups can be largely explained when including pertussis into the logistic regression model.

Discussion

In West Germany two groups of children with no pertussis vaccination have to be differentiated. One group got neither DPT nor DT vaccination. This group was not well educated and the percentage of foreigners was high. The lower prevalence of allergies and sensitisation in this group could mostly be explained by confounding with social factors. The second group got a DT but no DPT vaccination. This group was best educated which possibly reflects the negative discus-

Table 2. Effect of social characteristics and pertussis on differences in allergies, symptoms and sensitisation between differently vaccinated groups in West Germany[a]

DPT	DT Vaccination/ compared to DPT	No DT or DPT vaccination compared to DPT	% Change in OR towards the 1 when including education and nationality		% Change in OR towards the 1 when including pertussis	
			DT/DPT	NO/DPT	DT/DPT	NO/
Diagnosed:						
Bronchial asthma	1.31 (0.94–1.83)	1.20 (0.51–2.82)	2.3	–	11.0	2.6
Hay fever	0.92 (0.70–1.23)	0.74 (0.32–1.71)	4.2	–	–	–
Eczema	1.23 (1.05–1.44)	0.34 (0.17–0.66)	8.8	29.2	8.8	
Symptoms:						
Wheezing ever	1.22 (1.03–1.44)	0.76 (0.43–1.35)	4.3	28.3	13.0	–
Wheezing l. 12 m.	1.21 (0.88–1.65)	0.96 (0.30–3.16)	–	14.3	9.0	–
Sneezing/ red eyes l. 12 m.	1.18 (0.92–1.51)	0.74 (0.34–1.61)	2.6	14.0	8.3	–
Itchy skin rash ever	1.28 (0.99–1.64)	0.61 (0.19–1.99)	5.8	20.2	1.6	–
Itchy skin rash l.12 m	1.23 (0.87–1.74)	0.82 (0.20–3.44)	–	13.7	1.7	–
Atopic eczema at day of investigation	1.40 (1.07–1.85)	1.03 (0.41–2.61)	3.7		2.9	1.0
Sensitisation against:						
Birch pollen	0.94 (0.71–1.24)	0.48 (0.15–1.54)	–	20.0	–	–
Grass pollen	0.89 (0.72–1.10)	0.24 (0.08–0.77)	–	17.2	–	–
Mugwort pollen	0.88 (0.60–1.30)	0.31 (0.04–2.30)	–	13.9	–	–
House dust mite	0.86 (0.70–1.07)	0.87 (0.44–1.71)	–			
Total IgE >180 kU/l	0.83 (0.66–1.05)	1.52 (0.83–2.77)	1.2	18.8	2.4	

[a]Children with information on all covariates; odds ratio (OR) with 95% confidence limits.

sions about pertussis vaccination and the recommendation, that people with a poor socio-economic background should be vaccinated against pertussis. The prevalence of asthma and wheezing was higher not lower in this group than in the DPT vaccinated group. This could be explained when including pertussis into the logistic regression model. This means that DPT vaccination protects young children from asthma and wheezing by protecting from pertussis. We conclude that pertussis vaccination is not associated with more allergies in 6-year-old children from West Germany. This is in accordance with the results of two cohort studies [5, 6] but not with other cross sectional studies [1–4]. Two possible explanations could be given for this discrepancy. First, the negative effect of pertussis vaccination might be visible in older children only as have been investigated in the other cross sectional studies. Secondly social factors, which could not be accounted for in the studies in the U.S. and New Zealand because of the very small number of children not vaccinated, might be responsible for the low prevalence of allergies in this group, as it has been demonstrated in our study. Social factors as nationality and education determine life style which is known to influence the prevalence of allergies and sensitisation.

References

1. Kemp T, Pearce N, Fitzharris P, Crane J, Fergusson D, George IS, Wickens K, Beasley R Is infant immunization a risk factor for childhood asthma or allergy? Epidemiology 1997; 8:678–680
2. Hurwitz EL, Morgenstern H Effects of diphteria-tetanus-pertussis or tetanus vaccination on allergies and allergy-related respiratory symptoms among children and adolescents in the United States. J Manipulative Physiol Ther 2000; 23:81–90
3. Odent MR, Culpin EE, Kimmel T Pertussis vaccination and asthma: Is there a link? JAMA 1994; 272:592–593
4. Farooqi IS, Hopkin JM Early childhood infection and atopic disorder. Thorax 1998; 53:927–932
5. Henderson J, North K, Griffith M, Harvey I Pertussis vaccination and wheezing illnesses in young children:prospective cohort study. Brit Med J 1999; 318:1173–1176
6. Nilsson L, Kjellman N-I, Björksten B A randomized controlled trial of the effect of pertussis vaccines on atopic disease. Arch Pediatr Adolesc Med 1998; 152:734–738
7. Forastiere F, Agabiti N, Corbo G, Dell'Orco V, Porta D, Pistelli R, Levenstein S, Perucci C Socioeconomic status, number of siblings, and respiratory infections in early life as determinants of atopy in children. Epidemiology 1997; 8:678–680
8. Wickens KL, Crane J, Kemp T, Lewis S, D'Souza W, Sawyer G, Stone L, Tohill S, Kennedy J, Slater T et al. Family size, infections, and asthma prevalence in New Zealand children. Epidemiology 1999; 10:566–570
9. Bodner C, Godden D, Seaton A, Agabiti N Family size, childhood infections, and atopic disease. Thorax 1998; 53:28–32
10. Strachan DP, Harkins LS, Johnston IDA, Anderson HR Childhood antecedents of allergic sensitization in young british adults. J Allergy Clin Immun 1997; 99:6–12
11. Spiess A. Impfkompendium. Thieme, 1987

5   Human Allergogeneticists Should Listen to Their Dog's Barking

A.L. DE WECK, M. GRIOT-WENK, H. SCHNEIDER, B. SCHIESSL,
B. ZEEMANN, P. MAYER, E. LIEHL

Summary

A colony of Beagle dogs was used within the last 6 years to develop an allergic dog model. The dogs were sensitized to various allergens, such as recombinant Betv1 (birch) and Phl p5 (timothy), ovalbumin, peanut and many others. The first observation was that dogs clearly segregated into high and low IgE responder dogs when immunized for the first time by intradermal or subcutaneous injections of allergen within 1 month of birth. Characteristic for the high IgE response was the possibility to boost it at any time later in life and to extend it later to other allergens, like is usually the case in atopic man. Low IgE responder dogs showed a low response which was not boostable and could not be extended to other allergens later on. Numerous breeding experiments over 5 years demonstrated clearly that the high IgE response is inherited as a dominant trait.

However, it was then found that this trait does not express itself if first immunization of high IgE responders occurs later than the 3rd month of life. In that case, a potent suppressor mechanism for IgE takes over and the animal presents phenotypically later as a low IgE responder. The mode of sensitization is also crucial for later phenotypic expression. Sensitization by inhalation to the same allergens is obviously regulated by some additional gene(s) since only part of the high IgE responder litters may be sensitized by inhalation. A similar phenomenon was observed in the spontaneous occurrence of IgE to house dust mites or pollens in the dog colony.

These results show clearly that genetic studies based, like is still the case in man, on the spontaneous occurrence of IgE responses to ubiquitous allergens and phenotypes detected long after birth would lead to entirely wrong genetic conclusions.

Definition and Genetics of Atopy in Man

The concept and definition of „atopy" and „atopic diseases" in man was first coined by Coca [1]. This definition rests on the one hand on the hereditary character of some of the atopic diseases, on the other hand on their association with a special class of antibodies, the so-called atopic reagins, which were found 50 years later to be a special class of immunoglobulins, denominated IgE. Originally, atopic diseases or the atopic syndrome were defined as follows: „This group comprises bronchial asthma, hay fever, and the condition sometimes called infantile eczema (atopic dermatitis), which are subject to a common he-

New Trends in Allergy V
J. Ring, H. Behrendt (Eds.)
© Springer-Verlag Berlin, Heidelberg 2002

reditary cause. It is, indeed, this hereditary character of these clinical conditions which unites them in one group and separates them from the other categories" [2].

The association of reagins, later IgE, with this group of diseases, on the other hand, has been for a long time subject of controversies. This may be due, on the one hand, to the fact that IgE-mediated allergic reactions and diseases (e.g. anaphylactic shock, urticaria) frequently occur in the absence of any hereditary syndrome. On the other hand, some cases of atopic dermatitis appear not to be associated with abnormally high levels of IgE. Therefore, a number of authors have been reluctant to summarily associate high levels of IgE with atopy.

In fact, observations of nature, IgE levels and the notion of atopy can be reconciled if one considers that there are two types of IgE-mediated allergies or allergic diseases:
a) the classical hereditary atopic syndrome and
b) the non hereditary selective IgE response.

In the first case, the high IgE response usually appears already in infancy, is directed against several ubiquitous allergens and shows a trend to broaden its scope and the number of allergens involved with time. Clinically, the high IgE response manifests itself mostly as asthma, rhinitis or atopic dermatitis. There is a marked hereditary trend. In the case of selective IgE response, there is no indication for a hereditary trend, the high IgE response is usually directed against a restricted number of allergens (e.g. drugs, foods), does not expand with time and may occur at any age. It may be considered that this type of allergic IgE response is the result of an interruption of the normal IgE suppressor mechanism, described by Katz experimentally as „allergic breakthrough" [3].

Coca believed that atopy was restricted to man; in fact, the occurrence of hereditary IgE-mediated allergic reactions has been now well documented in dogs and horses.

Despite the possibility brought about by the discovery of IgE to define an objective marker of atopic disease and intensive research during the past 20 years, the genetics of these diseases have made relatively little progress [4–8]. This is due mainly to the fact that:
a) the phenotypes defining atopic diseases are not so clear cut as to make identification of affected individuals failproof;
b) IgE by itself may be a misleading marker, as discussed above;
c) numerous environmental factors appear to influence the phenotypic expression of atopy-related genes.

The recent development of molecular genetics and of tools enabling to identify structure and location of genes has not yet brought clarification, maybe even on the contrary, since candidate genes for atopy have multiplied [4–9] and the field seems more obscure than ever.

The general consensus of human allergogeneticists working on genetics of atopy is that we are dealing here with a complex gene disorder, one in which multiple genes are involved, both in terms of origin of the disease and its severity, some of which may interact [4]. This complexity has been described not only for the clinical asthma phenotype, but also for the human IgE response, which as such should be a more simple and objective marker [9].

The IgE Response in Dogs: Early Findings

Although first reagin-like antibodies, later identified as IgE, had been described in dogs in the early fifties and appeared associated with a relatively frequent hereditary skin eczematous condition described as atopic dermatitis, little was known about regulation of the IgE response in dogs when we started to study that response in a colony of Beagle dogs in 1993. These investigations were made possible by development of very specific monoclonal anti-IgE antibodies [10] since the polyclonal antibodies used heretofore were not sufficiently IgE-specific and also recognized dog IgG.

One of the very first observations, following immunization by injection of minute amounts of allergen (in the microgram range) in aluminium hydroxide, a classical IgE-fostering adjuvant, was that some dogs developed a long lasting allergen-specific IgE response, which declined when allergen was no longer injected but remained boostable at any time later on [11,12]. On the other hand, other dogs failed almost completely to produce IgE under similar conditions, In both cases, injections of allergen started at birth and were continued at biweekly or monthly intervals. Therefore, it became clear from the onset that dogs could be divided into high and low IgE responders. At the start, we were immunizing puppies without knowing the IgE status of their parents but since responders and non responders clustered clearly in high or low IgE response litters [12, Fig. 17.1], it became clear early that the IgE response in the dog was under genetic control.

This was soon confirmed by breeding experiments. A surprise, however, was that the status of high IgE responder appeared inherited as a dominant trait (Table 1), as shown also by some cross-breedings in which the same non IgE responding females were mated to high or low IgE responding males [12, Fig. 17.2]. As will be discussed below, however, the possibility of a dominant high IgE response gene in man and experimental animals has been evoked before.

Role of Early Immunization in the Expression of the High IgE Response Gene

As already observed in early immunization experiments, the high IgE response gene becomes manifest when the dogs receive their first injection of allergen and

Table 1. Genetics of IgE response in Beagle dogs

	Matings	Offspring	High responders (HR)	Low responders (LR)
HR×HR	26	124	124	0
HR×LR	5	29	29	0
LR×LR	5	30	0	30

adjuvant soon after birth. Subsequently, it has been found that this first injection may be delayed up to 4 weeks. If, however, the first injection of allergen is delayed for 3–4 months, an IgE different response pattern develops. Following the first 2–3 biweekly injections of allergen, a short burst of allergen-specific IgE may be shown in the serum, to then disappear forever, despite repeated allergen injections. It looks as if some potent suppressor mechanism has taken over.

These results were confirmed and extended by more formal experiments in which litters from high IgE responder parents were split into early-immunized and late-immunized puppies [13]. In that case, the early-immunized animals developed a high, prolonged and boostable IgE response, while the late-immunized animals produced a low, transient and non boostable IgE response.

Interestingly, the concomitant allergen-specific IgG response showed the opposite and was higher in animals showing a low IgE response. This pattern of response was identical for all allergens tested, such as milk proteins, ovalbumin and peanuts.

It was also similar when many months later, a new allergen, recombinant Phl p5 from timothy grass was injected. The early-immunized dogs developed a high and boostable IgE response and low IgG response to Phl p5, while the late immunized animals developed a low, non boostable IgE response and a high IgG response to Phl p5.

It appears, therefore, that early immunization primes the dogs for high and boostable IgE response for a long period of time to a large variety of allergens, while at the time of late immunization, the immune system has switched permanently to another balance in which IgG predominates over IgE and the IgE response appears permanently suppressed. Although no formal proof has yet been available in our system, it is tempting to assume that this change of predominance from IgE to IgG reflects a switch from a Th2 response to a Th1 response [14]. It has been shown in man [15] that the early immune response at or near birth may be skewed towards an IgE response. As observed, this may also be true in dogs.

Role of Allergen Feeding in the Expression of the High IgE Response Gene

While feeding with cow milk puppies immunized at birth with various allergens, including milk proteins, it was found [16] that feeding allergen at an early age induced a state of „split IgE tolerance", i.e. a suppression of the IgE response only but not of IgG, a phenomenon also called by some immune deviation [17]. When animals immunized with ovalbumin at birth were followed over a long period of time, the IgE response to ovalbumin which was high and boostable during the first few months spontaneously became lower, stable and no longer boostable by allergen. In addition, animals showing a high IgE response to various allergens but injected with ovalbumin only after 1 year of life could not be induced to produce IgE to ovalbumin, although they were capable at the same time to produce IgE against other food allergens obviously absent from the diet (e.g. shrimp). This phenomenon was interpreted as the expression of IgE tolerance induced by repeated amounts of allergen fed with the diet.

A probably similar experiment of nature has been observed in various populations of atopic dogs throughout the world. Dogs presenting with atopic dermatitis usually possess IgE antibodies against house dust mites, particularly *Dermatophagoides farinae*. In such animals, in Europe or Australia, the presence of IgE against food allergens (e.g. soya, wheat, meat) is very rare. In Japan, however, in a similar population, IgE against various food allergens is quite frequent, up to 40%. One possible explanation for this difference is the difference of pattern in feeding puppies, which in the Far East are still mostly fed from the table rather than by industrial foods.

So, according to our experience, early feeding with allergens may interfere with IgE production and affect the IgE phenotype, when examined at 1 year of age or later [18]. In some systematic experiments not reported here, it has been found that the window of opportunity enabling the induction of IgE tolerance lasts in the dog for about 6 months. Later on, induction of IgE tolerance seems less efficient. There are also differences in the ability of various allergens to induce IgE tolerance. While this is readily achieved with ovalbumin and milk proteins, it seems more difficult to achieve it in the dog with peanut. The possibility to achieve spontaneously IgE tolerance (due to allergen feeding?) in allergic infants by the age of 2–3 years to milk and egg but the difficulty to observe the same with peanuts is well documented [19].

Other Factors Affecting the Expression of the High IgE Response Gene

In man, several other environmental factors have been postulated to affect the outcome of IgE sensitization. Among these are hygienic conditions, the occurrence of bacterial or viral infections, particularly mycobacterial infections [20] have been described. The IgE suppressing effect of heat-killed *Listeria monocytogenes* in dogs [21] has also been described.

Although few formal experiments have yet been performed in the allergic dog model, it is likely that a number of environmental conditions affecting the Th1-Th2 equilibrium also influence the IgE response in the dog.

Role of the Mode of Administration

All results reported up to now concern dogs sensitized by intradermal or subcutaneous injection of allergens. In such animals possessing high levels of serum IgE, administration of allergen by inhalation causes allergic symptoms in the form of bronchial constriction (asthma), detected by alteration of pulmonary functions (increased resistance and compliance) and by the occurrence of a bronchial eosinophilic and lymphocytic exudate (BALF: bronchial alveolar fluid) In the eye, administration of allergen causes an acute conjunctivitis and intradermal injection the classical wheal and erythema skin reaction, particularly well visible in the dog when preceded by an intravenous injection of Coomassie blue [10].

Table 2. IgE response to injected or inhaled allergens

Dog no.	Allergen Bet V1 injected[a]	Allergen Ara A injected[a]	Allergen OVA inhaled[b]
140	39.6[c]	38.3	33.8
141	35.7	32.4	0[d]
142	35.0	34.4	0[d]
143	36.3	32.5	2.1
144	37.8	29.8	0[d]
145	38.3	27.9	27.6

[a] 10 µg allergen birch (Bet V1) or peanut (Ara A) injected subcutaneously for the first time at birth.
[b] 1% ovalbumin (OVA) administered for the first time at birth by aerosol.
[c] Specific IgE response in arbitrary units 4 months after first immunization.
[d] These negative animals were later successfully immunized with OVA by injection.

It has been asked, however, whether administration of allergen by inhalation (aerosol) causes sensitization in dogs with high IgE responder genetic background. To our surprise (Table 2), not all animals responding with high IgE levels to injection of allergens could be sensitized by allergen aerosols administered at birth or later on [22]. In a limited experiment, none of the low IgE response dogs could be sensitized by inhalation. This points to some additional control of sensitization by inhalation, probably genetic. However, appropriate breeding experiments have not yet been performed to demonstrate the existence of additional, probably recessive, „asthma gene(s)". If confirmed, it would indicate that the high IgE responder dog may also be looked at as a model for polygenic control of asthma, as suspected in man [4].

Similarly to the restricted pattern of experimental IgE sensitization by inhalation detected in our high IgE responders, spontaneous IgE sensitization to ubiquitous inhalation allergens such as house dust mites and pollens point to additional controls beyond the high IgE response gene(s). In our dog colony, IgE antibodies against house dust mites (particularly *Dermatophagoides farinae*) appeared irregularly in the 4–6 months following birth. While first sporadic and transient, probably reflecting exposure, the IgE response usually increased with age, becoming permanent and with an increasing titer. In the same litter, kept at the same time under similar conditions of exposure, the IgE response to house dust mites appeared only in some animals, reflecting again some additional individual control. None of the low IgE responder animals in the same colony developed IgE to house dust mites (Table 3). By contrast, practically all animals, including the low IgE re-

Table 3. Spontaneous IgE and IgG responses to house dust mites in high IgE responder Beagle dogs[a]

Total	Number of litters	IgE pos.	IgG pos.	First appearance IgE	IgG
95	20	29/95 30%	82/82 100%	day 107–653	day 58–118

[a] Dogs observed for 175–756 days, 10–47 blood samples during observation period.

sponders, developed IgG to the same allergen, confirming indirectly the universality of exposure. In the very clean environment of our experimental dog kennel, the presence of house dust mite allergen in the air filter dust could not be confirmed and it cannot therefore be excluded that exposure to the house dust mite allergen occurred by other ways, e.g. by food contamination.

Limited similar observations were made with IgE to the PP5 pollen allergen: only some animals of the same high IgE litter appeared to develop spontaneously pollen-specific IgE after 4–6 months of life and appropriate season of exposure.

Genetic Control of Atopic Dermatitis

Atopic dermatitis in the form of a pruriginous eczema appearing during the first year of life with characteristic localizations (paws, belly, perinasal and periorbital) and association with high levels of serum IgE is a frequent manifestation of atopy in dogs [10]. In the first years of experimental breeding for the high IgE response trait, this disease was not observed in our dog colony.

However, following extensive breeding for that trait and high IgE sensitization to some allergens present in the food (particularly ovalbumin). first cases of a dermatitis strongly resembling the natural variety occurred. This skin disease, called first „atopic-like dermatitis", was shown, also histologically, to resemble very much the natural disease but caution is still required, since the experimental variety appears to be non or little pruriginous. The atopic-like dermatitis usually starts within the first 3–6 months of life and shows clear flare-ups following administration of allergens, but takes then often an apparently non-allergen dependent course

Following breeding among animals showing the dermatitis, prevalence of the skin disease, which had first appeared sporadically in some litters, increased dramatically (Table 4). This again suggests an additional control, beyond possession of the high IgE response gene, for the occurrence of atopic-like dermatitis. None of the low IgE responder dogs ever developed the skin disease.

Table 4. Genetics of atopic dermatitis

Mating	Number of matings	Offspring number	AD number
LR×LR	5	30	0
HR #17 (AD)×HR (non AD)	7	28	2
HR #17 (AD)×HR (AD)	1	1	0
HR #128 (non AD)×HR (non AD)	1	6	2
HR #128 (non AD)×HR (AD)	1	6	6
HR #24 (AD)×HR #25 (AD)	4	13	13
HR #24 (AD)×HR #18 (AD)	2	9	8
HR #24 (AD)×HR #185 (AD)	1	4	4
HR #141 (AD)×HR # 184 (AD)	1	4	4

AD, atopic dermatitis; HR, high IgE responder; LR, low IgE responder.

In man, it is also obvious that atopic dermatitis is under some kind of genetic control: children from parents with high IgE and atopic dermatitis show an increased incidence of atopic dermatitis as clinical manifestation of the atopic syndrome.

Conclusion

The main finding of our breeding experiments for the high IgE type of response in Beagle dogs is that this type of response is inherited as a dominant trait, but with variable penetrance depending upon various environmental factors, such as the age of the animal at the time of first encounter with IgE sensitizing allergen and the mode of allergen administration. Even in dogs starting to produce IgE, environmental factors such as allergen feeding may modify the apparent phenotype.

From the analysis of events in our dog colony, it become obvious that mere phenotypic observation at a later age, including objective determination of IgE and allergen-specific IgE levels, does not reflect the true genetic background of the animals in terms of high or low IgE response and of the potential atopic state. If we had only observed the spontaneous development of IgE-mediated sensitivity and IgE levels in that colony, we would never have come to the conclusion that a dominant gene is at play but we would rather have concluded to the involvement of multiple recessive genes.

This is precisely the conclusion that current human allergogeneticists draw from clinical phenotypic observations of families including some IgE allergic individuals [4]. It should be recalled. however, that the hypothesis of autosomal dominant inheritance of the atopic syndrome, but with low penetrance, has been raised many times by authors describing genetic interpretation of allergic families data, including the very first large study by Cooke in 1916. In view of our clear-cut findings in dogs, we feel that this dominant hypothesis should no longer be summarily discarded, as still occurs nowadays.

Furthermore, the hypothesis of a dominant, but often non expressed gene, should also be considered when discussing the marked increase in prevalence of atopic diseases within the past 30–40 years and even before. It is clear at this stage that IgE-mediated atopic diseases were rather rare in ancient times, even up to the beginning of the 20th century. Rapid changes in the environmental factors, such as hygienic conditions, which repress the high IgE response gene, may be of more recent date and explain the dramatic increase of the disease in a population where the gene, multiplied in a dominant manner, may be much more frequent than assumed merely from the clinical occurrence of the IgE-mediated disease.

Beyond the IgE high response gene, other genes appear involved in IgE sensitization by inhalation or in the occurrence of atopic dermatitis, so that in the end, the whole picture of atopic diseases remains complex and subject to the influence of multiple genes. Nevertheless, confirmation in man of a basic requirement for a single high IgE response gene would be a major step and its identification a cornerstone in future diagnostic and early prevention of atopy.

Genetic material and cells available from our dog colony and families of high and low IgE responder dogs provide a suitable basis for molecular genetic studies, although studies of the dog genome are still in their infancy. However, search for dominant traits in our high IgE litters and in backcross breedings could soon provide new gene candidate markers. Considering that genes and proteins expressed by man and dog usually express 70–80% homology, IgE molecular genetic studies in dogs could provide a sizeable shortcut to molecular genetic understanding of atopy in man.

References

1. Coca A., Cooke R.A. On the classification of the phenomena of hypersensitiveness. J. Immunology, 8: 163–182 1923
2. Coca A., Grove E.F. Studies in hypersensitiveness. XIII. A study of atopic reagins. J. Immunol., 10: 445–464, 1925
3. Katz D.H. The allergic phenotype: Manifestation of „allergic breakthrough" and imbalance or normal „damping"of IgE production. Immunol. Rev. 41: 77–104, 1978
4. Holgate S.T., Wahn U. The genetics of atopy and asthma. Clin. Exp. Allergy 29 (Suppl.4): 1–59, 1999
5. Cookson W.O.C.M. Genetic aspects of atopy. In Epidemiology of Clinical Allergy (Burr M.L. Ed), Monographs in Allergy, Karger, Basle, 31: 171–189, 1993
6   Marsh D.G. Genetic studies of IgE responsiveness and asthma. In „From Genetics to Quality of Life" (Chanes P., Bousquet J., Michel F.B., Godard P. Eds) Hogrefe & Huber, Göttingen, 1996, pp. 9–14
7. Hopkin J.M., Shirakawa T. The genetics of atopy. In „Prediction and Prevention of Childhood Allergy" (Sasaki S., Miyamoto T., Hopkin J.M. Eds) Churchill-Livingstone, Osaka, 1995, pp 7–15
8. Wilkinson J., Thomas N.S., Morton N., Holgate S.T. Candidate gene and mutational analysis in asthma and atopy. Int. Arch. Allergy Immunol. 118: 265–267, 1999
9. Marsh D.G., Neely J.D., Breaseale D.R. et al. Linkage analysis of IL-4 and other chromosome 5q31.1 markers and total serum immunoglobulin E concentrations. Science, 264: 1152–1156 m 1994
10. de Weck A.L., Derer M., Mayer P., Stumper B., Schöni B., Haemmerling R., Kristensen F., Itaya H., Yamasita Y., Hasegawa A. Perspectives of diagnostics of canine allergies – a new serologic method for determination of allergen-specific IgE with strip tests. Prakt. Tierarzt, 79: 6–23, 1998
11. de Weck A.L. What can we learn from the allergic zoo ? Int. Arch. Allergy Immunol., 107, 13–18, 1995
12. de Weck A.L, Derer M., Mayer P., Stumper B. Allergy starts early in life: clinical and experimental evidence. In „Prediction and Prevention of Childhood Allergy" (Sasaki S., Miyamoto T., Hopkin J.M. Eds) Churchill-Livingstone, Osaka, 1995, pp 181–197
13. Schiessl B., de Weck A.L., Hodgkin-Pickart L., Zuni M., Zemann B., Mayer P., Liehl E. Importance of early allergen contact for the development of sustained immunoglobulin E response in Beagle dogs. Clin.Exp. Allergy, submitted
14. Ricci M., Rossi O., Bertoni M., Matucci A. The importance of Th2-like cells in the pathogenesis of of airway allergic inflammation . Clin. Exp. Allergy 23: 360–369, 1993
15. Romagnani S. Induction of Th1 and Th2 responses: a key role for the „natural" immune response ? Immunol. Today 13: 379–381, 1992
16. de Weck A.L. Food allergy, problems, fiction and hard facts. In „Highlights in Food Allergy" (Wühtrich B., Ortolani C., Eds) Karger, Basel,1998, pp 1–8
17. Holt .P.G., McMenamin D., Nelson D. Ptimary sensitization to inhalant allergens during infancy. Pediatr. Allergy Immunol. 1: 3–13, 1990
18. Zemann B., Griot-Wenk M.E., Schiessl B., Nefzger M., Mayer P., Liehl E, Schneider H., de Weck A.L. Induction of primary IgE oral tolerance to bb- lactoglobulin in an allergic dog model. Clin. Exp. Allergy, submitted

19. Bock S.A., Atkins F.M. The natural history of peanut allergy. J. Allergy Clin. Immunol. 83: 900–904, 1989
20. Shirakawa T., Enornoto T., Shimazu S., Hopkin J.M. The inverse association between tuberculin responses and atopic disorders. Science, 275:77–79, 1997
21. Umetsu D. Protective immunity in asthma and allergy. Congress Swiss Society of Allergology and Immunology, Lausanne, April 2001
22. de Weck A.L., Mayer P., Stumper B., Schiessl B., Pickart L. Dog allergy, a model for allergy genetics. Int. Arch. Allergy Immunol. 113: 55–57, 1997

Pathophysiology

6 Neuro-Immune Interaction in Allergy and Asthma

A. Braun, H. Renz

Abstract

Allergic bronchial asthma (BA) is characterized by chronic airway inflammation, development of airway hyperreactivity (AHR) and recurrent reversible airway obstruction. T-helper (Th) 2 cells and their products were shown to play an important role in this process. In contrast, the mechanisms by which T cells interact with the cells residing in lung and airways, such as neurons, epithelial or smooth muscle cells, still remains uncertain. Sensory and motor neurons innervating the lung exhibit a great degree of functional plasticity in BA defined as „neuronal plasticity". These neurons control development of airway hyperresponsiveness and acute inflammatory responses resulting in the concept of „neurogenic inflammation". Such quantitative and/or qualitative changes in neuronal functions are mediated to a great extent by a family of cytokines, the neurotrophins, which, in turn, are produced by activated immune cells, among others in BA. Therefore, we have developed the hypothesis that neuronal alterations in asthma are – at least in parts – due to inflammatory cells infiltration into the lung.

The Role of T Cells in Allergic Asthma

Allergic bronchial asthma (BA) is characterized by chronic airway inflammation that plays an important role in the development of acute symptoms. There is no doubt that T cells play a central role in allergic BA [1]. Multiple evidence supports the notion that Th2 cells orchestrate allergic inflammation driven by the effector function of B cells, mast cells and eosinophils. Th2 cells produce a cytokine profile that includes predominantly IL-4, IL-5 and IL-13. While IL-4 is mainly responsible for isotype switching in B cells towards IgE, IL-5 has pro-inflammatory properties by its function on growth, differentiation and recruitment of eosinophils. A further hallmark in the pathogenesis of BA is the development of airway hyperresponsiveness (AHR) which sometimes precedes airway inflammation. Acute asthma attacks are characterized by reversible broncho-obstruction due to airway smooth muscle constriction, inflammation and edema. To date, no satisfying concept linking inflammation with persistent symptoms of asthma is available. Therefore, the mechanisms by which inflammatory cells and their mediators interact with the resident lung cells, e.g. neurons, smooth muscle cells, and epithelial cells, await further elucidation.

New Trends in Allergy V
J. Ring, H. Behrendt (Eds.)
© Springer-Verlag Berlin, Heidelberg 2002

Neuronal Changes in Allergic Asthma

Human airways are innervated via efferent and afferent autonomic nerves, which regulate many aspects of airway function, including airway smooth muscle tone, mucus secretion, bronchial circulation, microvascular permeability and the recruitment and subsequent activation of inflammatory cells [2]. The innervation of the lung can be subdivided into cholinergic, adrenergic and non-adrenergic non-cholinergic (NANC) pathways, which are not strictly anatomically separated. At least certain NANC effects are mediated by the release of neuropeptides from classical cholinergic or adrenergic nerves [2]. The NANC system has been subdivided into e-NANC and i-NANC system. The e-NANC system is excitatory, bronchoconstrictory, C-fiber-mediated and tachykinin-dependent. In contrast, the i-NANC system is an inhibitory bronchodilatory pathway, located within parasympathetic nerves, mediating its effects mainly by nitric oxide (NO) and vasoactive intestinal peptide (VIP) [2].

In the last decade, growing evidence indicates neuronal dysregulation on several levels in allergic BA [3]. Since parasympathetic cholinergic nerves represent the dominant bronchoconstrictory pathway and anticholinergic drugs are very effective bronchodilators in acute severe asthma, cholinergic mechanisms must be considered in the development of AHR. These possible mechanisms include enhanced cholinergic reflex activity, increased acetylcholine (ACh) release, enhanced sensitivity of smooth muscle to ACh, and increased density of muscarinic receptors on airway smooth muscle.

The sympathetic adrenergic nervous system is less prominent than the parasympathetic nervous system within the human airways. It should be highlighted that there is a lack of sympathetic innervation of the human airway smooth muscle compared with other species [4–6]. Its main neurotransmitters are noradrenaline (NA) and neuropeptide Y (NPY). Guinea pig models indicate that antigen challenge induces a mast-cell mediated long lasting increase in synaptic efficacy [7]. In asthmatic airways, no difference in the number of NPY-immunoreactive nerves has been found as compared to healthy controls [8].

The e-NANC system seem to have a high degree of plasticity in inflammatory conditions. SP and NKA, preferentially released by sensory C-fibers, are members of a family of closely related neuropeptides termed tachykinins. They are synthesized preferentially in cell bodies of the sensory ganglia by a complex biosynthetic pathway. These neuropeptides are transferred via axonal transport not only to presynaptic axon endings in the spinal cord and the nucleus of the solitary tract, but also to peripheral sensory nerve endings [9]. Upon stimulation with mechanical, thermal, chemical (capsaicin, nicotine) or inflammatory stimuli (bradykinin, histamine, prostaglandins), tachykinins are released from nerves through a local (axon) reflex mechanism [10]. Tachykinins act in a dual fashion, as afferent neurotransmitters to the central nervous system as well as efferent neurosecretory mediators diffusing into the peripheral tissue. Increased levels of the neuropeptide SP have been detected in the lung of asthmatic patients [11]. Additionally, allergen challenge increased neurokinin A (NKA) levels in bronchoalveolar lavage fluid (BALF) of asthmatic patients [12]. Nerve fibers containing substance P (SP) have been described in and around bronchi, bronchioles, the more distal airways and occasionally extending into the alveoli. The fibers occur beneath and within the airway epithelium, around blood vessels and sub-mucosal glands, within the bronchial smooth muscle layer and around the local tracheo-bronchial ganglion cells [13]. In some studies, an increase in both the number and the length of SP immunoreactive nerve fibers was found in airways from subjects with asthma when compared with airways from subjects without asthma [14], while others detected no difference in SP like immunoreactivity [15]. However, the later finding may reflect augmented neuropeptide release. In a guinea pig model, it has been shown that sensory innervation of the airways is altered by allergic inflammation [16]. The increase of SP and NKA in the lung in response to allergen challenge has been related to an increased production of these neuropeptides in neurons of the nodose ganglion [17]. Impaired degradation of tachykinins could further enhance their local activity [18]. In addition, antigen-induced functional changes in sensory neurons including depolarization of the resting membrane potential, changes in membrane resistance, increases in mechanosensitivity (of Ad vagal afferent airway nerves) and enhanced response to SP were described [19, 20].

These data exemplify the dramatic changes observed on sensory and motor neurons in BA. It is plausible that these nerves not only trigger development of AHR, but also control important aspects of the acute inflammatory response in the airways. The alterations observed in these neurons are characterized by the term „neuronal plasticity", which emphasizes the great degree of modulatory capacity of these cells. On the cellular and molecular level „neuronal plasticity" may be due to nerve fiber growth, altered neuropeptide and tachykinine production, and release changes in receptor expression and lowering of the triggering threshold of neurons (Table 1). What causes these effects in BA? In this regard neurotrophins represent attractive candidate molecules.

Table 1. Experimental evidence for neuronal plasticity of lung and airway innervating nerves in BA

Functional changes	Species
Tachykinin upregulation in BAL	Human, guinea pig
Tachykinin upregulation in cell bodies of ganglion	Guinea pig
Nodosum Ad fibers	Guinea pig, human
Tachykinin upregulation in lung nerve fibers	Human, mouse
Neurotrophin upregulation	Mouse
Acetylcholine release	Guinea pig, human
Loss of function of inhibitory M2 muscarinic receptors on the airway parasympathetic nerves	Guinea pig
Increased mechanosensitivity in sensory Ad fibers	Guinea pig
Increased excitability of sensory neurons	Guinea pig
Increased response of sensory neurons to SP	Guinea pig
Increased sympathetic efficacy	Guinea pig

Biology of Neurotrophins and Their Receptors

The neurotrophins nerve growth factor (NGF), brain-derived neurotrophic factor (BDNF), neurotrophin-3 (NT-3) and neurotrophin-4/5 (NT-4) all belong to a family of homologous proteins that exert their effects primarily as target-derived, paracrine or autocrine neurotrophic factors. The role of the neurotrophins in survival, differentiation and maintenance of neurons is well defined [21]. They exhibit partially overlapping but distinct patterns of expression and cellular targets. In addition to their effects in the central nervous system (CNS), neurotrophins also affect peripheral afferent and efferent neurons. The biological effects of neurotrophins are mediated by binding either to high affinity (Kd -10^{-11}) tyrosine kinase receptors (trkA, trkB, trkC) or the low affinity (Kd -10^{-9}) panneurotrophin receptor (p75^{NTR}). Substantial biological effects of neurotrophins are mediated through the high affinity tyrosine kinase receptors. TrkA is the high affinity receptor for NGF, trkB for BDNF and NT-4, and trkC for NT-3. Neurotrophin receptors are widely expressed in the neurons of the peripheral and the central nervous system, both during development and in adults [21]. However, Trk receptors as well as p75^{NTR} are also expressed on non-neuronal cells including immune cells, muscle cells and epithelial cells.

Neurotrophins in BA

In inflammatory processes, NGF is produced by a wide range of immune cells including mast cells, macrophages, T cells and B cells (for review [22]). In a murine model of allergic lung inflammation, T cells, B cells and macrophages represent sources of enhanced NGF production. In vitro, allergen stimulation of mononuclear cells from sensitized mice resulted in enhanced NGF synthesis [23]. In addition, NGF production was enhanced by antigen stimulation in murine and human Th2 cell clones [24, 25]. BDNF synthesis has been detected in activated human T cells, B cells, macrophages, mast cells, and in thrombocytes [26, 27]. In addition to the constitutive production of BDNF by respiratory epithelial cells, we have demonstrated that activated murine macrophages and T cells, but not B cells, produce BDNF during allergic inflammation [27]. Histological analysis of the inflamed lung revealed strong NGF and BDNF production in cells of the peribronchial inflammatory infiltrate [23, 27].

Patients with allergic BA display enhanced levels of NGF in serum and BAL [16, 28]. In addition, increased neurotrophin production in response to allergen provocation was demonstrated in airways of subjects with allergic rhinitis or mild allergic asthma [29, 30]. After segmental allergen provocation in mild asthmatic patients neurotrophin content in BAL increased markedly in allergen exposed lung segments. Notably, this upregulation was seen during late phase response, but not in the early phase [30].

There is overwhelming evidence that sensory neurons innervating the lung are responsive to neurotrophins since local increase of neurotrophins in the lung could mediate similar neuronal changes in animal models as seen after allergic inflammation [16, 31]. It has been well established that visceral sensory neurons, localized in the nodose and dorsal root ganglia require neurotrophins for survival during development [32]. In adults, also functional properties of neurons are affected by neurotrophins [33]. NGF was shown to upregulate neuropeptide production in sensory neurons and contribute to inflammatory hypersensitivity [34]. Though cultured nodose ganglion neurons do not require NGF for survival, their SP production is regulated by NGF [35]. In transgenic mice overexpressing NGF in lung specific Clara-cells, marked sensory and sympathetic hyper-innervation and increased neuropeptide production was observed in projecting sensory neurons [36]. In addition, these mice demonstrated AHR to capsaicin. In a guinea pig model, tracheal injection of NGF induced SP production in mechanically sensitive „Ad" fibers that do not produce SP under physiological conditions [31]. These NGF induced effects are comparable with the neuronal changes that were seen acute airway inflammation [16]. The induction of neuropeptides in mechanically sensitive neurons may lead to exaggerated reflex response to innocuous stimuli [31]. Therefore, it is not surprising that NGF treatment induces AHR in the guinea pig. Interestingly, de Vries and colleagues were able to block NGF induced AHR to histamine by the NK-1 specific tachykinin antagonist SR 140333, pointing again to a central role for tachykinins in this condition [37]. In a murine model of allergic airway inflammation, we were able to demonstrate that the blocking of NGF by local treatment with anti-NGF antibody prevented the development of AHR [23]. Taken together these date provide further evidence that neurotrophins are central signaling molecules for immune cell-nerve communication as it occurs in pathophysiological conditions including BA.

Conclusion

There is emerging evidence that many cell types and mediators are involved in the complex network between immune and nervous system. Interaction between the two systems occurs on several levels: (1) Lung and airways are innervated via cholinergic, adrenergic, and non-adrenergic non-cholinergic pathways. (2) The neurotrophins NGF and BDNF are produced in increasing concentration by both immune and non immune cells in the asthmatic patient. (3) The predominant effect of neurotrophins on peripheral nerves is described by the term „neuronal plasticity". This is defined as qualitative or/and quantitative changes in the functional activity and capacity of peripheral neurones. One result of these alterations is the development of airway hyperresponsiveness in bronchial asthma. We propose the concept that neurotrophins act by aggravating and amplifying the pathology of bronchial asthma with all clinical consequences. Neurotrophins function as intermediate and long-term modulators of neuronal and immune functions.

We are just at the beginning of unraveling the complex interaction between neural and immune system. The above developed concepts now await further exploration, particularly in suitable in-vivo models. Ultimately, this concept requires to be proven using suitable intervention strategies.

References

1. Kay AB. Pathology of mild, severe, and fatal asthma. Am J Respir Crit Care Med 1996;154: S66–69
2. van der Velden VH, and A. R. Hulsmann. Autonomic innervation of human airways: structure, function, and pathophysiology in asthma. Neuroimmunomodulation 1999;6:145–159
3. Joos GF, Germonpre PR, Pauwels RA. Role of tachykinins in asthma. allergy 2000;55:321–337
4. Barnes PJ. Overview of neural mechanisms in asthma. Pulm Pharmacol 1995;8:151–159
5. Casale TB. Neurogenic control of inflammation and airway function, vol. 1. St. Louis, USA: Mosby, 1996
6. Joos GF, Germonpre PR, Pauwels RA. Neural mechanisms in asthma. clin exp allergy 2000;30 Suppl 1:60–65
7. Weinreich D, Undem BJ, Taylor G, Barry MF. Antigen-induced long-term potentiation of nicotinic synaptic transmission in the superior cervical ganglion of the guinea pig. journal of neurophysiology 1995;73:2004–2016
8. Howarth PH, Springall DR, Redington AE, Djukanovic R, Holgate ST, Polak JM. Neuropeptide-containing nerves in endobronchial biopsies from asthmatic and nonasthmatic subjects. american journal of respiratory cell and molecular biology 1995;13:288–296
9. Brimijoin S, Lundberg JM, Brodin E, Hokfelt T, Nilsson G. Axonal transport of substance P in the vagus and sciatic nerves of the guinea pig. Brain-Res 1980;191:443–457
10. Barnes PJ. Neuroeffector mechanisms: the interface between inflammation and neuronal responses. J Allergy Clin Immunol 1996;98:S73–81
11. Baumgarten CR, Witzel A, Kleine Tebbe J, Kunkel G. Substance P enhances antigen-evoked mediator release from human nasal mucosa. Peptides 1996;17:25–30
12. Heaney LG, Cross LJ, McGarvey LP, Buchanan KD, Ennis M, Shaw C. Neurokinin A is the predominant tachykinin in human bronchoalveolar lavage fluid in normal and asthmatic subjects. Thorax 1998;53:357–362
13. Lundberg JM, Hokfelt T, Martling CR, Saria A, Cuello C. Substance P-immunoreactive sensory nerves in the lower respiratory tract of various mammals including man. Cell Tissue Res 1984;235:251–261
14. Ollerenshaw SL, Jarvis D, Sullivan CE, Woolcock AJ. Substance P immunoreactive nerves in airways from asthmatics and nonasthmatics. Eur-Respir-J 1991;4:673–682
15. Lilly CM, Bai TR, Shore SA, Hall AE, Drazen JM. Neuropeptide content of lungs from asthmatic and nonasthmatic patients. american journal of respiratory and critical care medicine 1995;151:548–553
16. Undem BJ, Hunter DD, Liu M, Haak-Frendscho M, Oakragly A, Fischer A. Allergen-induced sensory neuroplasticity in airways. Int Arch Allergy Immunol 1999;118:150–153
17. Fischer A, McGregor GP, Saria A, Philippin B, Kummer W. Induction of tachykinin gene and peptide expression in guinea pig nodose primary afferent neurons by allergic airway inflammation. J Clin Invest 1996;98:2284–2291
18. van der Velden VHJ, Hulsmann AR. Peptidases: structure, function and modulation of peptide-mediated effects in the human lung. Clin Exp Allergy 1999;29:445–456
19. Undem BJ, Hubbard W, Weinreich D. Immunologically induced neuromodulation of guinea pig nodose ganglion neurons. journal of the autonomic nervous system 1993;44:35–44
20. Weinreich D, Moore KA, Taylor GE. Allergic inflammation in isolated vagal sensory ganglia unmasks silent NK-2 tachykinin receptors. journal of neuroscience 1997;17:7683–7693
21. Lewin GR, Barde YA. Physiology of the neurotrophins. Annu Rev Neurosci 1996;19:289–317
22. Braun A. Neurotrophins a new family of cytokines. Mod. Asp. Immunobiol. 2000;1:8–9
23. Braun A, Appel E, Baruch R, Herz U, Botchkarev V, Paus R, Brodie C, Renz H. Role of nerve growth factor in a mouse model of allergic airway inflammation and asthma. european journal of immunology 1998;28:3240–3251
24. Lambiase A, Bracci Laudiero L, Bonini S, Bonini S, Starace G, MM DE, De Carli M, Aloe L. Human CD4+ T cell clones produce and release nerve growth factor and express high-affinity nerve growth factor receptors. J Allergy Clin Immunol 1997;100:408–414

25. Otten U, Scully JL, Ehrhard PB, Gadient RA. Neurotrophins: signals between the nervous and immune systems. Prog Brain Res 1994;103:293–305
26. Kerschensteiner M, Gallmeier E, Behrens L, Leal VV, Misgeld T, Klinkert WE, Kolbeck R, Hoppe E, Oropeza-Wekerle RL, Bartke I, et al. Activated human T cells, B cells, and monocytes produce brain-derived neurotrophic factor in vitro and in inflammatory brain lesions: a neuroprotective role of inflammation? J Exp Med. 1999;189:865–870
27. Braun A, Lommatzsch M, Mannsfeldt A, Neuhaus-Steinmetz U, Fischer A, Schnoy N, Lewin GR, Renz H. Cellular sources of enhanced Brain-Derived Neurotrophic Factor (BDNF) production in a mouse model of allergic inflammation. Am. J. Respir. Cell Mol. Biol. 1999;21:537–546
28. Bonini S, Lambiase A, Bonini S, Angelucci F, Magrini L, Manni L, Aloe L. Circulating nerve growth factor levels are increased in humans with allergic diseases and asthma. proceedings of the national academy of sciences of the united states of america 1996;93:10955–10960
29. Sanico AM, Stanisz AM, Gleeson TD, Bora S, Proud D, Bienenstock J, Koliatsos VE, Togias A. Nerve growth factor expression and release in allergic inflammatory disease of the upper airways. am j respir crit care med 2000;161:1631–1635
30. Virchow JC, Julius P, Lommatzsch M, Luttmann W, Renz H, Braun A. Neurotrophins are increased in bronchoalveolar lavage fluid after segmental allergen provocation. american journal of respiratory and critical care medicine 1998;158:2002–2005
31. Hunter DD, Myers AC, Undem BJ. Nerve Growth Factor-Induced Phenotypic Switch in Guinea Pig Airway Sensory Neurons. Am J Respir Crit Care Med 2000;161:1985–1990
32. Snider WD. Functions of the neurotrophins during nervous system development: what the knockouts are teaching us. Cell 1994;77:627–638
33. Chalazonitis A, Peterson ER, Crain SM. Nerve growth factor regulates the action potential duration of mature sensory neurons. Proc-Natl-Acad-Sci-U-S-A 1987;84:289–293
34. Donnerer J, Schuligoi R, Stein C. Increased content and transport of substance P and calcitonin gene-related peptide in sensory nerves innervating inflamed tissue: evidence for a regulatory function of nerve growth factor in vivo. Neuroscience 1992;49:693–698
35. MacLean DB, Lewis SF, Wheeler FB. Substance P content in cultured neonatal rat vagal sensory neurons: the effect of nerve growth factor. Brain-Res 1988;457:53–62
36. Hoyle GW, Graham RM, Finkelstein JB, Nguyen KPT, Gozal D, Friedman M. Hyperinnervation of the airways in transgenic mice overexpressing nerve growth factor. American Journal of Respiratory Cell and Molecular Biology 1998;18 (2):149–157
37. de Vries A, Dessing MC, Engels F, Henricks PA, Nijkamp FP. Nerve growth factor induces a neurokinin-1 receptor- mediated airway hyperresponsiveness in guinea pigs. american journal of respiratory and critical care medicine 1999;159:1541–1544

7 Cadherin Biology of Langerhans Cells

T. Jakob

Langerhans cells (LC) are members of a family of highly specialized antigen presenting cells termed dendritic cells, that are widely distributed as minor cell populations in lymphoid tissue as well as in non-lymphoid organs such as the skin. LC are derived from cells originating in the bone marrow [1] that home via the peripheral blood to the basal and suprabasal layers of all stratified epithelia where they form a network of antigen presenting cells to monitor the epithelium as sentinels of the immune system. Positioned at the interface of environment and organism they are capable of taking up complex antigen and processing it into fragments that can be recognized by cells of the adaptive immune response. LC comprise all accessory cell activity that is present in normal uninflamed epidermis and are essential for the initiation and propagation of immune responses directed against epicutaneously applied antigens. The unique migratory ability allows them to shuttle antigen from the epidermis to the regional lymph node where they can initiate systemic immune responses by presenting surface-bound processed antigen to resting T lymphocytes [reviewed in 2].

LC Activation, Maturation and Mobilization

It is well recognized that LC like other dendritic cells undergo, morphological, phenotypical and functional changes in their life history before they turn into the potent antigen presenting cell in the regional lymph node. Resting LC that are located in the uninflamed epidermis are well suited for antigen uptake and processing, however express only low levels of MHC class I and II and costimulatory molecules and are poor stimulators of unprimed T cells [3]. Perturbation of the epidermal homeostasis by allergens, irritants, microbial infection or other factors results in the local activation of LC which exit the epidermis and migrate via the afferent lymphatics to the regional lymphoid tissue. In the course of this process LC lose their capacity for antigen uptake and processing, upregulate MHC class I and II antigens and various costimulatory molecules and turn into the most potent stimulators of unprimed T cells that have been identified [3–5].

Since LC play a pivotal role in the induction of cutaneous immune responses considerable interest has focused on mechanisms that regulate the functional maturation of immature epidermal LC and on factors that control the trafficking of LC in and out of the skin [reviewed in 6]. The turnover (half life) of epidermal LC under steady state conditions has been calculated to be in the order of 15 days [7]. Although LC appear almost stationary as compared to DC in other

New Trends in Allergy V
J. Ring, H. Behrendt (Eds.)
© Springer-Verlag Berlin, Heidelberg 2002

epithelial tissues (e.g. airway epithelium, half life approx. 2 days), there still seems to be a slow but consistent turnover of LC in normal uninflamed skin. Studies analyzing the numbers of LC in the afferent lymph draining normal human epidermis, demonstrate that considerable numbers of LC are continuously leaving the epidermis, even in the absence of inflammatory stimuli [8]. Local activation by inflammatory stimuli such as contact allergens leads to a dramatic increase of LC in the afferent lymphatics suggesting that under these conditions LC are actively mobilized from the skin. Several groups of investigators have studied the contact allergen-induced activation of epidermal LC and identified initial cytokine-dependent changes that lead to the mobilization of LC from the epidermis. One of the earliest events is the local production of epidermal proinflammatory cytokines such as IL-1 and TNFα [9]. Both cytokines induce a rapid activation and maturation of LC in situ and induce a rapid emigration of LC from the epidermis [10, 11]. Studies performed on cytokine or cytokine receptor knockout mice suggest that both cytokines are directly involved in this process and cross-inhibition studies with neutralizing antibodies imply that both cytokines may act in concert to mobilize LC from their epidermal environment [12]. It is now recognized that the steady state turnover of LC in the epidermis is tightly controlled by a fine balance of a number of local mediators, some of which retain the cells in an immature state (e.g. TGF-β, IL-10) within the epidermis and others that promote the activation and mobilization (e.g. IL-1, TNFα).

A side from local mediators that control the activation status of LC, research efforts focused on mechanisms regulating the adhesion of LC to keratinocytes. While attempting to identify adhesion molecules that might retain LC in their epidermal environment, Tang et al. [13] demonstrated that freshly isolated LC expressed high levels of E (epithelial)-cadherin and that E-cadherin mediated the binding of LC to keratinocytes in vitro. This observation was somewhat surprising since at the time members of the cadherin family were not know to be expressed by leukocytes.

Mechanisms of Cadherin-Mediated Adhesion

E-Cadherin belongs to a supergen family of calcium-dependent homophilic adhesion molecules that play important roles in morphogenesis and maintenance of tissue integrity [14]. A number of cadherin family members are expressed in the epidermis and mediate intercellular adhesion between keratinocytes. E-cadherin is present on the basal and suprabasal keratinocytes whereas P (placental)-cadherin is restricted to the basal keratinocytes. Both represent the major adhesive component in adherens junctions of keratinocytes. In contrast, other epidermal cadherins such as desmocollins and desmogleins are restricted to desmosomal binding structures.

Much of what we know about the regulation of cadherin-mediated adhesion comes from studies performed on epithelial cells. Cadherins that mediate high affinity adhesion are concentrated in adherens junctions and are linked to the actin filaments of the cytoskeleton by a group of cytoplasmic adapter proteins termed catenins [14]. This catenin-mediated linkage to the cytoskeleton is required for stable cadherin-mediated adhesion [15, 16]. Mutation analysis demonstrated that the C-terminal cytoplasmic tail of cadherins contain conserved domains that directly bind β-catenin, γ-catenin/plakoglobin and p120^{CAS} [17–19]. The binding sites for each of these proteins are in close proximity, suggesting that steric hindrance accounts for their mutually exclusive association with a single cadherin molecule. Both β-catenin and γ-catenin/plakoglobin mediate the binding to α-catenin [20], which in turn directly or indirectly via α-actinin binds to the actin filaments of the cytoskeleton [21, 22]. The role of p120^{CAS} in this process is less well defined. p120^{CAS} does not seem to bind α-catenin [18, 19], suggesting that it may act as a negative regulator, that blocks the binding of cadherins to the cytoskeleton. An alternative role has recently been suggested, in which p120^{CAS} is involved in the lateral clustering of cadherin molecules in the plane of the cell membrane [23]. In addition, cadherin-mediated adhesion is regulated by associated kinases and phosphatases. Phosphorylation of serine residues in the cytoplasmic tail of E-cadherin induces increased β-catenin binding [24], while tyrosine phosphorylation of β-catenin leads to the dissociation of the cadherin/catenin complex from the cytoskeleton [25]. Cadherin-associated membrane phosphatases such as PTPμ are likely to act as counter regulator, by reducing tyrosine phosphorylation of catenins and thus stabilizing the linkage of cadherins to the cytoskeleton [26].

The N-terminal extracellular domain of E-cadherin mediates the homophilic binding to E-cadherin on neighbouring cells. Crystal structure analysis and functional studies of the extracellular cadherin domain suggest, that cadherin form dimers in the plane of the cell membrane [27, 28]. Dimers from one cell connect

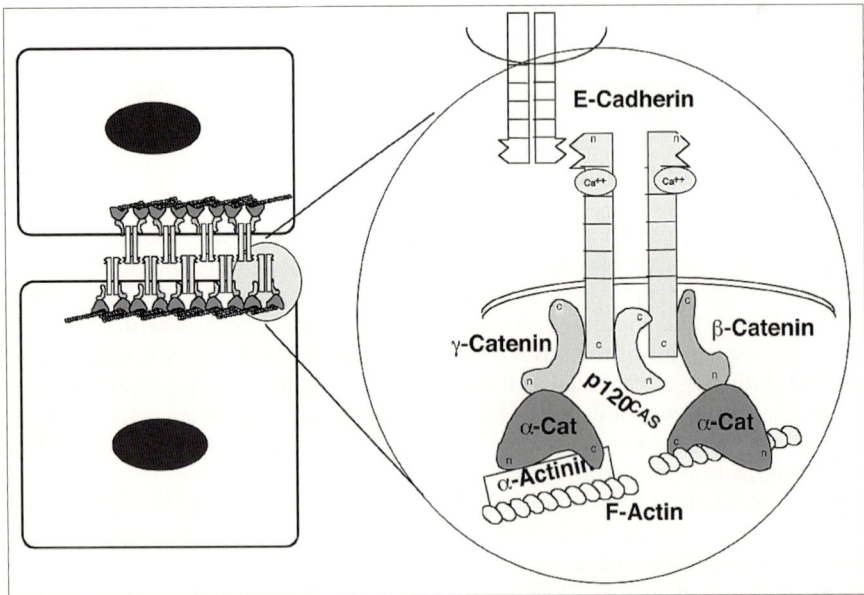

Fig. 1. Adherens junctions and the cadherin/catenin complex (for details see text)

to those for opposing cells by relatively weak adhesive bonds, and subsequent lateral recruitment of additional cadherin dimers into the binding site leads to the formation of a zipper-like structure in which multiple low affinity bonds accumulate to mediate high avidity binding [29] (Fig. 1) This lateral clustering is mediated by a juxtamembrane region of the cadherin cytoplasmic tail and it has been suggested that p120[CAS] is involved in the process [23]. Morphologically these cadherin clusters represent adherens junctions like they have been described in polarized and non polarized epithelial cells.

E-Cadherin Biology of LC

The demonstration of high levels of E-cadherin on murine and human LC [13, 30] and the observation of E-cadherin-mediated adhesion of LC to keratinocytes in vitro suggested that similar mechanisms may also be responsible for the retention of LC in the epidermis in vivo. The results of several series of experiments are consistent with this concept. First, among DC, E-cadherin is expressed only by LC and a subpopulation of skin draining lymph node DC that may be derived from LC [31]. Second, application of contact allergens that mobilize LC from skin induced a decrease in E-cadherin expression on a substantial subset (~40%) of activated LC in situ [32]. E-cadherin levels on activated LC (i.e. LC expressing increased levels of MHC class II antigens) were only 15–20% of those expressed by LC in normal skin, and were similar to levels on LC that migrated from skin explants [32] and lymph node DC that may be derived from LC [31]. Although these data suggested that E-cadherin-mediated LC-keratinocyte adhesion may decrease as a consequence of LC activation, and that decreased adhesion may result from reduced E-cadherin expression, direct evidence in support of this concept was lacking.

Studies of LC E-cadherin biology have been hampered by the lack of availability of large numbers of cells with appropriate characteristics. We recently described a primary culture system that allowed the expansion of Langerhans cell-like DC from fetal murine skin that resembled LC in terms of morphology, phenotype and function and that exhibited E-cadherin dependent homophilic adhesion [33–40]. Like LC [3], these cells spontaneously matured into interdigitating DC-like cells in vitro, manifested by a characteristic surface phenotype, cytokine profile and acquisition of potent allostimulatory activity. This in vitro maturation, like that of LC [13], was accompanied by decreased E-cadherin surface expression and by loss of E-cadherin-mediated adhesion [34].

Generation of LC-like DC from fetal murine skin provided a suitable model for functional and biochemical studies of LC cadherin biology, since large numbers of cells that displayed E-cadherin-mediated adhesion could be generated [34,35,40]. Immunoprecipitation of nonionic detergent FSDDC lysates with anti-E-cadherin mAb allowed insight into the association of E-cadherin with cytoplasmic proteins. Using this approach, we demonstrated that E-cadherin in FSDDC was associated with all known catenins (β-catenin, γ-catenin, p120[CAS] and α-catenin), suggesting that E-cadherin-expressing leukocytes might utilize the same mechanisms as epithelial cells in forming intercellular attachments [39].

As previously described for epithelial cells [41, 42], a fraction of total cellular E-cadherin and β-catenin was detected in the triton-insoluble fraction of the cell lysate, suggesting association with actin filaments of the cytoskeleton [39].

Since cadherins that mediate high affinity adhesion accumulate via lateral clustering in adherens junctions [14], we hypothesized that LC may form similar contacts with keratinocytes. Classical adherens junctions have initially been described in lateral apical membranes of polarized intestinal epithelial cells as part of the junctional complex consisting of tight junctions, adherens junctions and desmosomes [43–45]. Adherens junctions that were not associated with junctional complexes have been described in polarized and nonpolarized epithelia as button-like stuctures in areas of close membrane apposition [45–48]. Ultrastructurally, these adherens junctions differed from desmosomes in that membrane-associated intracellular plaques were less electron dense and plaques associated with microfilaments rather than intermediate filaments. Using similar criteria, keratinocyte adherens junctions were described initially in vitro [47, 48] and subsequently also in vivo [49].

Our ultrastructural analysis of cell-cell contacts in LC like DC demonstrated multiple junctional structures with a morphology similar or identical to adherens junctions described in non-polarized epithelial cells [39]. Immunogold localization of β-catenin to junctional structures supported the concept that LC-like DC form adherens junctions at sites of cell-cell adhesion [39], since β-Catenin, like E-cadherin, is a component of adherens junctions but not of desmosomes, hemidesmosomes or focal adhesions [50, 51].

Analysis of heterotypic cell-cell adhesion between LC like DC and KC yielded similar results [39]. DC exhibited multiple focal accumulations of E-cadherin in areas of contact with KC. E-cadherin accumulations were found at the end of spike-like cellular protrusions that stained positive for F-actin, suggesting linkage of these sites with actin filaments of the cytoskeleton. Finally, E-cadherin and β-catenin appeared to colocalize in sites of cell-cell contact and electron microscopy revealed adherens junction-like structures in areas of contact between LC-like DC and KC [39].

Formation of junctional structures was influenced by the maturational stage of the DC. Only LC-like cells with an immature phenotype displayed multiple focal accumulations of E-cadherin in areas of cell contact with keratinocytes, while DC with a mature phenotype did not. The inability of mature DC to form adherens junctions with KC was consistent with our hypothesis that E-cadherin-mediated adhesion is downregulated during LC maturation allowing the LC to detach from KC prior to emigration from epidermis.

Regulation of E-Cadherin-Mediated Adhesion

Previous in vivo studies implicated IL-1, TNFα and LPS in the activation and mobilization of LC from the epidermis, but did not allow mechanisms, or even targets, of action of these inflammatory mediators to be precisely determined [10–12, 32, 52]. LC from adult epidermis are not suitable for these kinds of studies for several reasons. First, the spontaneous activation and maturation that accompanies preparation of LC from epidermis precluded in vitro studies of the LC stimulatory properties of proinflammatory cytokines. Second, routine isolation of keratinocyte-free LC in quantities sufficient to study the regulation of E-cadherin-mediated adhesion was not possible.

Making use of LC-like DC expanded from fetal murine skin [34] we demonstrated that inflammatory mediators (IL-1, TNFα, LPS) that mobilize LC from the epidermis in vivo act directly on these cells and induced a reduction of E-cadherin expression and a loss of E-cadherin-mediated adhesion [35]. Because the same stimuli did not influence keratinocyte E-cadherin expression, we concluded that cadherin expression and function in leukocytes and epithelial cells can be differentially regulated. Loss of E-cadherin-mediated adhesion was accompanied by the development of dendritic morphology, upregulation of MHC class II Ag and costimulatory molecules and decreased expression of E-cadherin on LC-like DC in vitro. Activation of LC in vivo results in similar changes in surface phenotype within a similar time frame [10, 12, 32]. Changes in cellular morphology and in surface phenotype did not occur in cells in which E-cadherin-mediated homophilic adhesion was inhibited by a mAb (ECCD-1) [53], indicating that loss of E-cadherin-mediated adhesion is a consequence of activation and maturation of LC-like DC, and not a trigger of this process [35].

Studies in epithelial cells had demonstrated that E-cadherin mediated adhesion can be regulated at the level of tyrosine phosphorylation of β-catenin [25]. Using a sequential immunoprecipitation protocol we could demonstrate that in LC-like DC some of the E-cadherin associated β-catenin was indeed phosphorylated at tyrosine residues [33]. Since stimulation with IL-1, TNFα or LPS resulted in a decrease in E-Cadherin surface expression, we speculated that this also may be regulated at the transcriptional level. Northern blot analysis indicated that IL-1 and TNFα treatment induced a rapid reduction in steady state E-cadherin levels that preceded decreases in cell surface E-cadherin. E-cadherin mRNA levels decreased by ~50% within 2 h after addition of IL-1 or TNFα, while cell surface E-cadherin protein levels began to decrease only several h later. Subsequent changes in E-cadherin levels occurred with a time course compatible with the 5 h half-life previously reported for completely processed E-cadherin in epithelial cells [54] and resulted in the complete loss of E-cadherin-mediated adhesion (Fig. 2). This implies that E-cadherin expression and function in LC-like DC may be primarily (or entirely) regulated at the mRNA level. Currently we cannot differentiate effects of IL-1 and TNFα on E-cadherin transcription from those on mRNA stability. Based on prior studies, regulation at the transcriptional level seems likely.

In the past several years, cis-acting elements that regulate expression of murine and human E-cadherin genes have been identified and significant homologies have been noted. Particular emphasis has been placed on an upsteam pallindromic sequence termed E-pal, and E-pal binding proteins have been demonstrated in epithelial as well as mesenchymal cells. Deletion experiments suggest that E-pal binding proteins act as transcriptional activators in epithelial cells and repressors in mesenchymal cells, resulting in tissue specific expression of E-cadherin [55, 56]. Other studies indicate that the E-cadherin promoter is often silenced in carcinoma cells by hypermethylation of CG-rich regions [57, 58].

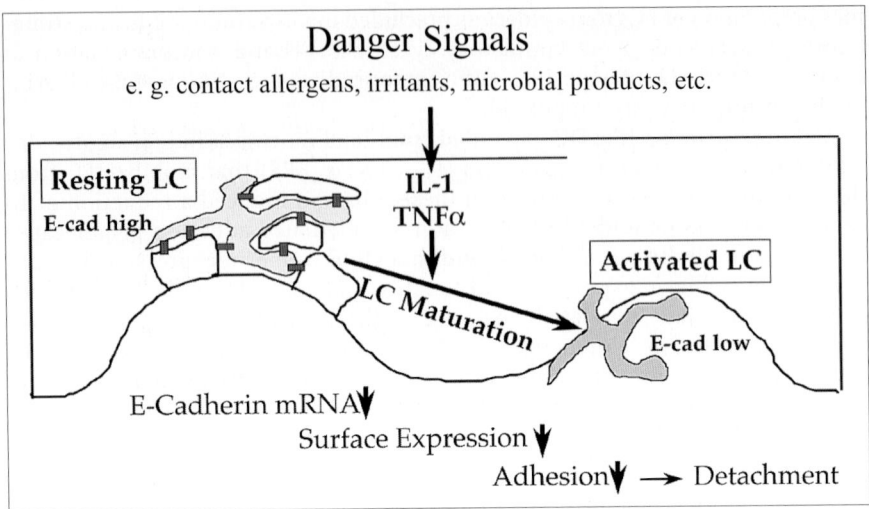

Fig. 2. Modulation of E-cadherin function on LC during the initial phase of LC mobilization (for details see text)

Overexpression of the transmembrane tyrosine kinase-encoding oncogene ERBB2 has been shown to decrease E-cadherin in mammary epithelial cells by inhibiting E-cadherin transcription, but it is not clear if this effect is mediated through DNA methylation [59]. Selective activation of AP-1 transcription factors (c-fos and c-jun) in mammary epithelial cells also results in decreased E-cadherin expression and/or function [60–62]. Since AP-1 is an important component of ERBB2, IL-1, TNFa and LPS signal transduction pathways, it is possible that increased expression or activation of this transcription factor complex in FSDDC is responsible for the downregulation of E-cadherin expression that we have observed. It will be of interest to determine if any, or all, of these pathways are activated in LC by IL-1, TNFα and LPS, or if LC E-cadherin expression is controlled via novel regulatory mechanisms.

References

1. Katz SI, Tamaki K, Sachs DH. Epidermal Langerhans cells are derived from cells originating in the bone marrow. Nature 1979; 282:324–326
2. Jakob T, Udey MC. Epidermal Langerhans cells: From neurons to nature's adjuvants. Adv. Dermatol. 1999; 14:209–258
3. Schuler G, Steinman RM. Murine epidermal Langerhans cells mature into potent immunostimulatory dendritic cells in vitro. J Exp Med 1985; 161:526–546
4. Steinman RM. The dendritic cell system and its role in immunogenicity. Ann Rev Immunol 1991; 9:271–296
5. Banchereau J, Steinman RM. Dendritic cells and the control of immunity. Nature 1998; 392:245–52
6. Jakob T, Ring J, Udey MC. Multistep Navigation of Langerhans/Dendritic cells in and out of the Skin. J Allergy Clin Immunol 2001; 108:688–696
7. Holt PG, Haining S, Nelson DJ, Sedgwick JD. Origin and steady-state turnover of class II MHC-bearing dendritic cells in the epithelium of the conducting airways. J Immunol 1994; 153:256–61

8. Brand CU, Hunziker T, Braathen LR. Studies on human skin lymph containing Langerhans cells from sodium lauryl sulphate contact dermatitis. J Invest Dermatol 1992; 99:109S-110 S

9. Enk AH, Katz SI. Early molecular events in the induction phase of contact sensitivity. Proc Natl Acad Sci USA 1992; 89:1398-1402

10. Enk AH, Angeloni VL, Udey MC, Katz SI. An essential role for Langerhans cell-derived IL-1b in the initiation of primary immune responses in skin. J Immunol 1993; 150:3698-3704

11. Cumberbatch M, Fielding I, Kimber I. Modulation of epidermal Langerhans cell frequency by tumour necrosis factor-a. Immunology 1994; 81:395-401

12. Cumberbatch M, Dearman RJ, Kimber I. Interleukin-1ß and the stimulation of Langerhans cell migration: comparison with TNF-alpha. Arch Dermatol Res 1997; 289:277-284

13. Tang A, Amagai M, Granger LG, Stanley JR, Udey MC. Adhesion of epidermal Langerhans cells to keratinocytes mediated by E-cadherin. Nature 1993; 361:82-85

14. Takeichi M. Cadherins: a molecular family important in selective cell-cell adhesion. Ann Rev Biochem 1990; 59:237-252

15. Ozawa M, Ringwald M, Kemler R. Uvomorulin-catenin complex formation is regulated by a specific domain in the cytoplasmic region of the cell adhesion molecule. Proc Natl Acad Sci U S A 1990; 87:4246-50

16. Takeichi M, Hirano S, Matsuyoshi N, Fujimori T. Cytoplasmic control of cadherin-mediated cell-cell adhesion. Cold Spring Harbor Symposia on Quantitative Biology 1992; 57:327-334

17. Ozawa M, Baribault H, Kemler R. The cytoplasmic domain of the cell adhesion molecule uvomorulin associates with three independent proteins structurally related in different species. EMBO J 1989; 8:1711-1717

18. Reynolds AB, Daniel J, McCrea PD, Wheelock MJ, Wu J, Zhang Z. Identification of a new catenin: the tyrosine kinase substrate p120cas associates with E-cadherin complexes. Mol Cell Biol 1994; 14:8333-42

19. Jou TS, Stewart DB, Stappert J, Nelson WJ, Marrs JA. Genetic and biochemical dissection of protein linkages in the cadherin-catenin complex. Proc Natl Acad Sci U S A 1995; 92:5067-71

20. Aberle H, Butz S, Stappert J, Weissig H, Kemler R, Hoschuetzky H. Assembly of the cadherin-catenin complex in vitro with recombinant proteins. J Cell Sci 1994; 107:3655-63

21. Rimm DL, Koslov ER, Kebriaei P, Cianci CD, Morrow JS. Alpha 1(E)-catenin is an actin-binding and -bundling protein mediating the attachment of F-actin to the membrane adhesion complex. Proc Natl Acad Sci U S A 1995; 92:8813-7

22. Knudsen KA, Soler AP, Johnson KR, Wheelock MJ. Interaction of alpha-actinin with the cadherin/catenin cell-cell adhesion complex via alpha-catenin. J Cell Biol 1995; 130:67-77

23. Yap AS, Niessen CM, Gumbiner B. The juxtamembrane region of the cadherin cytoplasmic tail supports lateral clustering, adhesive strengthening and interaction with p120ctn. J Cell Biol 1998; 141:779-789

24. Stappert J, Kemler R. A short core region of E-cadherin is essential for catenin binding and is highly phosphorylated. Cell Adhes Commun 1994; 2:319-27

25. Hoschuetzky H, Aberle H, Kemler R. Beta-catenin mediates the interaction of the cadherin-catenin complex with epidermal growth factor receptor. J Cell Biol 1994; 127:1375-80

26. Brady-Kalnay SM, Rimm DL, Tonks NK. Receptor protein tyrosine phosphatase PTPmu associates with cadherins and catenins in vivo. J Cell Biol 1995; 130:977-86

27. Shapiro L, Fannon AM, Kwong PD, et al. Structural basis of cell-cell adhesion by cadherins. Nature 1995; 374:327-37

28. Tomschy A, Fauser C, Landwehr R, Engel J. Homophilic adhesion of E-cadherin occurs by a co-operative two-step interaction of N-terminal domains. EMBO J 1996; 15:3507-3514

29. Yap AS, Brieher WM, Pruschy M, Gumbiner BM. Lateral clustering of the adhesive ectodomain: a fundamental determinant of cadherin function. Curr Biol 1997; 7:308-315

30. Blauvelt A, Katz SI, Udey MC. Human Langerhans cells express E-cadherin. J Invest Dermatol 1995; 104:293-296

31. Borkowski TA, Dyke BJV, Schwarzenberger K, McFarland VW, Farr AG, Udey MC. Expression of E-cadherin by murine dendritic cells: E-cadherin as a dendritic cell marker characteristic of epidermal Langerhans cells and related cells. Eur J Immunol 1994; 24:2767-2774

32. Schwarzenberger K, Udey MC. Contact allergens and epidermal proinflammatory cytokines modulate Langerhans cell E-cadherin expression in situ. J Invest Dermatol 1996; 106:553–558

33. Jakob T, Udey MC. E-cadherin associated proteins and tyrosine phosphorylation status in Langerhans cell-like dendritic cells. Faseb J 1996; 10:A1204

34. Jakob T, Saitoh A, Udey MC. E-cadherin-mediated adhesion involving Langerhans cell-like dendritic cells expanded from murine fetal skin. J Immunol 1997; 159:2693–701

35. Jakob T, Udey MC. Regulation of E-cadherin-mediated adhesion in Langerhans cell-like dendritic cells by inflammatory mediators that mobilize Langerhans cells in vivo. J Immunol 1998; 160:4067–4073

36. Jakob T, Walker P, Krieg A, Udey M, Vogel J. Activation of cutaneous dendritic cells by CpG-containing oligodeoxynucleotides: A role for dendritic cells in the augmentation of Th1 responses by immunostimulatory DNA. J Immunol 1998; 161:3042–3049

37. Jakob T. Regulation of E-cadherin function in skin-derived dendritic cells by proinflammatory epidermal cytokines: implications for the mobilization of Langerhans cells in vivo. J Am Acad Dermatol 1998; 39:274–5

38. von Stebut E, Belkaid Y, Jakob T, Sacks DL, Udey MC. Uptake of Leishmania major amastigotes results in activation and interleukin 12 release from murine skin-derived dendritic cells: implications for the initiation of anti-Leishmania immunity. J Exp Med 1998; 188:1547–52

39. Jakob T, Brown MJ, Udey MC. Characterization of E-cadherin-containing junctions involving skin- derived dendritic cells. J Invest Dermatol 1999; 112:102–8

40. Jakob T, Udey M. Generation of Langerhans Cell-like Dendritic Cells from Murine Fetal Skin. In: Robinson SP, editor, Dendritic Cell Protocols. Towata, NJ: Humana Press, Methods in molecular medicine. 2001; 64:231–241

41. Shores EW, Sharrow SO, Singer A. Presence of CD4 and CD8 determinants on CD4-CD8- murine thymocytes: Passive acquisition of CD8 accessory molecules. Eur J Immunol 1991; 21:973–977

42. Hinck L, Nathke IS, Papkoff J, Nelson WJ. Dynamics of cadherin/catenin complex formation: Novel protein interactions and pathways of complex assembly. J Cell Biol 1994; 125:1327–1340

43. Farquhar MG, Palade GE. Junctional complexes in various epithelia. J Cell Biol 1963; 17:375–412

44. Staehelin LA. Structure and function of intercellular junctions. Int Rev Cytol 1974;39:191–283

45. Geiger B, Schmid E, Franke WW. Spatial distribution of proteins specific for desmosomes and adherens junctions in epithelial cells demonstrated by double immunofluorescence microscopy. Differentiation 1983; 23:189–205

46. Drenckhahn D, Franz H. Identification of actin-, a-actinin-, and vinculin-containing plaques at the lateral membrane of epithelial cells. J Cell Biol 1986; 102:1843–1852

47. Green KJ, Geiger B, Jones JcR, Talian JC, Goldman RD. The relationship between intermediate filaments and microfilaments before and during the formation of desmosomes and adherens-type junctions in mouse epidermal keratinocytes. J Cell Biol 1987; 104:1389–1402

48. O'Keefe EJ, Briggaman RA, Herman B. Calcium-induced assembly of adherens junctions in keratinocytes. . J Cell Biol 1987; 105:807–817

49. Kaiser HW, Ness W, Jungblut I, A.Briggaman R, Kreysel HW, O'Keefe EJ. Adherens junctions: Demonstration in human epidermis. J Invest Dermatol 1993; 100:180–185

50. Cowin P, Burke B. Cytoskeleton-membrane interactions. Curr Op Cell Biol 1996; 8:56–65

51. Boller K, Vestweber D, Kemler R. Cell adhesion molecule uvomorulin is localized in intermediate junctions of adult intestinal epithelium. . J Cell Biol 1985; 100:327–332

52. Roake JA, Rao AS, Morris PJ, Larsen CP, Hankins DF, Austyn JM. Dendritic cell loss from nonlymphoid tissues after systemic administartion of lipopolysaccharide, tumor necrosis factor and interleukin 1. J Exp Med 1995; 181:2237–2247

53. Yoshida-Noro C, Suzuki N, Takeichi M. Molecular nature of the calcium-dependent cell-cell adhesion system in mouse teratocarcinoma and embryonic cells studied with a monoclonal antibody. Dev Biol 1984; 101:19–27

54. Shore EM, Nelson WJ. Biosynthesis of the cell adhesion molecule uvomorulin (E-cadherin) in Madin-Darby Canine Kidney epithelial cells. J Biol Chem 1991; 266:19672–19680

55. Behrens J, Lowrick O, Klein-Hitpass L, Birchmeier W. The E-cadherin promoter: Functional analysis of a GC-rich region and an epithelial cell-specific palindromic regulatory element. Proc Natl Acad Sci U S A 1991; 88:11495–11499

56. Hennig G, Lowrick O, Birchmeier W, Behrens J. Mechanisms identified in the transcriptional control of epithelial gene expression. J Biol Chem 1996; 271:595–602

57. Yoshiura K, Kanai Y, Ochiai A, Shimoyama Y, Sugimura T, Hirohashi S. Silencing of the E-cadherin invasion-suppressor gene by CpG methylation in human carcinomas. Proc Natl Acad Sci U S A 1995; 92:7416–7419

58. Graff JR, Herman JG, Lapidus RG, et al. E-cadherin expression is silenced by DNA hyper-methylation in human breast and prostate carcinomas. Cancer Res 1995; 55:5195–5199

59. D'Souza B, Taylor-Papadimitriou J. Overexpression of ERBB2 in human mammary epithelial cells signals inhibition of transcription of the E-cadherin gene. Proc Natl Acad Sci U S A 1994; 91:7202–7206

60. Reichmann E, Schwarz H, Deiner EM, et al. Activation of an inducible c-FosER fusion protein causes loss of epithelial polarity and triggers epithelial-fibroblastoid cell conversion. Cell 1992; 71:1103–1116

61. Hennig G, Behrens J, Truss M, Frisch S, Reichmann E, Birchmeier W. Progression of carcinoma cells is associated with alterations in chromatin structure and factor binding at the E-cadherin promoter in vivo. Oncogene 1995; 11:475–484

62. Fialka I, Schwarz H, Reichmann E, Oft M, Busslinger M, Beug H. The estrogen-dependent cJunER protein causes a reversible loss of mammary epithelial cell polarity involving destabilization of adherens junctions. J Cell Biol 1996; 132:1115–1132

8 CD8 T Cell–Dendritic Cell (DC) Interaction in the Regulation of IgE

D.M. Kemeny, M.J. Thomas

Introduction

During the past 15 years many of the molecules that regulate IgE have been identified. Interleukin (IL)-4 [1] and –13 [2] promote IgE class switching while interferon gamma (IFN-γ), interleukin 12 (IL-12) and transforming growth factor beta (TGF-β) are inhibitory [3, 4]. IL-4 and IL-13 are principally derived from T helper 2 (Th2) CD4 T cells while IFN-γ is produced by Th1, and TGF-β by T helper 3 (Th3), CD4 T cells [5, 6]. Whether Th1 or Th2 immune responses are produced in the first place is regulated both by specific cytokines, and by the strength of the T cell receptor (TcR) engagement with peptide-MHC.

IL-4 promotes the differentiation of Th2 cells [7] while IL-12 [8, 9] and IL-18 [10, 11] favor Th1 cells. IL-4 signals for IL-4 gene transcription via the signal transducer and activator of transcription-6 (STAT6). IL-4 gene expression is higher in T cells from STAT6 knockout mice than in Th1 cells from wild type mice indicating that another factor is involved. Introduction of GATA-3 into STAT6 deficient mice completely restored their capacity to produce IL-4 [12]. IFN-γ gene expression in CD4 and CD8 T cells require STAT4 and STAT2 signaling following IL-12/IL-18 ligation but only CD4 T cells require STAT4 for IFN-γ induction via the TcR pathway [13]. IL-12 is synthesized as two chains – p35 and p40. These combine to produce the active p70 heterodimer. Homologous combination of p40 chains forms a (p40)2 homodimer that binds to the IL-12 with comparable affinity to p70 but does not signal [14, 15] and so is a potent inhibitor of IL-12 [16]. IL-12 (p40)2 is produced endogenously following DC activation [17].

The strength of the T cell receptor (TcR)-peptide interaction has a profound effect on cytokine production. High affinity interactions favor Th1 cells [18–20], weaker signals give rise to Th2 cells. These different affinity signals alter intracellular signaling [21] and are able to override the effects of IL-4 and IL-12. This may explain how Th1 responses can occur in the presence of IL-4 and Th2 responses in the presence of IL-12 (e.g. Atopic dermatitis). Thus, in addition to the cytokine milieu, the type of antigen, the peptides generated and the efficiency of antigen processing and presentation will determine the nature of the immune response.

CD8 T Cell Regulation of IgE

In addition to CD4 T cells, CD8 T cells too have been shown to regulate the IgE responses. IgE inhibitory T cells can be activated following immunization with

New Trends in Allergy V
J. Ring, H. Behrendt (Eds.)
© Springer-Verlag Berlin, Heidelberg 2002

ovalbumin (OVA) [22]. These cells are cyclophosphamide [23] and radiation [24] sensitive and express the lymphocyte surface antigen Lyt2 (CD8α) [25]. IgE inhibitory CD8 T cells can be induced following inhalation of OVA aerosol [26]. These lung CD8 T cells expressed the γδ form of the TcR [27].

Much less evidence has been accumulated about the role of CD8 T cells in IgE regulation in humans. Comparable experiments to those carried out in rats and mice cannot be performed for obvious reasons. However, there is an allergic disease in which the normal regulatory processes that protect against allergy have broken down and both atopics and non-atopics become sensitized and CD8 T cells are implicated as inhibitors of IgE. Sensitization to castor bean dust occurs in practically all those who are exposed [28, 29]. The dust contains a toxic lectin, ricin. Ricin enhances IgE response to castor bean proteins or other bystander antigens such as ovalbumin or bee venom phospholipase A$_2$ [30]. Ricin was found to kill a population of IgE inhibitory CD8 T cells activated early in the immune response following parenteral immunization without antigen or with alum [31–35]. The importance of CD8 T cells was confirmed by depletion of CD8 T cells at a critical stage of the immune response which substantially increased serum IgE levels [36] and also enhanced the balance of Th2 over Th1 CD4 T cells [37].

IgE inhibitory CD8 T cells have been cloned. They express the αβ form of the TcR and are MHC class I restricted [38]. Interestingly, early-activated CD8 T cells were not detected in specific pathogen free (SPF) animals – supporting the view that activation of these cells may require certain pathogens. This supports the hygiene hypothesis that states that the increase in allergic sensitization in the latter part of the 20th century has occurred because people are exposed to less infections [39]. In this paper we will review recent work from our laboratory into the mechanism of CD8 T cell mediated IgE regulation.

IFN-γ

CD8 T cells constitutively make IFN-γ. They do not require IL-12, nor do they need to signal via STAT4 (see above). Since IFN-γ inhibits IgE and inhibits Th2 cells this it is a likely candidate. However the ability of OVA-specific rat αβ CD8 T cells, cloned following parenteral immunization, to inhibit IgE responses was unrelated to their capacity to make IFN-γ although IFN-γ was certainly involved as anti-IFN-γ antibody enhanced IgE in OVA immunized control animals [38].

To investigate the contribution of IFN-γ to CD8 T cell mediated IgE regulation, Tc1 and Tc2 CD8 T cells were generated in vitro from H-2K^b mice that expressed the transgene encoding the Vβ5.2 TcR that specifically binds the OVA peptide 257–264 when complexed to MHC class I H-2K. Both Tc1 and Tc2 CD8 T cells inhibited IgE [40, 46]. However Tc2 CD8 T cells make small amounts of IFN-γ, and IL-12 readily induces IFN-γ in Tc2 CD8 T cells [41]. To establish beyond doubt whether CD8 T cell IFN-γ was required, OVA-specific CD8 T cell from IFN-γ$^{-/-}$ mice were adoptively transferred to naïve wild type mice. These cells inhibited IgE to the same extent as IFN-γ competent CD8 T cells, indicating that CD8 T cells do not regulate IgE responses by secreting IFN-γ. Indeed, CD8 T cells that make IFN-γ are not able to inhibit B cell IgE synthesis directly, as Tc1 CD8 T cells had no effect on IgE production in IFN-γ knockout mice. However IFN-γ is involved, as CD8 T cells could inhibit IgE when transferred to IFN-γ$^{-/-}$ mice reconstituted with wild type CD4 T cells. Thus the cell that makes the IFN-γ that inhibits IgE in this system is the Th1 CD4 T cell. These data also show that CD8 T cells do not inhibit IgE by other direct effects on B cells such as cytotoxicity.

IL-12

We have observed that CD8 T cells from Vβ5.2 CD8 TcR transgenic mice (that recognize OVA peptide[257-264]) cultured with DC pulsed with relevant peptide stimulate IL-12 p40 secretion. The contribution of IL-12 was investigated in similar fashion to IFN-γ using IL-12$^{-/-}$ mice. CD8 T cell inhibition of IgE was completely dependent on the capacity of mice to make IL-12. Adoptive transfer of either Tc1 or Tc2 CD8 T cells to IL-12$^{-/-}$ mice completely failed to suppress the IgE response. Transfer of DC, derived from the periphery of wild type mice, to IL-12$^{-/-}$ mice completely restored the capacity of CD8 T cells to suppress IgE. Thus IL-12 is essential for CD8 T cells to inhibit IgE. As detailed above, IL-12 promotes the differentiation of naïve CD4 T cells into Th1 effector cells (Fig. 1).

Using DC from mice skin painted with a contact sensitizing agent, (trimellitic anhydride, TMA) that promotes Th2 CD4 T cell immune responses it was possible to skew Vβ5.2 CD8 T cells to a Tc2 phenotype. The key signals involved have yet to be identified but it is clear that immune skewing effects of CD8 T cells are mediated by their interaction with DC. IL-12 promotes differentiation of Th1 cells in synergy with IL-18 [42]. Indeed IL-18 is dependent on IL-12 which stimulates IL-18 receptor expression [43]. IL-18 receptor expression is higher on CD8 than on CD4 T cells [44] and on Th1 as compared with Th2 cells [45]. Although it is clear that IL-12 is the essential link between CD8 T cells and the suppression of the IgE response, and that IFN-γ producing CD4 T cells deliver the signal to the B cells that inhibits IgE synthesis, it has not yet been formally established that the IL-12 induced by CD8 T cells promotes Th1 and inhibits Th2 CD4 T cells. Fur-

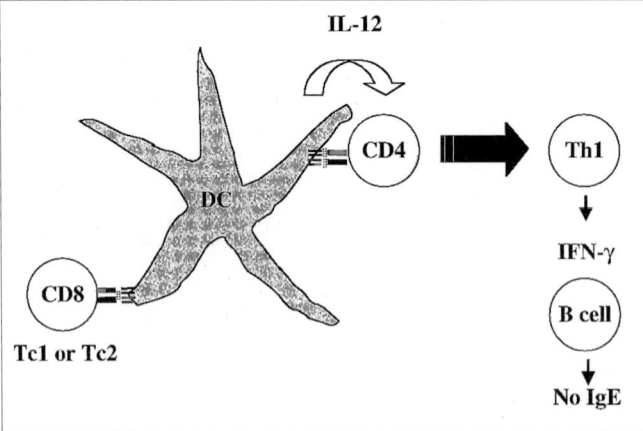

Fig. 1. DC recruit both Tc1 and Tc2 CD8 T cells through cognate interaction of CD8 T cell TcR and the DC MHC class I-peptide complex. This interaction stimulates synthesis of DC IL-12, which promotes Th1 over Th2 CD4 T cells. IFN-γ produced by Th1 cells inhibits B cell switching to IgE

thermore, we do not yet know what CD8 T cell signal(s) induce IL-12 synthesis by DC – although we do know that it is not simply IFN-γ. One family of candidate molecules is the chemokines that are preferentially produced by CD8 T cells. A recent report has demonstrated that signaling through CCR5 enhances DC IL-12 synthesis. During the next few years we expect to see the different elements of this pathway revealed.

References

1. Coffman, RL, Ohara, J, Bond, MW, Carty, J, Zlotnik, A, Paul, WE. B cell stimulatory factor-1 enhances the IgE response of lipopolysaccharide-activated B cells. J Immunol 1986;136(12):4538–4541
2. Punnonen, J, Aversa, G, Cocks, BG, McKenzie-ANJ, Menon, S, Zurawski, G, De-Waal-Malefyt, R, De-Vries, JE. Interleukin 13 induces interleukin 4-independent IgG4 and IgE synthesis and CD23 expression by human B cells. Proc Natl Acad Sci U S A 1993;90(8):3730–3734
3. Snapper, CM, Paul, WE. Interferon-γ and B cell stimulatory factor-1 reciprocally regulate Ig isotype production. Science. 1987;236:944–947
4. Gauchat, JF, Aversa, G, Gascan, H, De-Vries, JE. Modulation of IL-4 induced germline epsilon RNA synthesis in human B cells by tumor necrosis factor- alpha, anti-CD40 monoclonal antibodies or transforming growth factor- beta correlates with levels of IgE production. Int Immunol 1992;4(3):397–406
5. Miller, A, Lider, O, Roberts, AB, Sporn, MB, Weiner, HL. Suppressor T cells generated by oral tolerization to myelin basic protein suppress both in vitro and in vivo immune responses by the release of transforming growth factor beta after antigen-specific triggering. Proc Natl Acad Sci U S A 1992;89(1):421–5
6. Powrie, F, Carlino, J, Leach, MW, Mauze, S, Coffman, RL. A critical role for transforming growth factor-beta but not interleukin 4 in the suppression of T helper type 1-mediated colitis by CD45RB(low) CD4 T cells. J Exp Med 1996;183(6):2669–74
7. Swain, SL, Weinberg, AD, English, M, Huston, G. IL-4 directs the development of Th2-like helper effectors. J. Immunol. 1990;145(11):3796–3806
8. Manetti, R, Gerosa, F, Giudizi, MG, Biagiotti, R, Parronchi, P, Piccinni, MP, Sampognaro, S, Maggi, E, Romagnani, S, Trinchieri, G, et, a. Interleukin 12 induces stable priming for interferon gamma (IFN-gamma) production during differentiation of human T helper (Th) cells and transient IFN-gamma production in established Th2 cell clones. J Exp Med 1994; 179(4):1273–83
9. Gerosa, F, Paganin, C, Peritt, D, Paiola, F, Scupoli, MT, Aste-Amezaga, M, Frank, I, Trinchieri, G. Interleukin-12 primes human CD4 and CD8 T cell clones for high production of both interferon-gamma and interleukin-10. J Exp Med 1996;183(6):2559–69
10. Dao, T, Ohashi, K, Kayano, T, Kurimoto, M, Okamura, H. Interferon-gamma-inducing factor, a novel cytokine, enhances Fas ligand-mediated cytotoxicity of murine T helper 1 cells. Cell Immunol 1996;173(2):230–5
11. Yang, J, Murphy, TL, Ouyang, W, Murphy, KM. Induction of interferon-gamma production in Th1 CD4 T cells: evidence for two distinct pathways for promoter activation. Eur J Immunol 1999;29(2):548–55
12. Ouyang, W, Lohning, M, Gao, Z, Assenmacher, M, Ranganath, S, Radbruch, A, Murphy, KM. Stat6-independent GATA-3 autoactivation directs IL-4-independent Th2 development and commitment. Immunity 2000;12(1):27–37
13. Carter, LL, Murphy, KM. Lineage-specific requirement for signal transducer and activator of transcription (Stat)4 in interferon gamma production from CD4 versus CD8 T cells. J Exp Med 1999;189(8):1355–60
14. Ling, P, Gately, MK, Gubler, U, Stern, AS, Lin, P, Hollfelder, K, Su, C, Pan, YC, Hakimi, J. Human IL-12 p40 homodimer binds to the IL-12 receptor but does not mediate biologic activity. J Immunol 1995;154(1):116–27

15. Gillessen, S, Carvajal, D, Ling, P, Podlaski, FJ, Stremlo, DL, Familletti, PC, Gubler, U, Presky, DH, Stern, AS, Gately, MK. Mouse interleukin-12 (IL-12) p40 homodimer: a potent IL-12 antagonist. Eur J Immunol 1995;25(1):200–6

16. Moussavi, A, Dearman, RJ, Kimber, I, Daniel, KC, Kemeny, DM. Antigen-specific and non-specific determinants of cytokine production during topical sensitization of mice to chemical allergens. J All Clin Immunol 2000;106:357–368

17. Hochrein, H, O'Keeffe, M, Luft, T, Vandenabeele, S, Grumont, RJ, Maraskovsky, E, Shortman, K. Interleukin (IL)-4 is a major regulatory cytokine governing bioactive IL-12 production by mouse and human dendritic cells. J Exp Med 2000;192:823–833

18. Constant, S, Pfeiffer, C, Woodard, A, Pasqualini, T, Bottomly, K. Extent of T cell receptor ligation can determine the functional differentiation of naive CD4 T cells. J Exp Med 1995;182(5):1591–6

19. Tao, X, Constant, S, Jorritsma, P, Bottomly, K. Strength of TCR signal determines the costimulatory requirements for Th1 and Th2 CD4 T cell differentiation. J Immunol 1997;159(12):5956–63

20. Leitenberg, D, Boutin, Y, Constant, S, Bottomly, K. CD4 regulation of TCR signaling and T cell differentiation following stimulation with peptides of different affinities for the TCR. J Immunol 1998;161(3):1194–203

21. Noble, A, Vyas, B, Vuckmanovic-Stejic, M, Kemeny, DM. The balance of calcium and protein kinase c signalling directs T cell subset development. J Immunol 2000;164:1807–1813

22. Okumura, KO, Tada, T. Regulation of homocytotrophic antibody formation in the rat. IV. Inhibitory effect of thymocytes on the homocytotrophic antibody response. J. Immunol. 1971;107:1682–1689

23. Taniguchi, M, Tada, T. Regulation of homocytotropic antibody formation in the rat. IV. Effects of various immunosuppressive drugs. J Immunol 1971;107(2):579–85

24. Tada, T, Taniguchi, M, Okumura, K. Regulation of homocytotropic antibody formation in the rat. II. Effect of X-irradiation. J Immunol 1971;106(4):1012–8

25. Okumura, K, Takemori, T, Tokuhisa, T, Tada, T. Specific enrichment of the suppressor T cell bearing I-J determinants: parallel functional and serological characterizations. J Exp Med 1977;146(5):1234–45

26. Sedgwick, JD, Holt, PG. Suppression of IgE responses in inbred rats by repeated respiratory tract exposure to antigen: responder phenotype influences isotype specificity of induced tolerance. Eur J Immunol 1984;14(10):893–7

27. McMenamin, C, Pimm, C, McKersey, M, Holt, PG. Regulation of IgE responses to inhaled antigen in mice by antigen-specific gamma delta T cells. Science 1994;265(5180):1869–71

28. Thorpe, SC, Kemeny, DM, Panzani, R, Lessof, MH. Allergy to castor bean. I. Its relationship to sensitization to common inhalant allergens (atopy). J Allergy Clin Immunol 1988;82(1):62–6

29. Thorpe, SC, Kemeny, DM, Panzani, RC, McGurl, B, Lord, M. Allergy to castor bean. II. Identification of the major allergens in castor bean seeds. J Allergy Clin Immunol 1988;82(1):67–72

30. Thorpe, SC, Murdoch, RD, Kemeny, DM. The effect of the castor bean toxin, ricin, on rat IgE and IgG responses. Immunology 1989;68(3):307–11

31. Diaz-Sanchez, D, Kemeny, DM. The sensitivity of rat CD8 and CD4 T cells to ricin in vivo and in vitro and their relationship to IgE regulation. Immunology 1990;69(1):71–7

32. Diaz-Sanchez, D, Kemeny, DM. Generation of a long-lived IgE response in high and low responder strains of rat by co-administration of ricin and antigen. Immunology 1991;72(2):297–303

33. Noble, A, Staynov, DZ, Diaz-Sanchez, D, Lee, TH, Kemeny, DM. Elimination of IgE regulatory rat CD8 T cells in vivo increases the co- ordinate expression of Th2 cytokines IL-4, IL-5 and IL-10. Immunology 1993;80(2):326–9

34. Diaz-Sanchez, D, Noble, A, Staynov, DZ, Lee, TH, Kemeny, DM. Elimination of IgE regulatory rat CD8 T cells in vivo differentially modulates interleukin-4 and interferon-gamma but not interleukin-2 production by splenic T cells. Immunology 1993;78(4):513–9

35. Diaz-Sanchez, D, Lee, TH, Kemeny, DM. Ricin enhances IgE responses by inhibiting a subpopulation of early- activated IgE regulatory CD8 T cells. Immunology 1993;78(2):226–36

36. Holmes, BJ, MacAry, PA, Kemeny, DM. Depletion of CD8 T cells following primary immunization with ovalbumin results in a high and persistent IgE response. Int Arch Allergy Immunol 1997;113(1–3):160–2

37. Holmes, BJ, MacAry, PA, Noble, A, Kemeny, DM. Antigen-specific CD8 T cells inhibit IgE responses and interleukin-4 production by CD4 T cells. Eur J Immunol 1997;27(10):2657–65
38. MacAry, PA, Holmes, BJ, Kemeny, DM. Ovalbumin-specific, MHC class I-restricted, alpha beta-positive, Tc1 and Tco CD8 T cell clones mediate the in vivo inhibition of rat IgE. J Immunol 1998;160(2):580–7
39. von Mutius, E, Martinez, FD, Fritzsch, C, Nicolai, T, Roell, G, Thiemann, HH. Prevalence of asthma and atopy in two areas of West and East Germany. Am J Respir Crit Care Med 1994;149(2 Pt 1):358–64
40. Thomas, MJ, MacAry, PA, Noble, A, Askenase, PW, Kemeny, DM. Tc1 and Tc2 CD8 T cells both inhibit IgE responses. Int Arch Allergy Immunol 2001;124:187–189
41. Vukmanovic-Stejic, M, Vyas, B, Gorak-Stolinska, P, Noble, A, Kemeny, DM. Human Tc1 and Tc2/Tco CD8 T-cell clones display distinct cell surface and functional phenotypes. Blood 2000; 95(1):231–40
42. Tominaga, K, Yoshimoto, T, Torigoe, K, Kurimoto, M, Matsui, K, Hada, T, Okamura, H, Nakanishi, K. IL-12 synergizes with IL-18 or IL-1beta for IFN-gamma production from human T cells. Int Immunol 2000;12(2):151–60
43. Yoshimoto, T, Takeda, K, Tanaka, T, Ohkusu, K, Kashiwamura, S, Okamura, H, Akira, S, Nakanishi, K. IL-12 up-regulates IL-18 receptor expression on T cells, Th1 cells, and B cells: synergism with IL-18 for IFN-gamma production. J Immunol 1998;161(7):3400–7
44. Tomura, M, Maruo, S, Mu, J, Zhou, XY, Ahn, HJ, Hamaoka, T, Okamura, H, Nakanishi, K, Clark, S, Kurimoto, M, Fujiwara, H. Differential capacities of CD4, CD8, and CD4-CD8- T cell subsets to express IL-18 receptor and produce IFN-gamma in response to IL-18. J Immunol 1998;160(8):3759–65
45. Xu, D, Chan, WL, Leung, BP, Hunter, D, Schulz, K, Carter, RW, McInnes, IB, Robinson, JH, Liew, FY. Selective expression and functions of interleukin 18 receptor on T helper (Th) type 1 but not Th2 cells. J Exp Med 1998;188(8):1485–92
46 Thomas MJ, Noble A, Sawicka E, Askenase PW, Kemeny DM. CD8T cells inhibit IgE via dendritic cell Il–12 that promotes Th1 counter regulation. J Immunol 2002; 169:216–223

9 MHC Class II-Restricted T Cell Activation by Mouse and Human Mast Cells: Potential Clinical Implications

S. MÉCHERI

The mechanisms by which mast cells play a role in IgE-dependent allergic reactions and secrete histamine and other inflammatory mediators are known in considerable detail. Mast cells can also be regarded as a cell prototype that combine characteristics of both innate and acquired immune responses. For example, mast cells bind to mannose-specific lectin expressed on enterobacteria [1] and phagocytose and kill enterobateria, suggesting that they are capable of antigen-processing functions [1] classically ascribed to macrophages. Recent data demonstrating their capacity to promote specific immune responses suggest that mast cells may participate as an effector arm of both innate and acquired immune responses.

Mouse and Human Mast Cells Express Functional MHC II Molecules

In the past few years, the question of whether mast cells can initiate and eventually polarize specific immune responses in the absence of specific IgE and IgG antibodies has been addressed. Antigen presentation and activation of specific T cells requires the presence on antigen presenting cells of a complex between immunogenic peptides and MHC II products. The first indication came from the finding that mouse bone-marrow-derived mast cells (BMMCs) express major histocompatibility complex (MHC) class II molecules and present immunogenic peptides to CD4+ T-cell hybridomas [2, 3]. Similar findings were obtained with rat peritoneal mast cells which express MHC II molecules and activate PPD-specific T cell clones in the presence of the antigen [4]. The intracellular compartment where antigen processing takes place in mast cells has not been documented so far. In a recent study we addressed the question whether mast cell granules with lysosomal characteristics are the meeting point between MHC II molecules and immunogenic peptides [5]. In BMMC, the bulk of MHC II molecules was found in type I (multivesicular) and type II granules (which contain an electron-dense core surrounded by membrane vesicles) but not in type III granules. More importantly, in these secretory granules, MHC II molecules are associated with 60–80 nm vesicles termed exosomes which are secreted upon mast cell activation triggered by IgE-antigen complexes. This mechanism may provide mast cells with immunoregulatory properties in that a local inflammatory response may spread out and develop into loco-regional or systemic immune response.

To examine the position of MHC II-containing exosomes in the endocytic pathway, we analyzed the accessibility of this compartment to exogenous added anti-

New Trends in Allergy V
J. Ring, H. Behrendt (Eds.)
© Springer-Verlag Berlin, Heidelberg 2002

gen. Kinetic studies have shown that both type I and type II granules can be reached by bovine serumalbumin (BSA) conjugated to gold particles suggesting that these secretory granules are positioned in the endocytic pathway [5].

Studies on human mast cells suggest that these cells may function as antigen presenting cells [6]. In this report, it has been shown that the human mast cell line, HMC-1 expresses the costimulatory molecules B7–1, B7–2 and ICAM-1 as well as the MHC class II antigens HLA-DR, -DP and -DQ. More recently, it has been demonstrated that HLA-DR positive HMC-1 cells are able to present bacterial superantigens to T cells [7] and that staphylococcal enterotoxin A (SEA) can directly activate HMC-1 cells through HLA-DR molecules as demonstrated by ultrastructure changes [8]. In addition, when HMC-1 cells were cocultured with the Vβ3-expressing T cell hybridoma K25 in the presence of SEA, they trigger IL-2 secretion by these T cells [8]. Hence, these data support the concept that human mast cells can be activated via the MHC II signalling pathway and stimulate T cells upon presentation of superantigens.

MHC II Molecules Mediate Cytokine Gene Activation in Mast Cells

It is now clear that the presence of IL-4 and IL-12 during the development of naive T cells is critical for the differentiation of Th2 and Th1 cells respectively. Based on this concept, mast cells can be considered as a prototype APC that may contribute to the polarization toward the Th2 phenotype. Indeed, mast cells activated by IgE aggregation on the cell surface have been shown to produce a pattern of cytokines related to the Th2 phenotype [9, 10]. The MHC class II-dependent triggering of mast cell IL-4 release could be an alternative to IgE-mediated cytokine release. This hypothesis has been strengthened by using a quantitative RT-PCR technique showing that mRNA for IL-4, IL-5 and IL-10 can be specifically induced by stimulating mouse BMMC in the presence of specific T-cell hybridomas and the related peptide [11]. In standard assays, there was 200-fold increase in IL-4 transcripts. In addition, using anti-I-A and anti-I-E-coated beads on purified mast cells, it was established that MHC II molecules are the critical signalling molecules whose ligation results in IL-4 mRNA transcription. However, the mast-cell-induced T helper phenotype is becoming increasingly difficult to forecast. Indeed, Th1 responses could also be preferentially driven by mast cells that have been shown to produce IL-12 if they were exposed to SCF instead of IL-3 [12]. The concept put forward that mast cells play a dominant role in immediate hypersensitivity reactions by providing type 2 cytokines needs therefore to be reexamined. An alternative possibility such as the participation of mast cells in down-regulating Th2-mediated allergic responses should be taken into consideration. This dual mast cell function may occur at the level of mucosal sites where various pathogens have been shown to interact with receptors such as CD14, complement components or the mannose receptor for the production of IL-12 [13, 14] or with CD1 for the production of IL-4 [15, 16].

Specific antigen targeting to surface IgE and IgG on mouse bone marrow-derived mast cells enhances efficiency of antigen presentation

Earlier reports have demonstrated that cross-linking of FcεRI by immune complexes leads to immediate immobilization of the receptors, interactions with the cytoskeleton [17, 18] and to endocytosis of the immune complexes into coated-pits vesicles [19–21]. Recently, we have shown that internalization of antigen via FcγR or FcεRI by GM-CSF cultured mast cells upregulated their capacity to present antigen to specific T cells [22]. Internalization of Lol p 1 through various specific IgG mAbs resulted in the activation of Lol p 1-specific T cell hybridoma at concentrations about 100-fold less than that required for T cell stimulation by uncomplexed antigen. IgE-complexed Lol p 1, which facilitates trapping of antigen by mast cells, induced an accelerated and more efficient antigen presenting capacity of mast cells than that obtained with uncomplexed antigen [22]. On the other hand, IFN-γ which highly upregulates MHC class II expression on mast cells, completely inhibits their antigen presenting capacity. We have used this model to study the role of FcεRI- and FcγR-mediated antigen internalization in the regulation of the antigen presenting function of IFN-γ-treated mast cells. We found that FcεRI but not FcγR could reverse the IFN-γ-treated mast cells from inefficient to highly efficient antigen presenting cells [23]. Inhibition of the antigen presenting capacity by piceatannol, a PTK syk-specific inhibitor, indicates that this is an active process resulting from IgE-antigen-FcεRI engagement which involves tyrosines found in the immunoreceptor tyrosine-based activation motif (ITAM) embedded in the cytoplasmic tail of the FcεRI β and γ chains [23]. Antigen presenting function was also shown to require the activation of PI-3 kinase, downstream of PTK syk phosphorylation, since this activity was completely blocked by wortmannin, a PI3 kinase-specific inhibitor [23]. These data strongly demonstrate that FcεRI is actively involved in the antigen presentation process, not only as a vehicle for antigen entry but also by transmitting intracellular signals allowing optimal antigen processing.

Biological Significance and Clinical Implications

IgE-mediated antigen presentation by mast cells exposed to IFN-γ could be relevant physiologically. Mast cells which are present with high frequency in mucosal barriers such as the lung and the gut, are among the first antigen presenting cells that are exposed to many antigens and aggressive agents. During inflammatory reactions where IFN-γ concentrations are elevated, naturally occurring IgE-bearing mast cells could clear antigens more rapidly through specific endocytosis and induce vigorous immune responses via increased efficiency of antigen presentation to T cells. Major implications may result from mast cell-T cell interaction: IgE-antigen complex formation leads to aggregation of FcεRI and causes immediate release of inflammatory mediators and cytokines [12]. Furthermore, cytokine gene activation especially IL-4 has recently been shown also to occur through aggregation of mast cell MHC class II molecules [11]. This synergy between FcεRI- and MHC class II-mediated IL-4 production may occur during antigen presentation and could lead to the upregulation of specific IgE synthesis by inducing T helper cells to differentiate into Th2 phenotype. IgE-independent IL-4 production by mast cells as a result of cognate interaction with CD4 T cells could be critical for the development of Type 2 responses. This novel mechanism may contribute to the induction and/or amplification of specific IgE-mediated allergic responses. A hypothesis could be that following delivery of low dose of allergen within a peripheral tissue, under certain conditions where mast cells are recruited as APCs within lymphoid organs, naive CD4 T cells could specifically induce MHC class II-mediated mast cell activation resulting in IL-4 secretion. Produced IL-4 will, in turn, directly influence the polarization of allergen-reactive T cells toward the Th2 pathway. This mechanism may account for allergic disorders such as intrinsic asthma or some chronic idiopathic urticaria where inflammatory processes do not seem to implicate specific IgE antibodies.

References

1. Malaviya, R., E. A. Ross, J. I. MacGregor, T. Ikeda, J. R. Little, B. A. Jakschik, and S. N. Abraham. 1994. Mast cell phagocytosis of FimH-expressing enterobacteria. J Immunol 152:1907
2. Frandji, P., C. Tkaczyk, C. Oskéritzian, J. Lapeyre, R. Peronet, B. David, J. G. Guillet, and S. Mécheri. 1995. Cytokine-dependent regulation of MHC class II expression and antigen presentation of mast cells. Cell. Immunol 163:37
3. Frandji, P., C. Oskéritzian, F. Cacaraci, J. Lapeyre, R. Peronet, B. David, J. G. Guillet, and S. Mécheri. 1993. Antigen-dependent stimulation by bone-marrow-derived mast cells of MHC class II-restricted T cell hybridoma. J Immunol 151:6318
4. Fox, C. C., S. D. Jewell, and C. C. Whitacre. 1994. Rat peritoneal mast cells present antigen to a PPD-specific T cell line. Cell Immunol 158:253
5. Raposo, G., D. Tenza, S. Mécheri, R. Peronet, C. Bonnerot, and C. Desaymard. 1997. Accumulation of MHC class II molecules in mast cell secretory granules and their release upon degranulation. Molec Biol Cell 8:2631
6. Love, K. S., L. R. R., J. H. Butterfield, and C. C. Fox. 1996. INF-g-Stimulated Enhancement of MHC Class II Antigen Expression by Human Mast Cell Line HMC-1. Cell. Immunol. 170:85
7. Fox, C., K. Love, and R. Lakshmanan. 1997. Human mast cell mediated activation of T cells by staphylococcal exotoxins. J Allergy Clin Immunol 99:89 (Abstarct 363)
8. Dimitriadou, V., S. Mécheri, M. Koutsilieris, W. Fraser, R. Al-Dakkak, and W. Mourad. 1998. Expression of functional major histocompatibility complex class II molecules on HMC-1 human mast cells. J Leuk Biol 64:791
9. Plaut, M., J. H. Pierce, C. J. Watson, J. Hanley-Hyde, R. P. Nordan, and W. E. Paul. 1989. Mast cell lines produce lymphokines in response to cross-linkage of FceRI or to calcium ionophores. Nature 339:64
10. Burd, P. R., H. W. Rogers, J. R. Gordon, C. A. Martin, S. Jayaraman, S. D. Wilson, A. M. Dvorak, S. J. Galli, and M. E. Dorf. 1989. Interleukin 3-dependent and -independent mast cells stimulated with IgE and antigen express multiple cytokines. J Exp Med 170:245
11. Frandji, P., W. Mourad, C. Tkaczyk, B. David, J. H. Colle, and S. Mécheri. 1998. IL-4 mRNA transcription is induced in mouse bone marrow-derived mast cells through an MHC class II-dependent signalling pathway. Eur.J.Immunol 28;844
12. Smith, T. J., L. A. Ducharme, and J. H. Weis. 1994. Preferential expression of interleukin-12 or interleukin-4 by murine bone marrow mast cells derived in mast cell growth factor or interleukin-3. Eur J Immunol 24:822
13. Reiner, S. L., and R. A. seder. 1995. T helper cell differentiation in immune response. Curr Opin Immunol 7:360

14. Biron, C. A., and R. T. Gazzinelli. 1995. Effects of IL-12 on immune responses to microbial infections: a key mediator in regulating disease outcome. Curr Opin Immunol 7:485
15. Bendelac, A. 1995. Mouse NK1+ T cells. Curr Opin Immunol 7:367
16. Porcelli, S. A., and R. L. Modlin. 1995. CD1 and the expanding universe of T cell antigens. J Immunol 155:3709
17. Menon, A. K., D. Holowka, and B. Baird. 1986. Clustering, mobility, and triggering activity of small oligomers of immunoglobulin E on rat basophilic leukemia cells. J. Cell. Biol 102:534
18. Robertson, D., D. Holowka, and B. Baird. 1986. Cross-linking of immunoglobulin E-receptor complexes induces their interaction with the cytoskeleton of rat basophilic leukemia cells. J. Immunol 136:4565
19. Pfeiffer, J. R., J. C. Seagrave, B. H. Davis, G. G. Deanin, and J. M. Oliver. 1985. Membrane and cytoskeletal changes associated with IgE-mediated serotonin release from rat basophil leukemia cells. J. Cell. Biol 101:2145
20. Seagrave, J., J. R. Pfeiffer, C. Wofsy, and J. M. Oliver. 1991. Relationship of IgE receptor topography to secretion in RBL-2H3 mast cells. J. Cell. Physiol 148:139
21. Mao, S. Y., J. R. Pfeiffer, J. Oliver, and H. Metzger. 1993. Effects of subunit mutation on the localization to coated pits and internalization of cross-linked IgE-receptor complexes. J. Immunol 151:2760
22. Tkaczyk, C., M. Viguier, Y. Boutin, P. Frandji, B. David, J. Hebert, and S. Mécheri. 1998. Specific antigen targeting to surface IgE and IgG on mouse bone marrow-derived mast cells enhances efficiency of antigen presentation. Immunology 94:318
23. Tkaczyk, C., I. Villa, R. Peronet, B. David, and Mécheri. 1999. FceRI-mediated antigen endocytosis turns IFN-g-treated mouse mast cells from inefficient into potent antigen presenting cells. Immunology 97: 333

10 T Cell Reactivity Against Timothy Grass Pollen Allergens in Allergic Versus Non-Allergic Human Donors: Epitope Recognition and Cytokine Profile

R.L. Oropeza-Wekerle, E. Albert, U. Darsow, J. Ring, H. Behrendt

Introduction

Pollen from timothy grass (*Phleum pratense*) count among the most common allergens. In Europe they are the cause of 75% of all cases of allergy type I. The clinical importance of Phleum pollen provided an essential stimulus for research into its role in allergenic pathomechanisms. Structural genes encoding pollen components have been cloned, and expressed, making available recombinant proteins for identification of allergenic epitopes and the design novel therapeutic strategies [1].

It is clear that allergen-specific IgE antibodies are the decisive pathogenic factors in pollen-specific allergy. Complexed to pollen determinants, IgE is bale to activate the inflammatory mechanisms underlying clinical allergic disease. It is equally clear, however, that generation of pathological levels of allergenic IgE depends on the activity of allergen-specific helper T lymphocytes. In particular, Th2 lymphocytes are required to direct a pollen-specific B lymphocyte response to the production of IgE isoforms. Th2 lymphocytes are activated by immune-specific recognition of critical pollen epitopes presented on suitable antigen-presenting cells. Upon activation, the Th2 cells release cytokines (IL-4, IL-5, IL-13) which lead the pollen-specific B lymphocytes to selectively produce immuno-globulins of IgE isotype. Obviously, the sequential steps of interactions between antigen presenting cells, pollen-specific Th2 cells and IgE releasing B cells offer themselves as promising targets for selective therapy of allergy [2]. In an attempt to analyze these intercellular interactions, we have isolated allergen-specific T cell lines from MHC matched atopic and non-atopic donors to study their antigen specificity, MHC restriction, and most important, their cytokine production patterns.

Antigen-Specific T Cell Lines

We recruited a panel of atopic as well as non-atopic blood donors whose allergic status was determined using several methods. A CAP system to quantify allergen reactive IgE titers in serum, and skin reactivity was studied by prick testing. T cell lines were isolated from fresh blood samples by a primary limiting dilution system, which had been developed initially to select autoantigen-specific T cells from patients with multiple sclerosis. This technique is based on the establishment and screening of multiple parallel microcultures. This limiting dilution approach allows the high-yield identification of T cell lines ("clonoids") com-

New Trends in Allergy V
J. Ring, H. Behrendt (Eds.)
© Springer-Verlag Berlin, Heidelberg 2002

posed of very few, if not only one T cell clone [3]. In our present studies, we used both recombinant allergenic proteins and peptide fragments spanning the entire protein sequence. As controls, we isolated T cell lines reacting against tetanus toxoid and myelin basic protein (MBP), a candidate autoantigen in MS.

We compiled multiple T cell lines from 4 atopic and 4 non-atopic donors. Following our present protocol, we selected the allergen-specific T cell lines primarily by combinations of synthetic 20-meric peptides spanning the entire length of the Phl p5 protein in an overlapping fashion. Primary selection was followed in a second step by propagation driven by recombinant allergen (rPhlp5).

Examination of the fine specificity of allergen-specific T cell clones, from atopic with non-atopic donors was achieved using individual synthetic peptide analogs representing the dominant epitope of Phl p5. The peptides are gradually truncated at the N- and the C-terminus. So far we identified a core sequence of 12 amino acids, which was common to T cell clones from 2 unrelated atopic donors (HLA haplotypes DR4/DR6, and DR7/DR12). A comparable series of T cell clones from a non-atopic donor (DR2/DR14) had a core region of similar position, but required additional 3 amino acids to be fully recognizable.

Cytokine Production by Allergen-Specific T Cells from Allergic and Non-Allergic Donors

Cytokine production of allergen and control T cell lines was assessed combining ELISA (for cytokine secretion) with FACS analysis (for intracellular expression of cytokines). As assessed by ELISA, all lines showed a Th2-like cytokine secretion pattern, with IL-4 release stronger than IFN-γ. Cytoplasmic cytokine determination by cytofluorometry, which allows T cell analysis on single-cell level [4], however, yielded a more complex picture. This method revealed that all T cell lines were composed, at different proportions, of T cells secreting either IL-4 or IFN-γ alone, or in combination. FACS analyses did, however confirm a clear tendency towards Th2-like reactions in *Phleum pratense*-specific T cells both from allergic as well as from non-allergic donors. In striking contrast, T cell responses against tetanus toxoid, as a control antigen, were slanted towards Th1-like cytokine patterns in both groups of donors.

Conclusion

Our present data indicate that the immune repertoires of allergic and non-allergic humans contain T cell clones reactive against dominant epitopes of the allergenic protein Phl p5 of timothy grass. Interestingly, the epitope patterns of Phl p5 reactive T cells were strikingly similar between allergic and non-allergic donors. Furthermore, and possibly most importantly, the majority of all allergen-specific T cell clones produce cytokines in a Th2- or Th0-like manner. This pattern is seen in all allergen-specific T cell populations, irrespective of the donors' clinical status. Our results encourage further investigations into the factors, which may drive pollen-specific T cells into Th2-like differentiation.

Acknowledgements. We thank Ms. M. Klessinger for excellent technical assistance. This work was supported by grants from BMBF Klinische Forschergruppe „Molekulare und angewandte Allergotoxikologie".

References

1. Valenta,R., S.Vrtala, S.Laffer, S.Spitzauer, and D.Kraft. 1998. Recombinant allergens. Allergy 53:552–561
2. Leung,D.Y.M. 2000. Atopic dermatitis: New insights and opportunities for therapeutic intervention. J.Allergy Clin.Immunol. 105:860–876
3. Pette,M., K.Fujita, D.Wilkinson, D.M.Altmann, J.Trowsdale, G.Giegerich, A.Hinkkanen, J.T.Epplen, L.Kappos, and H.Wekerle. 1990. Myelin autoreactivity in multiple sclerosis: Recognition of myelin basic protein in the context of HLA-DR2 products by T lymphocytes of multiple sclerosis patients and healthy donors. Proc.Natl.Acad.Sci.USA 87:7968–7972
4. Schauer,U., T.Jung, N.Krug, and A.Frew. 1996. Measurement of intracellular cytokines. Immunol.Today 17:305–306

11 α1,3-Fucosyltransferase VII mRNA Expression Is Induced by Superantigens and Blocked by Inhibitors of NF-κB

M. Podda, H.A. Beschmann, A.M. Duijvestijn, U.H. v. Andrian, R. Kaufmann, T.M. Zollner

Introduction

Lymphocyte migration is an essential requirement for efficient surveillance of tissues for infectious pathogens and for recruitment of effector cells at sites of injury or infection. Although leukocyte recirculation functions in immune surveillance, excessive trafficking to extravascular locations can lead to serious tissue injury and destruction [1–3]. A role of inappropriate T-cell skin homing, via induction of T-cell cutaneous lymphocyte-associated antigen (CLA), has recently been suggested in the initiation and perpetuation of the inflammatory process of skin diseases [4–6]. CLA is a ligand for E-selectin expressed on human lymphocytes which can be induced by bacterial superantigens such as TSST-1 [6–8]. It is characterized by its reactivity with the antibody HECA-452 and expressed on the majority of T-cells in skin. Given the very initial role of carbohydrate-selectin interactions in the emigration process and the potential of excessive leukocyte extravasation for tissue injury, inhibition of carbohydrate-selectin interaction seems to be a promising tool for therapeutic intervention in inflammatory processes [2, 9].

Recently, the molecular nature of CLA has been partially clarified. There is strong evidence that CLA is produced by post-translational glycosylation of the constitutively expressed P-selectin glycoprotein ligand-1 (PSGL–) through α1,3-fucosyltransferase VII (FucT-VII) [10, 11]. The regulatory processes involved in T-cell CLA expression, however, are still largely unknown. The inducers of CLA expression have the activation of the transcription factor nuclear factor kappa B (NF-κB) in common [12, 13]. Putative NF-κB binding sites have been identified in the promoter of FucT-VII [14], but a direct role for NF-κB in FucT-VII transcription or CLA expression has not been shown so far. We analyzed the effects of TSST-1 on FucT-VII mRNA expression and the potential of NF-κB inhibitors to reduce TSST-1 mediated FucT-VII induction.

Materials and Methods

Cell Preparations and Reagents

PBMC were cultured in AIM-V medium in the absence or presence of TSST-1 (100 ng/ml). The antioxidant NAC (0–25 mM) was obtained from Sigma and lactacystin (0–25 μM) from Calbiochem-Novabiochem (Bad Soden, Germany).

RT-PCR detection of fucosyltransferase VII mRNA was performed as described previously with slight modifications . FucT-VII forward primer was 5´-CAC CTC

New Trends in Allergy V
J. Ring, H. Behrendt (Eds.)
© Springer-Verlag Berlin, Heidelberg 2002

CGA GGC ATC TTC AAC TG-3´ and the reverse primer 5´-CGT TGG TAT CGG CTC TCA TTC ATG-3´ [15].

Intravital microscopy was performed as described previously with slight modifications [16].

Statistical Analysis

Data are presented as mean±SD. For those data which satisfied the normality test, data were analyzed by one-way ANOVA with the Bonferroni correction. P values <0.05 were considered statistically significant.

Results

FucT-VII mRNA Is Induced by the Superantigen TSST-1

Induction of CLA by superantigens has been described by several groups. As CLA is produced by post-translational glycosylation of the constitutively expressed PSGL–1 through FucT-VII we analyzed the effect of TSST-1 on FucT-VII mRNA expression. Resting PBMC only weakly express FucT-VII mRNA. However, acti-

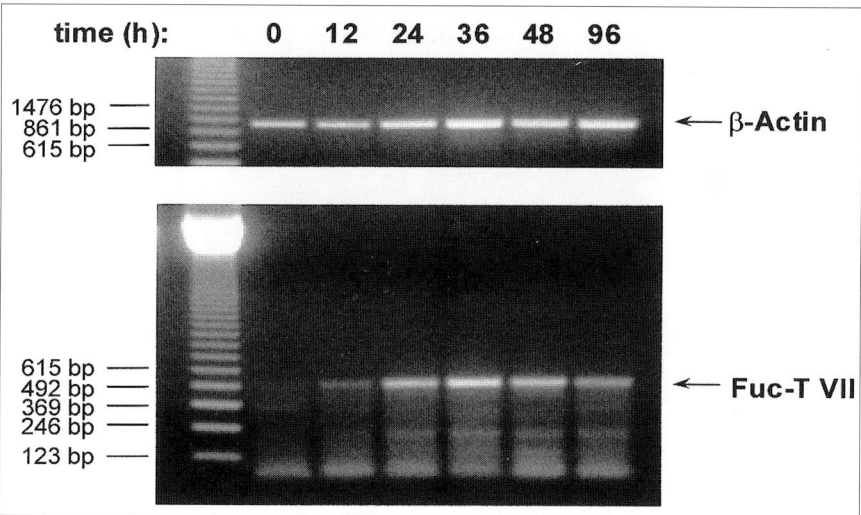

Fig. 1. FucT-VII mRNA expression in TSST-1-stimulated PBMC. PBMC were stimulated in AIM-V medium with TSST-1 (100 ng/ml) for up to 96 h. Total RNA was isolated at the indicated time points and RT-PCR for FucT-VII (*lower lanes*) and the house keeping gene β-actin (*upper lanes*) was performed as outlined in „Materials and Methods". RT-PCR products were visualized by agarose gel electrophoresis with ethidium bromide staining. For verification, PCR products were sequenced to confirm identity with the published FucT-VII cDNA sequence [15]. Experiments were also performed in the absence of RT to exclude contamination by genomic DNA. The results are representative of three independent experiments

vation of PBMC with the superantigen TSST-1 (100 ng/ml) induced in a time-dependent manner a marked upregulation of FucT-VII as determined by RT-PCR and identification by sequence analysis. FucT-VII mRNA expression reached a maximum after 36–48 h and declined thereafter (Fig. 1).

FucT-VII mRNA Induction by TSST-1 Can Be Reduced by NF-κB Inhibitors

In the promoter region of FucT-VII, putative NF-κB binding sites have been described. We therefore asked whether NF-κB inhibitors such as NAC or lactacystin can reduce the superantigen mediated induction of FucT-VII mRNA. We therefore stimulated PBMC with TSST-1 in the presence of NAC (0–25 mM) and lactacystin (0–25 µM) for up to 48 h and analyzed FucT-VII mRNA expression in the presence and absence of the NF-κB inhibitors. For both compounds, we found a dose-dependent inhibition of FucT-VII mRNA expression which reached a maximum at 25 mM NAC and 25 µM lactacystin (Fig. 2, and data not shown for lactacystin). These concentrations have been shown to be non-toxic by trypane blue exclusion test and propidium iodine staining (data not shown).

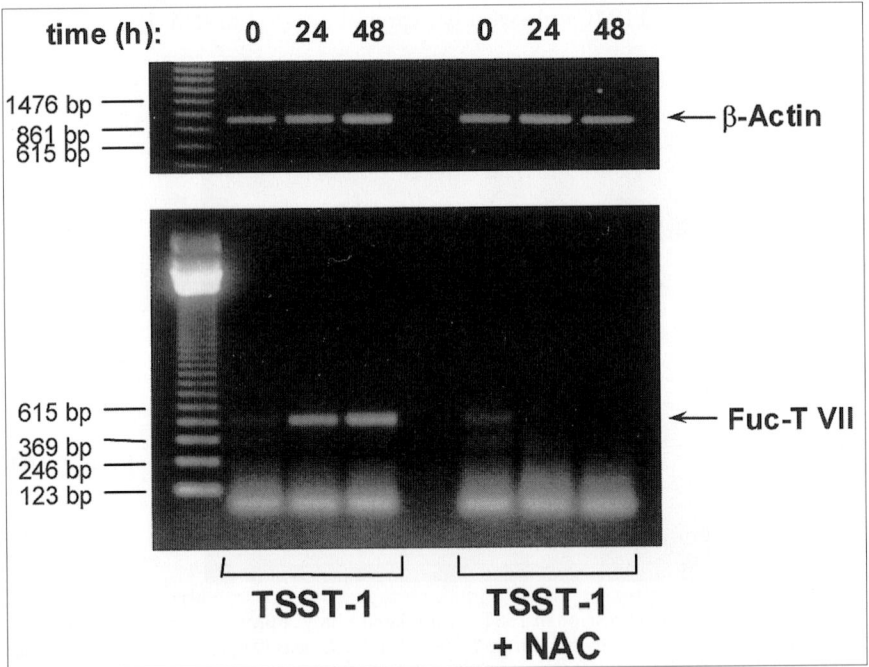

Fig. 2. NF-κB inhibitors suppress TSST-1-induced FucT-VII mRNA upregulation. PBMC were stimulated in AIM-V medium with TSST-1 (100 ng/ml) in the absence or presence of NAC and lactacystin (data not shown) for up to 48 h. Total RNA was isolated at the indicated time points and RT-PCR for FucT-VII (*lower lanes*) and the house keeping gene β-actin (*upper lanes*) was performed as outlined in „Materials and Methods"

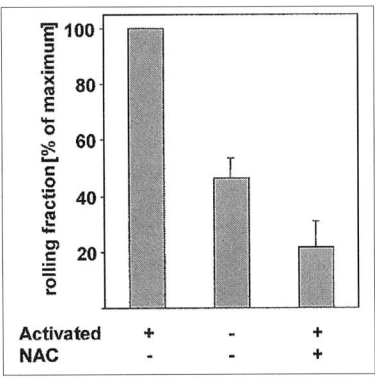

Fig. 3. Rolling of stimulated cells is inhibited by NF-κB inhibitors. After in vitro culture (see „Materials and Methods"), cells were labeled with BCECF and injected retrogradely into the right carotid artery. Cells were visualized by fluorescent microscopy and the rolling fraction was determined as percentage of rolling cells in the total flux. T-cell stimulation increased the rolling fraction in wild-type mice, whereas two NF-κB inhibitors, NAC (25 mM) and lactacystin (LC, 25 μM; data not shown), blocked this increase. Values shown are the mean±SD of 14 vessels in three wild-type mice

Suppression of T-Cell Rolling on Endothelial Selectins In Vivo by NF-κB Inhibitors

The intravital microscopy has made possible the direct observation of leukocyte interaction with postcapillary venular endothelium in vivo. The ability of human E- and P-selectin ligands to interact effectively with murine selectins allows human leukocytes to be studied in mouse microvessels [17]. Rolling of leukocytes on skin endothelium is exclusively mediated by P- and E-selectin and can be observed in mouse skin microcirculation without surgical manipulation of the tissue, thus allowing observation of basal interactions between leukocytes and non-inflamed endothelium. Based on our in vitro results, rolling of NF-κB inhibitor pretreated, stimulated T-cells on endothelial selectins is expected to be reduced as compared to stimulated T-cells. In three mice, fluorescently labeled T-cells were injected through the right common carotid artery into the aortic arch and observed directly in the microcirculation of the left ear. In total, 14 vessels were examined for rolling lymphocytes. Stimulated T-cells showed a more than 2-fold increase in the frequency of rolling interactions as compared to resting T-cells (Fig. 3). Treatment of stimulated T-cells with NAC or lactacystin reduced the rolling fraction even below the ratio of resting T-cells.

Discussion

The recruitment of memory T-cells into the skin plays a pivotal role in cutaneous immune surveillance and in pathogenesis of T-cell mediated dermatoses. It is mediated by a complex multistep program which is initiated by the interaction of endothelial E- and P-selectin molecules with their ligands CLA and PSGL-1 on T-cells [18–20]. CLA is the key molecule responsible for the recruitment of T-cells into the skin and it promotes subsequent steps of the adhesion cascade. In this study, we further investigated the mechanism of CLA induction by bacterial superantigens. We found that CLA induction by superantigens is preceded by an induction of FucT-VII mRNA expression. We therefore assume that superantigens induce CLA expression on T-cells via induction of FucT-VII.

Additionally, we analyzed potential pharmacological agents for the inhibition of T-cell CLA expression. Since FucT-VII, the glycosyltransferase responsible for CLA production, has several putative NF-κB binding sites in its promoter region [14] and the known CLA inducers have the activation of NF-κB in common [12, 13] we examined the effect of two different compounds interfering with the activation of NF-κB. We report that (I) an antioxidant (NAC) known to inhibit IκB kinase activity and (II) a proteasome inhibitor (lactacystin) markedly suppress activation-induced T-cell FucT-VII mRNA expression, CLA expression and in vivo function.

It has been shown that T-cells are sufficient to induce T-cell dermatoses like psoriasis [21, 22]. Skin infiltrating T-cells are capable to induce skin diseases in non-inflamed skin dependent on a disease-prone genetic background. The primary event in these experimental models is the induction of a T-cell mediated dermatosis via interaction of skin seeking T-cells with non-inflamed endothelium. We analyzed regulatory mechanisms of this initial interaction of distinct T-cell populations with non-inflamed tissue. NF-κB inhibitors dramatically reduced this disease initiating interactions of activated skin seeking T-cells with non-inflamed endothelium. As recently reviewed, activation of NF-κB is of major importance for T-cell recirculation into the skin [4]. This report extends the functional role of NF-κB for the skin immune system as it indicates that CLA, E- and P-selectin binding of T-cells can be regulated by NF-κB inhibitors.

References

1. Albelda SM, Smith CW, Ward PA. Adhesion molecules and inflammatory injury. Faseb J 1994;8(8):504–12.
2. Lowe JB, Ward PA. Therapeutic inhibition of carbohydrate-protein interactions in vivo. J Clin Invest 1997;100(11 Suppl):S47–51.
3. Springer TA. Traffic signals for lymphocyte recirculation and leukocyte emigration: the multistep paradigm. Cell 1994;76(2):301–14.
4. Robert C, Kupper TS. Inflammatory skin diseases, T cells, and immune surveillance. N Engl J Med 1999;341(24):1817–28.
5. Boehncke WH, Dressel D, Zollner TM, Kaufmann R. Pulling the trigger on psoriasis. Nature 1996;379(6568):777.
6. Leung DY, Gately M, Trumble A, Ferguson-Darnell B, Schlievert PM, Picker LJ. Bacterial superantigens induce T cell expression of the skin-selective homing receptor, the cutaneous lymphocyte-associated antigen, via stimulation of interleukin 12 production. J Exp Med 1995;181(2):747–53.
7. Zollner TM, Munk ME, Keller T, et al. The superantigen exfoliative toxin induces cutaneous lymphocyte- associated antigen expression in peripheral human T lymphocytes. Immunol Lett 1996;49(1–2):111–6.
8. Zollner TM, Nuber V, Duijvestijn AM, Boehncke WH, Kaufmann R. Superantigens but not mitogens are capable of inducing upregulation of E-selectin ligands on human T lymphocytes. Exp Dermatol 1997;6(4):161–6.
9. Hynes RO, Wagner DD. Genetic manipulation of vascular adhesion molecules in mice. J Clin Invest 1996;98(10):2193–5.
10. Fuhlbrigge RC, Kieffer JD, Armerding D, Kupper TS. Cutaneous lymphocyte antigen is a specialized form of PSGL-1 expressed on skin-homing T cells. Nature 1997;389(6654):978–81.
11. Borges E, Pendl G, Eytner R, Steegmaier M, Zollner O, Vestweber D. The binding of T cell-expressed P-selectin glycoprotein ligand-1 to E- and P-selectin is differentially regulated. J Biol Chem 1997;272(45):28786–92.

12. Hong YH, Peng HB, La Fata V, Liao JK. Hydrogen peroxide-mediated transcriptional induction of macrophage colony-stimulating factor by TGF-beta1. J Immunol 1997;159(5):2418–23.
13. Baeuerle PA, Henkel T. Function and activation of NF-kappa B in the immune system. Annu Rev Immunol 1994;12:141–79.
14. Hiraiwa N, Hiraiwa M, Kannagi R. Human T-cell leukemia virus-1 encoded Tax protein transactivates alpha 1–>3 fucosyltransferase Fuc-T VII, which synthesizes sialyl Lewis X, a selectin ligand expressed on adult T-cell leukemia cells. Biochem Biophys Res Commun 1997;231(1):183–6.
15. Sasaki K, Kurata K, Funayama K, et al. Expression cloning of a novel alpha 1,3-fucosyltransferase that is involved in biosynthesis of the sialyl Lewis x carbohydrate determinants in leukocytes. J Biol Chem 1994;269(20):14730–7.
16. Weninger W, Ulfman LH, Cheng G, et al. Specialized contributions by alpha(1,3)-fucosyltransferase-IV and FucT- VII during leukocyte rolling in dermal microvessels. Immunity 2000;12(6):665–76.
17. Robert C, Fuhlbrigge RC, Kieffer JD, et al. Interaction of dendritic cells with skin endothelium: A new perspective on immunosurveillance. J Exp Med 1999;189(4):627–36.
18. Berg EL, Yoshino T, Rott LS, et al. The cutaneous lymphocyte antigen is a skin lymphocyte homing receptor for the vascular lectin endothelial cell-leukocyte adhesion molecule 1. J Exp Med 1991;174(6):1461–6.
19. Catalina MD, Estess P, Siegelman MH. Selective requirements for leukocyte adhesion molecules in models of acute and chronic cutaneous inflammation: participation of E- and P- but not L-selectin. Blood 1999;93(2):580–9.
20. Chu A, Hong K, Berg EL, Ehrhardt RO. Tissue specificity of E- and P-selectin ligands in Th1-mediated chronic inflammation. J Immunol 1999;163(9):5086–93.
21. Schon MP, Detmar M, Parker CM. Murine psoriasis-like disorder induced by naive CD4+ T cells. Nat Med 1997;3(2):183–8.
22. Nickoloff BJ, Wrone-Smith T. Injection of pre-psoriatic skin with CD4+ T cells induces psoriasis. Am J Pathol 1999;155(1):145–58.

12 Dendritic Cells and Tolerance

J. Saloga, I. Bellinghausen, U. Brand, K. Steinbrink, A.H. Enk,
J. Knop

Abstract

Dendritic cells (DC) as potent antigen presenting cells play a pivotal role in the
induction and elicitation of allergic immune responses. Due to their high antigen presenting capacity they may also be useful tools for the antigen/allergen-
specific modification of immune responses on the T cell level. Recently developed
culturing techniques of peripheral blood leukocytes make DC available in higher
amounts and allow distinct manipulations of their function.

For the experiments presented below we obtained immature DC with high
phagocytotic activity after cultivation of $CD14^+$ monocytes with GM-CSF and
IL-4 for uptake of allergens added to the cultures on day 7. For full maturation
leading to high antigen presenting capacity DC were incubated with TNF-α,
IL-1β and PGE_2 in the presence of varying modifiers described below for additional 2 days. Finally DC were cocultured with autologous T cells from atopic
donors with relevant sensitizations to the allergens used in vitro (birch pollen,
grass pollen and/or house dust mite) or control donors.

In naive and memory T cells allergen-loaded, but not control DC were able to
induce antigen-specific proliferative responses and cytokine production. Production of Th2 cytokines was much higher in atopic donors than in non-atopic donors,
especially concerning IL-4 production. Incubation of DC and T cells on collagen I
strongly enhanced the IL-12 production of DC and consecutively the production of
the Th1 cytokine IFN-γ of T cells in an allergen-specific way, while the production
of Th2 cytokines was inhibited. Incubation of DC with hydrocortisone during the
last 2 days of their maturation period strongly decreased their ability to induce the
production of Th1, but not of Th2 cytokines, partially due to a decreased IL-12 secretion of DC combined with the inhibition of the expression of HLA-DR and
costimulatory molecules, especially CD86. This inhibition was even stronger when
the DC were matured in the presence of IL-10 leading to an inhibition of induction
of Th1 as well as Th2 cytokine production in autologous T cells from sensitized atopic
donors. These T cells could not be stimulated to produce Th1 or Th2 cytokines even
when they were restimulated with regularly matured allergen-loaded DC. Only the
addition of compounds known to be able to break anergy of T cells, like IL-2, were
able to restore the responsiveness of the allergen-specific T cells. Enhancement of
apoptosis of T cells was not observed after stimulation with IL-10-treated DC.

These data indicate that DC loaded with allergens depending on their culture
conditions are able to deviate an already established allergic immune response
from a Th2- to a Th1-dominated response and to induce anergy in allergen-specific Th1 and Th2 cells in vitro.

New Trends in Allergy V
J. Ring, H. Behrendt (Eds.)
© Springer-Verlag Berlin, Heidelberg 2002

Introduction

Atopic diseases and IgE production are associated with exaggerated Th2 responses [1–3]. Therefore deviation of this Th2-dominated immune response towards a Th1 response and/or inhibition of such an immune response as it both occurs during specific immunotherapy appears to be an option for the treatment of such diseases [4–9]. Vaccination with peptide or DNA/RNA pulsed dendritic cells (DC) may represent a new form of immunotherapy, as DC are the most potent antigen-presenting cells specialized for the induction of primary immune responses in naive T lymphocytes [10–13]. Advanced techniques have been established to generate mature DC in large numbers from blood precursors in vitro [14] and these DC are already used in clinical trials for cancer therapy [15, 16]. Additionally, results from several groups suggest that distinct DC subsets control the developing immune response [17–19]. Therefore, we were interested to investigate the immune response of naive and memory T cells from atopic compared to nonatopic donors which were stimulated with allergen-pulsed DC. In the following we describe some of the results we obtained concerning this issue and how modification of these allergen-pulsed DC influences the allergen-specific immune response.

Patients and Methods

Heparinized blood was obtained from nonatopic control subjects and atopic donors with allergic rhinoconjunctivitis or asthma to grass pollen, birch pollen, rye pollen, or house dust mite (*Dermatophagoides pteronyssinus*). Specific sensitization was documented by positive skin prick test to the respective allergen, and detection of allergen-specific IgE in the sera [radioallergosorbent test (RAST) class ≥ 2].

PBMC were isolated from heparinized blood by Ficoll-Paque 1.077 density centrifugation. To enrich $CD14^+$ monocytes by adherence, 1×10^7 PBMC per well were incubated in a 6-well plate in RPMI 1640 supplemented with 3% autologous serum at 37°C. After washing the nonadherent cells, the remaining monocytes were incubated in 3 ml/well X-VIVO 15 supplemented with 1% heat-inactivated autologous serum, 800 U/ml GM-CSF, and 1000 U/ml IL-4. After 7 days of culture the resulting immature DC were pulsed with 10 µg/ml grass pollen, birch pollen, rye pollen, or house dust mite allergen extracts (ALK-SCHERAX, Hamburg, Germany) and fully matured by the addition of 1000 U/ml TNF-α, 2000 U/ml IL-1β, and 1 µg/ml PGE_2. For some experiments 20 ng/ml IL-10 (DNAX, Palo Alto, CA) or 5×10^{-6} M hydrocortisone (Sigma, Deisenhofen, Germany) were also added to the culture. Mature DC were harvested 48 h after stimulation, washed twice and used for T-cell stimulation assays.

Autologous $CD45RA^+$ (naive) and $CD45Ro^+CD4^+$ (memory) T cells were purified from PBMC of the same donor with use of antibody-coated paramagnetic MicroBeads (MACS, Miltenyi Biotec, Bergisch Gladbach, Germany) according to the protocol of the manufacturer. Separation was controlled by flow cytometry (purity of >98% $CD4^+$ T cells, >95% $CD45RA^+CD4^+$ T cells, and >95% $CD45Ro^+CD4^+$ T cells).

For cytokine production assays, 5×10^5 CD45RA[+] or CD45Ro[+]CD4[+] T cells were cocultured in 48-well-plates with 5×10^4 autologous allergen-pulsed DC, pretreated with IL-10 or HC, or untreated, in 1 ml X-VIVO 15. In some experiments, the plates were coated with 50 μg per well of collagen type I from human placenta (Sigma) before coculture. After 1 week of coculture, T cells were restimulated with newly generated allergen-pulsed DC, IL-10- or HC-treated, or untreated. Supernatants were collected 24 h later, and analyzed for IL-4, IL-5, and IFN-γ content by ELISA as previously described [20].

Results and Discussion

Dendritic Cells Are Able to Induce Th2 Responses in Naive and Memory T Helper Cells from Atopic Individuals

As in-vitro generated monocyte-derived dendritic cells (DC) are potent inducers of antigen-specific Th1 responses due to their production of IL-12, we analyzed which immune response is induced by DC in atopic compared to nonatopic persons. In Fig. 1 is demonstrated that naive (CD45RA[+]) and especially memory (CD45Ro[+]) CD4[+] T cells from atopic donors produced significantly higher amounts of IL-4 and IL-5 after stimulation with autologous allergen-pulsed DC

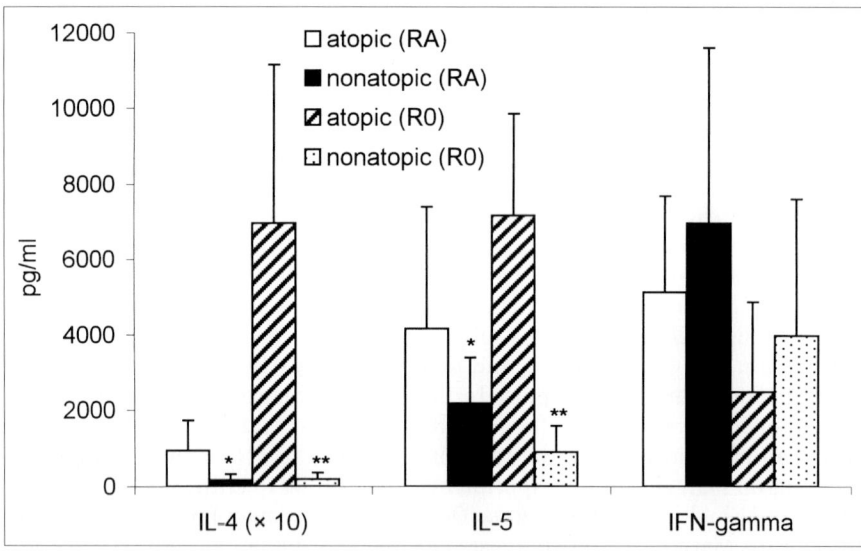

Fig. 1. Comparison of the cytokine production by naive and memory T helper cells from atopic and nonatopic donors after stimulation with autologous allergen-pulsed DC. 5×10^5 CD45RA[+] (naive) or CD45Ro[+] (memory) CD4[+] T cells were stimulated with 5×10^4 autologous allergen-pulsed DC. T cells were restimulated weekly with 5×10^4 newly generated DC of the same donor. Supernatants were collected 24 h after the second restimulation and analyzed for IL-4, IL-5 and IFN-γ content by ELISA. Shown are the means±SD from 16 atopic and 15 nonatopic donors. *$p \leq$ 0.05 and **$p \leq$ 0.01 indicates statistically significant differences between atopic and nonatopic subjects

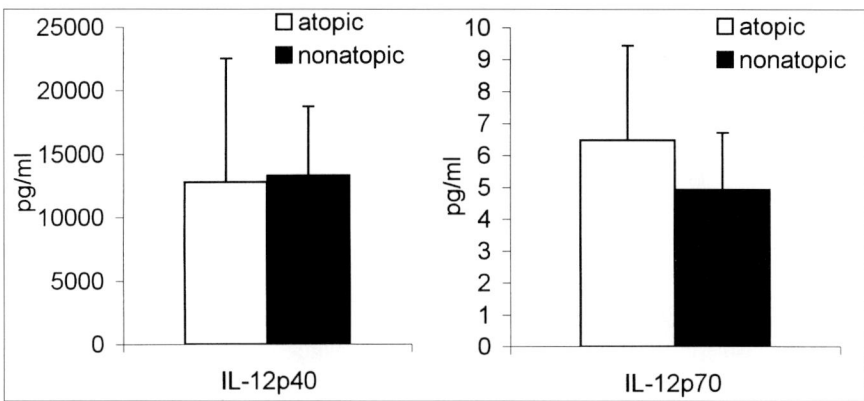

Fig. 2. Cytokine production of allergen-pulsed mature DC from atopic compared to nonatopic donors. Supernatants were harvested on day 9 of DC culture for assessment of IL-12p40 and IL-12p70 production by ELISA. The results represent the means±SD of 10 independent experiments

compared with T cells from nonatopic donors [20]. While IL-4 was expressed in 91.6% of the atopic individuals, it was only detectable in 35% of the examined nonatopic controls. However, the production of IFN-γ was slightly but not significantly reduced in the atopic group. These results are in line with other reports showing that DC can also promote Th2 responses and play an important role in allergic diseases [21–26]. The induction of Th2 cytokines was not due to a diminished secretion of IL-12 by DC from atopic donors because they produce equal amounts of IL-12p40 and bioactive IL-12p70 compared with DC from nonatopic controls (Fig. 2), and addition of neutralizing anti-IL-12 mAb only diminished IFN-γ but did not further enhance IL-4 or IL-5 production [20]. Furthermore, there is no difference in phenotype or T-cell stimulatory capacity by DC derived from atopic or nonatopic donors on day 9 of the described in-vitro culture [20]. Thus, other reasons may explain our observations, probably the inherent property of T helper cells from atopic donors to produce Th2 cytokines [27, 28].

Induction of a Th2 to Th1 Shift in T Helper Cells from Atopic Individuals by Collagen Type I

Previously, we have shown that cultivation of DC on collagen type I induces an increased production of TNF-α, which in turn leads to their maturation characterized by expressing high levels of MHC class II, the costimulatory molecules CD80 and CD86, and the DC-specific marker CD83 [29]. Furthermore, we observed an enhanced production of IL-12 by DC after exposure to collagen type I [30]. As DC from atopic donors did not lead to an exclusive Th1 response (Fig. 1), we investigated the influence of DC on allergen-specific T cells in the presence of collagen type I using the coculture system described above. In these experiments, the production of IFN-γ was strongly increased, and IL-5 production was significantly decreased, while IL-4 production was not significantly diminished

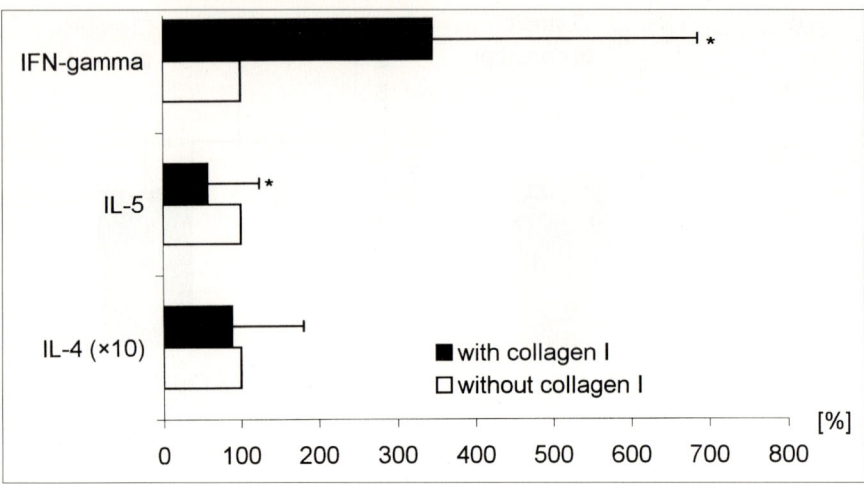

Fig. 3. Influence of collagen type I on cytokine production of T helper cells stimulated with allergen-pulsed DC. 5×10^5 CD4$^+$ T cells were stimulated with 5×10^4 autologous allergen-pulsed DC in 48-well plates coated with 50 μg per well of collagen type I. Supernatants were collected 48 h after the second stimulation and analyzed for IL-4, IL-5 and IFN-γ content by ELISA. Shown are the means±SD from 15 independent experiments. *$p\leq0.05$ indicates statistically significant differences between collagen type I coated and uncoated wells

(Fig. 3; [30]). This effect was only partially inhibited by the addition of blocking anti-IL-12 mAb, as collagen type I also directly activates T cells to increase proliferation and IFN-γ production [30, 31]. This indicates that collagen type I not only induces a preferential development of Th1 cells, but also leads to a Th2/Th1 shift in allergen-specific T cells from atopic donors.

Inhibition of Allergen-Specific Th2 Responses by IL-10 but not by HC-Treated Dendritic Cells

Prior studies have shown that DC, which were treated with the antiinflammatory agents IL-10 or HC during the last 2 days of their maturation phase, inhibit alloantigen- and peptide-specific proliferation of Th1 cells [32–37]. As the influence of IL-10- or GC-treated DC on Th2 cell functions has not been investigated so far, we used our allergen-specific setting to investigate this question. In Fig. 4 we demonstrate that exposure of DC to IL-10 or HC differentially influences human allergic immune responses. The use of IL-10-treated allergen-pulsed DC for T cell stimulation resulted in decreased production of Th1 (IFN-γ) as well as of Th2 (IL-4, IL-5) cytokines by naive and memory CD4$^+$ T cells from atopic individuals, whereas HC-treated DC only inhibited Th1, but enhanced IL-4 production, while IL-5 production was not significantly affected (Fig. 4, [38]). Both effects were long-lasting and stable as cytokine production remained low or increased especially among the naive T cell population even after restimulation with fully matured

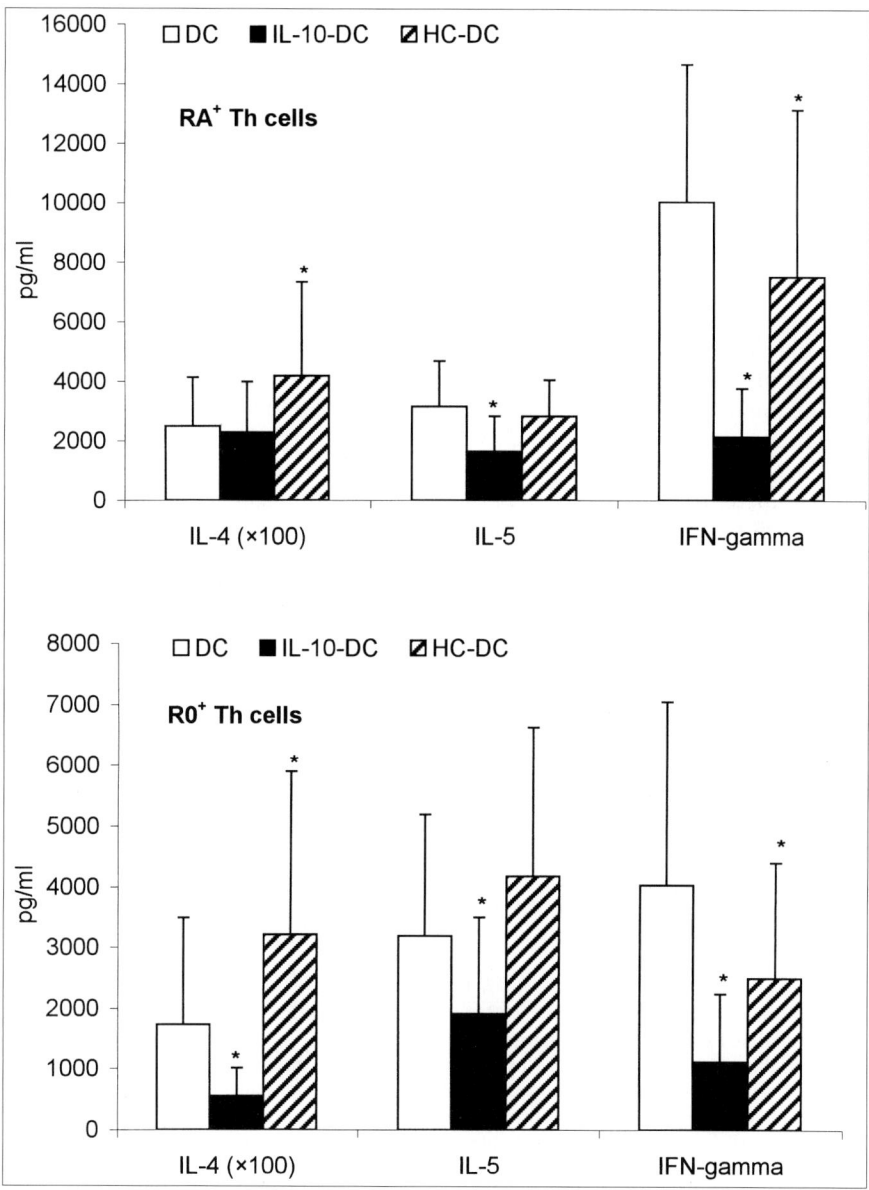

Fig. 4. IL-10- or HC-treated DC differentially modulate cytokine production of naive and memory Th cells from atopic donors. 5×10[5] CD45RA[+] or CD45Ro[+] CD4[+] T cells were stimulated with 5×10[4] autologous allergen-pulsed DC, pretreated with IL-10 or HC, or untreated. After 1 week of culture, T cells were restimulated with 5×10[4] newly generated DC or IL-10- or HC-treated DC of the same donor. Supernatants were collected 24 h later and analyzed for IL-4, IL-5 and IFN-γ content by ELISA. Shown are the means±SD from 19 (for IL-10-treated DC) and 16 (for HC-treated DC) independent experiments. * Indicates statistically significant differences ($p \leq 0.05$) between untreated and IL-10-or HC-treated DC

DC [38]. These long-lasting inhibitory effects of IL-10- or HC-treated DC are not due to enhanced cell death, but to functional hyporesponsiveness, as they could be reversed by the addition of IL-2 [38]. However, the fact, that memory Th cells still respond to regular DC after primary stimulation with IL-10- or HC-treated DC, favors other mechanisms than anergy probably the induction of regulatory T cells [39]. This possibility remains to be investigated in further studies.

Concluding Remarks

Taken together, the described culture system of allergen-pulsed DC and T helper cells may be exploited for the further analysis of human allergic immune responses in vitro. Factors of the extracellular matrix such as collagen type I or the antiinflammatory agents IL-10 and HC are shown to inhibit allergen-specific proliferation and except of HC they also inhibit allergen-specific Th2 responses. This may be exploited for the design of new forms of immunotherapy for allergic diseases, as in-vitro cultured DC are already used in clinical trials to stimulate cellular immune responses against cancer [15, 16]. In this respect IL-10- or collagen type I-treated DC may be useful for the downregulation of allergic immune responses of atopic individuals.

References

1. Wierenga EA, Snoek M, de Groot C, Chretien I, Bos JD, Jansen HM, Kapsenberg ML. Evidence for compartmentalization of functional subsets of CD2+ T lymphocytes in atopic patients. J Immunol 1990; 144:4651–4656.
2. Abbas AK, Murphy KM, Sher A. Functional diversity of helper T lymphocytes. Nature 1996; 383:787–793.
3. O'Garra A. Cytokines induce the development of functionally heterogeneous T helper cell subsets. Immunity 1998; 8:275–283.
4. Secrist H, Chelen CJ, Wen Y, Marshall JD, Umetsu DT. Allergen immunotherapy decreases interleukin 4 production in CD4+ T cells from allergic individuals. J Exp Med 1993; 178:2123–2130.
5. Jutel M, Pichler WJ, Skrbic D, Urwyler A, Dahinden C, Muller UR. Bee venom immunotherapy results in decrease of IL-4 and IL-5 and increase of IFN-gamma secretion in specific allergen-stimulated T cell cultures. J Immunol 1995; 154:4187–4194.
6. Bellinghausen I, Metz G, Enk AH, Christmann S, Knop J, Saloga J. Insect venom immunotherapy induces interleukin-10 production and a Th2-to-Th1 shift, and changes surface marker expression in venom-allergic subjects. Eur J Immunol 1997; 27:1131–1139.
7. Durham SR, Till SJ. Immunologic changes associated with allergen immunotherapy. J Allergy Clin Immunol 1998; 102:157–164.
8. Bellinghausen I, Knop J, Saloga J. Role of interleukin 10-producing T cells in specific (allergen) immunotherapy. Allergy Clin Immunol Int 2000; 12:20–25.
9. Akdis CA, Blesken T, Akdis M, Wüthrich B, Blaser K. Role of Interleukin 10 in specific immunotherapy. J Clin Invest 1998; 102:98–106.
10. Inaba K, Metlay JP, Crowley MT, Steinman RM. Dendritic cells pulsed with protein antigens in vitro can prime antigen-specific, MHC-restricted T cells in situ [published erratum appears in J Exp Med 1990 Oct 1;172(4):1275]. J Exp Med 1990; 172:631–640.
11. Steinman RM. The dendritic cell system and its role in immunogenicity. Annu Rev Immunol 1991; 9:271–296.

12. Tuting T, Wilson CC, Martin DM, Kasamon YL, Rowles J, Ma DI, Slingluff CL, Jr., Wagner SN et al. Autologous human monocyte-derived dendritic cells genetically modified to express melanoma antigens elicit primary cytotoxic T cell responses in vitro: enhancement by cotransfection of genes encoding the Th1-biasing cytokines IL-12 and IFN-alpha. J Immunol 1998; 160:1139–1147.

13. Boczkowski D, Nair SK, Snyder D, Gilboa E. Dendritic Cells Pulsed with RNA are Potent Antigen-presenting Cells In Vitro and In Vivo. J Exp Med 1996; 184:465–472.

14. Romani N, Reider D, Heuer M, Ebner S, Kampgen E, Eibl B, Niederwieser D, Schuler G. Generation of mature dendritic cells from human blood. An improved method with special regard to clinical applicability. J Immunol Methods 1996; 196:137–151.

15. Nestle FO, Alijagic S, Gilliet M, Sun Y, Grabbe S, Dummer R, Burg G, Schadendorf D. Vaccination of melanoma patients with peptide- or tumor lysate-pulsed dendritic cells. Nat Med 1998; 4:328–332.

16. Fong L, Brockstedt D, Benike C, Wu L, Engleman EG. Dendritic cells injected via different routes induce immunity in cancer patients. J Immunol 2001; 166:4254–4259.

17. Banchereau J, Briere F, Caux C, Davoust J, Lebecque S, Liu YJ, Pulendran B, Palucka K. Immunobiology of dendritic cells. Annu Rev Immunol 2000; 18:767–811.

18. Rissoan MC, Soumelis V, Kadowaki N, Grouard G, Briere F, de Waal Malefyt R, Liu YJ. Reciprocal control of T helper cell and dendritic cell differentiation. Science 1999; 283:1183–1186.

19. Pulendran B, Smith JL, Caspary G, Brasel K, Pettit D, Maraskovsky E, Maliszewski CR. Distinct dendritic cell subsets differentially regulate the class of immune response in vivo. Proc Natl Acad Sci U S A 1999; 96:1036–1041.

20. Bellinghausen I, Brand U, Knop J, Saloga J. Comparison of allergen-stimulated dendritic cells from atopic and nonatopic donors dissecting their effect on autologous naive and memory T helper cells of such donors. J Allergy Clin Immunol 2000; 105:988–996.

21. Kalinski P, Hilkens CM, Snijders A, Snijdewint FG, Kapsenberg ML. IL-12-deficient dendritic cells, generated in the presence of prostaglandin E2, promote type 2 cytokine production in maturing human naive T helper cells. J Immunol 1997; 159:28–35.

22. Lambrecht BN, Salomon B, Klatzmann D, Pauwels RA. Dendritic cells are required for the development of chronic eosinophilic airway inflammation in response to inhaled antigen in sensitized mice. J Immunol 1998; 160:4090–97.

23. Stumbles PA, Thomas JA, Pimm CL, Lee PT, Venaille TJ, Proksch S, et al. Resting respiratory tract dendritic cells preferentially stimulate T helper cell type 2 (Th2) responses and require obligatory cytokine signals for induction of Th1 immunity. J Exp Med 1998; 188:2019–31.

24. Roth R, Spiegelberg HL. Activation of cloned human CD4+ Th1 and Th2 cells by blood dendritic cells. Scand J Immunol 1996; 43:646–651.

25. Sung SJ, Taketomi EA, Smith AM, Platts Mills TA, Fu SM. Efficient presentation of house dust mite allergen Der p 2 by monocyte-derived dendritic cells and the role of beta 2 integrins. Scand J Immunol 1999; 49:96–105.

26. Lambrecht BN. The dendritic cell in allergic airway diseases: a new player to the game. Clin Exp Allergy 2001; 31:206–218.

27. Marsh DG, Neely JD, Breazeale DR, Ghosh B, Freidhoff LR, Ehrlich Kautzky E, Schou C, Krishnaswamy G et al. Linkage analysis of IL4 and other chromosome 5q31.1 markers and total serum immunoglobulin E concentrations. Science 1994; 264:1152–1156.

28. Anderson GG, Cookson WO. Recent advances in the genetics of allergy and asthma. Mol Med Today 1999; 5:264–273.

29. Brand U, Bellinghausen I, Enk AH, Jonuleit H, Becker D, Knop J, Saloga J. Influence of extracellular matrix proteins on the development of cultured human dendritic cells. Eur J Immunol 1998; 28:1673–1680.

30. Brand U, Bellinghausen I, Enk AH, Jonuleit H, Becker D, Knop J, Saloga J. Allergen-specific immune deviation from a TH2 to a TH1 response induced by dendritic cells and collagen type I. J Allergy Clin Immunol 1999; 104:1052–1059.

31. Tschoetschel U, Schwing J, Frosch S, Schmitt E, Schuppan D, Reske Kunz AB. Modulation of proliferation and lymphokine secretion of murine CD4+ T cells and cloned Th1 cells by proteins of the extracellular matrix. Int Immunol 1997; 9:147–159.

32. Steinbrink K, Wolfl M, Jonuleit H, Knop J, Enk AH. Induction of tolerance by IL-10-treated dendritic cells. J Immunol 1997; 159:4772–4780.

33. Steinbrink K, Jonuleit H, Muller G, Schuler G, Knop J, Enk AH. Interleukin-10-treated human dendritic cells induce a melanoma-antigen-specific anergy in CD8(+) T cells resulting in a failure to lyse tumor cells. Blood 1999; 93:1634–1642.

34. Caux C, Massacrier C, Vanbervliet B, Barthelemy C, Liu YJ, Banchereau J. Interleukin 10 inhibits T cell alloreaction induced by human dendritic cells. Int Immunol 1994; 6:1177–1185.

35. Vieira PL, Kalinski P, Wierenga EA, Kapsenberg ML, de Jong EC. Glucocorticoids inhibit bioactive IL-12p70 production by in vitro-generated human dendritic cells without affecting their T cell stimulatory potential. J Immunol 1998; 161:5245–5251.

36. Piemonti L, Monti P, Allavena P, Sironi M, Soldini L, Leone BE, Socci C, Di Carlo V. Glucocorticoids affect human dendritic cell differentiation and maturation. J Immunol 1999; 162:6473–6481.

37. de Jong EC, Vieira PL, Kalinski P, Kapsenberg ML. Corticosteroids inhibit the production of inflammatory mediators in immature monocyte-derived DC and induce the development of tolerogenic DC3. J Leukoc Biol 1999; 66:201–204.

38. Bellinghausen I, Brand U, Steinbrink K, Enk AH, Knop J, Saloga J. Inhibition of human allergic T cell responses by interleukin-10-treated dendritic cells: differences to hydrocortisone-treated dendritic cells. J Allergy Clin Immunol 2001; 108:242–249.

39. Groux H, O'Garra A, Bigler M, Rouleau M, Antonenko S, de Vries JE, Roncarolo MG. A CD4+ T-cell subset inhibits antigen-specific T-cell responses and prevents colitis. Nature 1997; 389:737–742.

13 Eosinophils Maintain Their Capacity to Degranulate upon Repetitive Stimulation with the Same Agonist

H.-U. Simon, F. Levi-Schaffer

Introduction

Inflammatory disorders are characterized by an expansion of hematopoietic effector cells. In allergic and parasitic diseases, the cellular infiltrate consists mainly of eosinophils. Several mechanisms are involved in this process, such as increased eosinophil production in the bone marrow, preferential recruitment and chemotaxis to the site of inflammation, as well as delayed apoptosis [1]. At the site of inflammation, eosinophils release toxic cationic proteins upon stimulation, a process thought to be important in host defense. Tissue damage caused by eosinophil granule proteins may also be important in the pathophysiology of asthma, atopic dermatitis, and other chronic allergic diseases.

There have been a number of studies describing eosinophil activation mechanisms. Hematopoietins, such as IL-3, IL-5, and GM-CSF, increase functional responses of eosinophils to various agonists, including lipid mediators, complement factors, or chemokines. This effect of hematopoietins, called „priming", is also observed in other granulocyte subtypes. Priming of eosinophils appears to be required for ligand-induced degranulation.

Most of the activation studies have focused on the response of eosinophils to a single step of activation. However, since the eosinophils may live in the inflamed tissue for more than a week [2], it is likely that the same ligand stimulates the cell repeatedly or continuously. Therefore, we have recently studied the effect of repetitive stimulation with the same agonist in an in vitro model of eosinophil activation [3]. We demonstrated that GM-CSF primed eosinophils can be activated by platelet-activating factor (PAF) or complement factor C5a to release eosinophil cationic protein (ECP) up to six times. Moreover, it was found that one major mechanism of temporary eosinophil unresponsiveness by agonist-induced stimulation appears to be receptor inactivation by the agonist itself.

Materials and Methods

Subjects

A group of 15 atopic dermatitis patients, two patients with the hypereosinophilic syndrome, and four healthy control individuals were studied.

New Trends in Allergy V
J. Ring, H. Behrendt (Eds.)
© Springer-Verlag Berlin, Heidelberg 2002

Eosinophil Purification

Human eosinophils were purified as previously described [4–6]. The resulting cell populations contained 99% eosinophils as determined by staining with Diff-Quik (Baxter, Düdingen, Switzerland) and light microscopy.

Eosinophil Cultures

Eosinophils were cultured at 1×10^6/ml in the presence or absence of GM-CSF, PAF, C5a, or eotaxin for the indicated times using complete culture medium at 37°C in 5% CO_2 in a humidified atmosphere. GM-CSF was used at a concentration of 50 ng/ml. PAF was used at 10^{-7} M, C5a at 10^{-8} M, and eotaxin at 100 ng/ml.

Intracellular Calcium Measurements

Intracellular ionized free calcium concentrations were assayed with a bulk spectrofluorometric assay as previously described [7].

ECP Measurements

ECP levels were measured in eosinophil lysates and supernatants using the Pharmacia UniCAP System for ECP (Pharmacia & Upjohn, Dubendorf, Switzerland) according to the manufacturer's instructions.

Results

ECP Levels Do Not Differ Between Blood Eosinophils Derived from Normal Control Individuals and Eosinophilic Patients

As shown in Figure 1, total ECP contents of purified eosinophil populations were compared. ECP expression did not differ between control individuals and patients

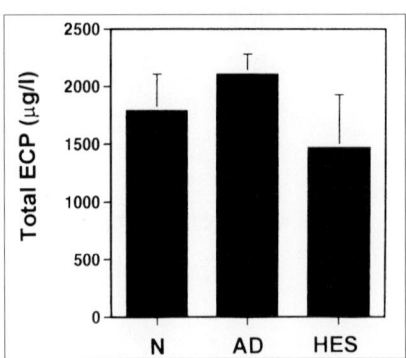

Fig. 1. The ECP content in blood eosinophils of normal controls (*N*, *n*=4), patients with atopic dermatitis (*AD*, *n*=15) or the hypereosinophilic syndrome (*HES*, *n*=2). Data are mean+SEM

with atopic dermatitis. In addition, purified eosinophils from two patients with the hypereosinophilic syndrome had similar cellular ECP levels.

PAF and C5a but Not Eotaxin Release ECP
from GM-CSF Primed Eosinophils

We next searched for a system for ECP release from peripheral blood eosinophils using physiologic agonists. Significant ECP release was observed when eosinophils were pretreated with GM-CSF and subsequently stimulated with optimal concentrations of PAF or C5a. If these three agonists were used alone, no significant release of ECP was observed. Interestingly, activation with PAF and subsequent stimulation with GM-CSF was not associated with an increased ECP release. In contrast to PAF and C5a, eotaxin did not induce a significant ECP release from GM-CSF primed eosinophils. In preliminary experiments, we established the optimal time for GM-CSF priming (20 min) and subsequent PAF or C5a stimulation (both 25 min). 10 min- and 40 min-incubations for priming or degranulation stimulation were clearly less effective.

Eosinophils Release ECP upon a Second Stimulation
with the Same Agonist

Stimulation of cells by agonists is usually followed by a time period of unresponsiveness, also called „desensitization". In this time period, cells do not show a func-

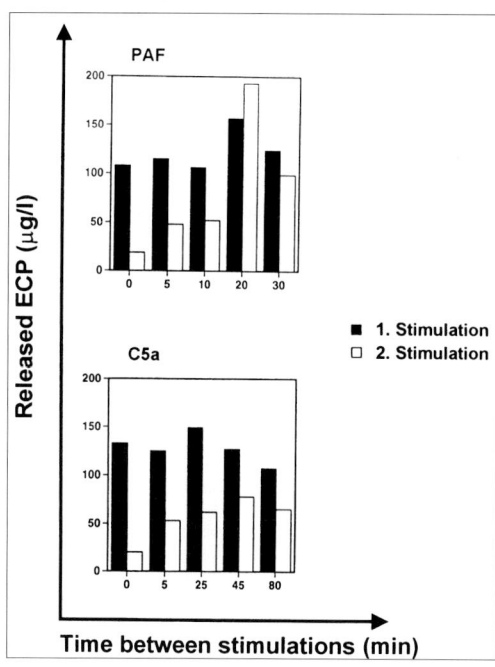

Fig. 2. Release of ECP from eosinophils upon repeated stimulation. GM-CSF primed eosinophils were stimulated with either PAF or with C5a twice. Time periods between stimulations included a washing step and varied from 0–30 min (PAF) and 0–80 min (C5a). No significant ECP releases upon second stimulation were observed within these time periods without a washing step after the first stimulation (ECP concentrations always <15 µg/l). Results of one representative out of five independent experiments is shown in each case

tional response upon stimulation either with the same or another ligand, which binds to the same or different receptors with same signal transductions pathways. However, as shown in Figure 2, eosinophils could be triggered to a second ECP release by the same agonist when the cells were washed after the first stimulation. Already 5 min after the first stimulation, eosinophils responded to either PAF or C5a activation. The response to the second PAF stimulation after 20 min was as high as the first response. The second C5a response reached its maximum after 45 min, but was always less in comparison to the ECP levels released upon the first stimulation. We stimulated GM-CSF primed eosinophils with PAF up to six times within 5 h and always observed a significant release of ECP. After six stimulations, the eosinophils still contained more than 50% of the original ECP content.

A Second Stimulation with the Same Agonist Increases Cytosolic Free Calcium

We next investigated agonist-induced changes in intracellular calcium levels to evaluate receptor-mediated signaling mechanisms. Both PAF and C5a led to rapid, transient, and dose-dependent changes in intracellular free calcium concentrations. Peak calcium levels were observed within 1 min of addition of 10^{-7}M PAF or 10^{-8}M C5a. The inactive metabolite lyso-PAF had no effect in this system.

Sequential activation with the same agonist did not induce an increase in intracellular calcium, even when the time period between the first and second stimulation was more than 1 h. However, when eosinophils were washed using complete culture medium after the first PAF stimulation, cells responded to second stimulation with the same ligand already after 5 min with a calcium rise (Fig. 3). In contrast, if cells were washed in medium containing 10^{-7}M PAF, no second calcium response was observed, implying that washing with medium alone might have removed PAF from its receptor (see below). The investigation of

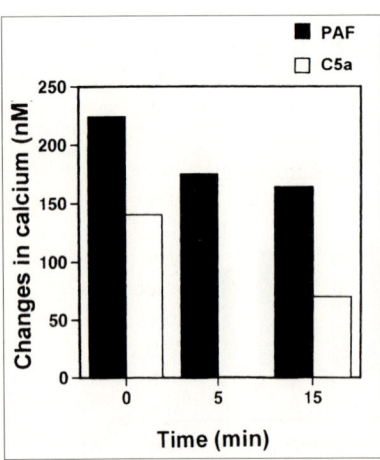

Fig. 3. Intracellular calcium changes in eosinophils in response to repeated stimulation with PAF or with C5a. Calcium signals were measured by Fura-2 fluorescence. The cells were washed between the applications of the agonists. „0" means freshly purified cells that had been stimulated with the indicated agonists for the first time. The time interval (5 and 15 min) between the applications is indicated and includes the washing step. Five minutes after the first stimulation, a second PAF stimulation was associated with rapid calcium response, which was only slightly less compared to the first response. In contrast, complete homologous desensitization was observed in the case of C5a, since the second C5a stimulation did not result in an increase of intracellular free calcium levels at this time point. Results of one representative out of five (C5a) or six (PAF) independent experiments is shown

shorter time periods between stimulations was technically impossible. In contrast to the PAF experiments, the second C5a response was abrogated within the first 5 min after initial stimulation. However, significant increases in cytosolic free calcium were observed when the second C5a stimulation was performed 15 min after the first stimulation (Fig. 3). C5a stimulations at later time periods (up to 1 h) did not give higher responses.

PAF Stimulation Does Not Result in a Complete Loss of PAF Receptors on the Surface of Eosinophils

To understand the responsiveness of eosinophils towards the same agonist following a washing step, we performed ligand-binding studies. Using fluorescent PAF and fluorescent lyso-PAF (which also binds to the PAF receptor), we performed flow cytometric and microscopic studies. Fluorescent PAF bound to freshly purified eosinophils confirming earlier studies on the presence of PAF surface receptors on these cells. The signal was blocked by the specific PAF receptor antagonist WEB 2086, suggesting that the majority of fluorescent PAF binding likely occurred via PAF surface receptors. Moreover, washing the cells resulted in a complete loss of the signal when they were incubated with labeled PAF at 4°C, indicating that fluorescent PAF was removed by this procedure. In contrast, a small remaining signal was observed when eosinophils were exposed before washing to fluorescent PAF at 37°C, implying at least partial internalization of ligand/receptor complexes. When cells were incubated a second time with fluorescent PAF, a strong signal was seen, independent from the temperature of incubation. Similar results were obtained using fluorescent microscopy. Taken together, these data suggest that some PAF/PAF receptor complexes are internalized following PAF stimulation. However, a significant proportion of PAF receptors remains on the surface and is immediately available for second stimulation as long as the agonist from the previous stimulation has been removed.

Discussion

The purpose of this study was to investigate whether an eosinophil can be repetitively stimulated by the same agonist, a mechanism, which is likely to occur in long-living eosinophils in vivo. As an in vitro model for eosinophil degranulation, we used peripheral blood eosinophils primed with GM-CSF. After optimal stimulation with PAF or C5a, primed eosinophils released large amounts of ECP into the supernatant.

Similar to earlier studies where eosinophils were stimulated by chemokines, we found that PAF- or C5a-induced calcium responses were attenuated following previous stimulation with the same agonist in vitro. Several mechanisms may be responsible for abrogation of the second response, including receptor occupancy, down regulation due to internalization, or uncoupling from downstream effector mechanisms. In our experiments, we found that upon washing the cells, the full recovery of the PAF response to repeated application of the ligand takes some

20 min. This probably excludes receptor occupancy as a sole mechanism for the desensitization. Receptor internalization and recycling may take some time, which is in agreement with our findings. We found some degree of internalization at 37°C. However, a significant proportion of PAF receptors were not internalized. Thus, this mechanism is unlikely to account for the complete loss of the response upon repeated application of the ligand. In our study, we found that receptor occupancy induces long-lasting changes in signal transduction, e.g. the diminished calcium signal.

After C5a stimulation of eosinophils, we observed a complete unresponsiveness in a short period of time as well as reduced calcium rises and less released ECP at later time points. This suggests that the proportion of ligand-induced receptor internalization may play a larger role in this compared to the PAF system, or that under our experimental conditions the efficiency of the washing step was lower in the C5a compared to the PAF system. Nevertheless, a significant proportion of C5a receptors is still available for a rapid second stimulation as soon as the previous ligand has been removed.

The possibility to immediately re-sensitize eosinophils following PAF stimulation enabled us to stimulate them for at least six times within a few hours with the same agonist. Each time, agonist-mediated stimulation resulted in the release of significant amounts of ECP. Following such repetitive stimulation, the ECP content was in average 57% of the level observed in unstimulated cells. Since no desensitization even in the absence of a washing step was observed when eosinophils were first stimulated with PAF and subsequently activated with C5a (or vice versa), we used both reagents for further and more rapid reduction of cellular ECP contents. When eosinophils were simultaneously stimulated with PAF and C5a for three times, they contained in average 48.5% of the original ECP content. Such eosinophils did not resynthesize ECP even in the presence of eosinophil hematopoietins (not presented).

In conclusion, we have shown that eosinophils maintain their capacity to degranulate upon repetitive stimulation with the same agonist as long as the receptor is not occupied from a previous stimulation. The cellular content of ECP appears to be no limiting factor in the case of repetitive stimulation, implying that mature eosinophils may not require ECP resynthesis.

Acknowledgements. This work was supported by grants from the Swiss National Science Foundation (Grant No. 31–58916.99), Helmut Horten Foundation (Madonna del Piano), Novartis Foundation (Basel), EMDO Foundation (Zurich), and The Aimwell Charitable Trust (UK).

References

1. Simon HU: Eosinophil apoptosis in allergic diseases – an emerging new issue. Clin Exp Allergy 28(1998), 1321–1324
2. Simon HU, Yousefi S, Schranz C, Schapowal A, C. Bachert C, Blaser K: Direct demonstration of delayed eosinophil apoptosis as a mechanism causing tissue eosinophilia. J Immunol 158(1997), 3902–3908

3. Simon HU, Weber M, Becker E, Zilberman Y, Blaser K, Levi-Schaffer F: Eosinophils maintain their capacity to signal and release eosinophil cationic protein upon repetitive stimulation with the same agonist. J Immunol 165(2000), 4069–4075
4. Simon HU, Yousefi S, Dommann-Scherrer CC, Zimmermann DR, Bauer S, Barandun J, Blaser K: Expansion of cytokine-producing CD4⁻CD8⁻ T cells associated with abnormal Fas expression and hypereosinophilia. J Exp Med 183(1996), 1071–1082
5. Simon HU, Yousefi S, Dibbert B, Levi-Schaffer F, Blaser K: Anti-apoptotic signals of granulocyte-macrophage colony-stimulating factor are transduced via Jak2 tyrosine kinase in eosinophils. Eur J Immunol 27(1997), 3536–3539
6. Simon HU, Yousefi S, Dibbert B, Hebestreit H, Weber M, Branch DR, Blaser K, Levi-Schaffer F, Anderson GP: Role for tyrosine phosphorylation and Lyn tyrosine kinase in Fas receptor-mediated apoptosis in eosinophils. Blood 92(1998), 547–557
7. Simon HU, Tsao PW, Siminovitch KA, Mills GB, Blaser K: Functional platelet-activating factor receptors are expressed by monocytes and granulocytes but not by resting or activated T and B lymphocytes from normal individuals or patients with asthma. J Immunol 153(1994), 364–377

14 Mast Cells as Initiators and Effectors of Allergic Inflammation

A. Solomon, A.M. Piliponsky, J. Pe'er, F. Levi-Schaffer

Introduction

Mast cells are recognized as the key cells of allergic inflammatory reactions. They are derived from precursors that originate in the bone marrow, circulate through the blood and migrate into tissues where they mature in the presence of stem cell factor (SCF) [1]. In addition to their role in allergy, they are also implicated in the pathogenesis of a number of chronic inflammatory diseases, in wound healing, in fibrosis and in native immunity [2]. These cells possess on their membrane FcεRI and contain prominent cytoplasmic granules that store several preformed mediators, such as histamine, neutral proteases and proteoglycans [3]. Following activation mast cells release preformed mediators and synthesize and release phospholipid metabolites and an array of cytokines [4]. Activators of mast cells include allergens (via allergen-specific IgE bound to FcεRI), complement factors (e.g. C5a), cytokines, chemokines and neuropeptides [5].

In rodents, two main mast cell subtypes have been described according to their tissue localization: the mucosal-type mast cell (mucosa of the gastrointestinal tract, the lamina propia of the respiratory tract), and the connective tissue-type mast cell (submucosa of the gastrointestinal tract, skin and peritoneum) [6]. In humans, there are two main mast cell phenotypes distinguishable by their neutral protease content, one containing only tryptase (MC_T) and the other one containing both tryptase and chymase (MC_{TC}). MC_T (intestinal mucosa, lung) appear to be immune system-related, whereas MC_{TC} (skin, intestinal submucosa) appear to have functions in angiogenesis and tissue remodeling [6]. Both phenotypes express FcεRI and participate in IgE-mediated reactions. MC_{TC} are responsive to basic compounds (IgE-independent activation) and to a number of neuropeptides while MC_T are not [7]. Human mast cells are also heterogeneous in respect to cytokine content. Interleukin (IL)-4 is distributed between both phenotypes. In contrast, IL-5 and IL-6 are restricted almost exclusively to the MC_T subset [8].

The triggering of mast cells by an IgE-dependent mechanism starts the early phase of the allergic reaction, by releasing preformed mediators, synthesis and release of arachidonic acid metabolites and at later hours of cytokines. The late phase occurs several hours after mast cell degranulation, and is characterized by penetration and activation of granulocytes, and specifically eosinophils, and of mononuclear cells into the tissue. If the inflammatory event is not self-limiting, chronic inflammation, tissue damage, and consequent fibrosis take place. During the late phase of the allergic reaction, both mast cells and eosinophils are in a state of continued and repeated activation. This prolonged activation leads to

New Trends in Allergy V
J. Ring, H. Behrendt (Eds.)
© Springer-Verlag Berlin, Heidelberg 2002

extended survival of both mast cells and eosinophils, recruitment of other inflammatory cells, and further secretion of inflammatory mediators resulting in tissue damage.

Mast cell-eosinophil interactions take place once the eosinophils have infiltrated into the tissue. Several lines of evidence suggest that these two cell types interact during the late phase reaction by a cross-talk due to the release of several mediators. This interaction perpetuates the allergic inflammatory condition. We have observed that in this complex network of interactions, mast cells possess a dual stand. On one hand, mast cells influence eosinophils through production and secretion of an array of cytokines and mediators [9, 10]. On the other hand, mast cells can be activated by eosinophils to release mediators that affect the target cells in tissues. Therefore, we have hypothesized that mast cells are not only initiators of the early and the late phase response, but also effector cells that deliver the end-products to the inflamed tissue. Mast cells seem also to be involved in the reparative stage that follows the inflammatory reaction, by promoting angiogenesis and regulating fibrotic processes.

Mast Cells Are Regulators of Allergic Inflammation: Effects of Mast Cells on Eosinophils

Activation of mast cells by cross-linking of receptor bound IgE molecules causes secretion of preformed and newly synthesized cytokines and arachidonic acid metabolites, which have effects on recruitment, activation and survival of eosinophils.

Tumor Necrosis Factor (TNF)-α appears to be a major mediator of the mast cell-eosinophil cross talk, since it is both preformed and newly synthesized in activated mast cells. This potent inflammatory cytokine has multiple effects on eosinophils alone and in synergy with other mediators. TNF-α is released from mast cells following IgE-dependent activation [11]. Mast cell expression of TNF-α in nasal biopsies showed a 7-fold increase following allergen challenge [12], thereby demonstrating that the IgE-specific activation of mast cells that initiates the immediate phase of an allergic reaction also induces the production of TNF-α. Moreover, anti-IgE triggering of dispersed lung cells has been shown to cause TNF-α release at levels that can affect eosinophils and neutrophils in vitro [13]. Therefore, TNF-α may contribute to the inflammatory processes that lead to the late phase allergic reaction. Eosinophils constitutively express either, or both, the two known TNF-α receptors (TNF-αRI, TNF-αRII) [14, 15], and therefore, can respond directly to TNF-α. Indeed TNF-α can stimulate superoxide production [14, 16], matrix metalloproteinase-9 (MMP-9) secretion [17], cytokines (e.g. IL-12 [18] and IL-8 [19]) and chemokines (e.g. eotaxin) [20] production by human eosinophils. Moreover we have demonstrated that mast cell derived TNF-α enhances eosinophil survival and induces their degranulation releasing Eosinophil Cationic Protein (ECP) and IL-8 [21, 22]. In addition, TNF-α increases eosinophil adhesion to Vascular Cell Adhesion Molecule-1 (VCAM-1), Intercelullar Adhesion Molecule-1 (ICAM-1) and IgG [22, 23]. Interestingly, of all these TNF-α effects, only TNF-α induced IL-8 release was inhibited by dexamethasone [22].

Several mediators that are secreted by activated mast cells can increase the intracellular concentration of calcium in human eosinophils. Both platelet activating factor (PAF) and prostaglandin D_2 (PGD_2) are potent stimuli for calcium mobilization, while leukotriene B_4 (LTB_4) and histamine were also active, although higher concentrations of histamine were required to detect a response. The effects of PGD_2 and histamine were found to be specific for eosinophils, while LTB_4 and PAF increased calcium in both neutrophils and eosinophils [24]. Interestingly, of the various mast cell mediators, LTB_4 and PAF were found to be the most potent stimulators of ECP release from eosinophils [25].

Several other cytokines that are produced by mast cells were found to influence eosinophil survival and activation. These include IL-4, IL-6, and specifically the so-called „eosinophil survival cytokines", IL-3, IL-5 and Granulocyte-Macrophage Colony-Stimulating Factor (GM-CSF) [8,12]. Both IL-5 and GM-CSF were found to be produced and released by mast cells triggered with anti-IgE and SCF, and were shown to be responsible for ECP secretion by eosinophils [9, 26]. In addition, IL-5 has a prominent effect on eosinophil survival, degranulation, and adhesion to the vascular endothelium.

Nerve Growth Factor (NGF) is becoming acknowledged as an important factor associated with allergic inflammation. It was recently shown to have a significant role in mast cell-eosinophil cross talk [27]. NGF can be produced by both mast cells [28] and eosinophils [29] and can have divergent effects on eosinophils: it induces Eosinophil Peroxidase (EPO) release from eosinophils [29] but not of IL-6, and it can also inhibit LTC_4 release from these cells [30].

Stem Cell Factor (SCF) is yet another cytokine that is produced by mast cells and influences eosinophils [31]. SCF was found in conjunctival mast cells and in the culture supernatants of isolated lung mast cells. However, cross-linkage of FcεRI on the lung mast cells in culture did not alter SCF expression. In addition, the levels of SCF mRNA expression in conjunctival mast cells were similar between normal subjects and patients with seasonal allergic conjunctivitis, showing that the production of SCF by mast cells may be regulated via mechanisms other than IgE receptor-mediated pathways [31] The receptor for SCF, c-Kit, was found also in eosinophils. SCF increased eosinophil adhesion to FN40, a fragment of plasma fibronectin, and to VCAM-1. The SCF/c-Kit adhesion effect was mediated by Very Late Antigen-4 (VLA-4). Taken together, these data show that mast cells can activate eosinophils for VLA-4-mediated adhesion, which contributes to the emigration of these cells from the blood, their tissue localization, and their prominence in allergic inflammatory responses [32].

Mast Cells Are Effectors of Allergic Reactions: Effects of Eosinophils on Mast Cells

Traditionally, mast cells have been considered to be initiators of the allergic response, whereby the first trigger, namely the allergen, activates these cells, which thereafter produce and secrete various mediators. Subsequently, mast cells have been proposed to affect eosinophils or other inflammatory cells, secreting mediators that cause the late phase or chronic stage symptomatology. Recently, it became evident that mast cells can also be influenced by eosinophils and other cells, and serve as the effector cells that express and secrete some of the mediators responsible for later stages of allergy.

Eosinophil granule proteins (ECP and MBP, but not EDN or EPO) were found to stimulate the release of histamine and tryptase and the production of PGD_2 from human heart mast cells [33, 34]. This finding was not established, however, for human skin mast cells, in which these cationic proteins inhibited histamine release induced by Substance P [35]. The release of histamine and tryptase from mast cells can also act as a positive feedback loop, whereby histamine induces eosinophil chemotaxis and activation, and tryptase activate complement, the products of which (C3a and C5a) can further activate mast cells to induce mediator release [36].

Several cytokines that are pre-stored in eosinophil granules or produced by Th2 lymphocytes are known to regulate the functions of human mast cells. These include IL-3 (Th2-derived cytokine) and IL-4, IL-5 and IL-6, (secreted by both eosinophils and Th2 lymphocytes). These cytokines prolonged mast cell survival in a dose-dependent manner [37]. In addition, IL-4, IL-5, or IL-6 enhance histamine release from mast cells, whereas IL-3 has a negligible effect [37].

Of these cytokines, IL-5 has a cardinal role in regulating mast cells as effector cells. Human Cord Blood-Derived Mast Cells (CBMC) express functional receptors for IL-5. IL-5 stimulates mast cells to express and secrete TNF-α, IL-5, IL-13, Macrophage Inflammatory Protein-1α (MIP-1α), and GM-CSF. IL-5 has therefore an autocrine effect on mast cells, as well as a paracrine effect, being released from both cell types, and this effect may amplify the allergic inflammatory responses [38].

We have recently demonstrated that eosinophils produce and secrete SCF [39]. SCF has several important effects on mast cell growth and activity. This cytokine can induce immature mast cells to mature and to acquire multiple characteristics of MC_{TC}, and is responsible for mast cell differentiation and proliferation [40, 41]. In addition, it was found to induce mast cell chemotaxis [42] and regulate mast cell adhesion to fibronectin [43]. SCF enhances IgE-dependent mediator release at concentrations 10–100 times lower than that required to promote cell proliferation, including the release of histamine and LTC_4 and PGD_2, and increases intracellular Ca^{2+} concentrations [44, 45]. SCF does not induce mediator release per se, but increases the sensitivity of mast cells to anti-IgE receptor stimulation and also enhances mediator release to maximally effective concentrations of anti-IgE receptor antibody [44].

NGF was recently found to be produced by eosinophils [29]. This growth factor was found to enhance mast cell survival, promote differentiation [46], cause mast cell degranulation and induce PGD_2, PGE_2 and IL-6 production [47].

One of the interesting characteristics of mast cell activation is that mast cells can be activated by eosinophils once they are desensitized to IgE-dependent challenge. This can lead to the persistence and the chronicity of the allergic inflammatory responses. We have recently shown that rat peritoneal mast cells that have been previously challenged by IgE-dependent stimuli, can be reactivated to release histamine following incubation with eosinophil sonicate, or purified Major Basic Protein (MBP) [48]. Previously, we had demonstrated that continuous in vitro exposure to compound 48/80 results in mast cell degranulation and se-

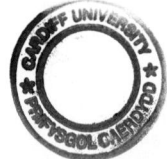

cretion of histamine. This continuous exposure does not adversely affect the ability of mast cells to synthesize histamine and to respond to repeated stimuli for a long period of time in vitro [49].

Besides the fact that mast cells can be activated several times, it is important to point out that the viability of these cells is not affected after multiple IgE-dependent or IgE-independent repeated stimuli. From this observation, we believe that mast cell activation might also be related to the prolonged survival of these cells. Indeed, IL-3-dependent murine mast cells are rescued from apoptosis in the absence of IL-3 by IgE-dependent activation, an effect suppressed by the addition of glucocorticoids [50].

Mast Cell Regulation of Fibrotic Processes

The presence of mast cells in tissue repair processes and early fibrosis and their participation in fibrotic diseases with different pathologies is well known [51,52]. The overall effect of mast cells on fibrotic responses is not well understood as yet, as there are contradictory effects of mast cells mediators on fibroblast functions.

Several mediators released by mast cells can modulate fibroblasts functions, and thereby contribute to tissue repair. Histamine, for example, stimulates the proliferation of human skin fibroblasts [53] and increases collagen synthesis by guinea pig fibroblasts [54]. We added histamine to 3T3 fibroblasts in an in-vitro wound model, and had found a stimulatory effect of histamine on fibroblast proliferation, that was abrogated by the addition of the H2-antagonist cimetidine [55].

The mast cell proteases, tryptase and chymase, have been shown to degrade collagen type IV and V, laminin and fibronectin. In addition, mast cells can also produce MMP-9, which is an extracellular matrix degrading enzyme [56]. Moreover, mast cell tryptase enhances the proliferation of normal lung and skin fibroblasts, and stimulates the production of type I collagen [57–59].

Heparin, another important mast cell mediator, has been shown to inhibit a protein kinase C dependent induction of the proto-oncogenes c-fos and c-myc, which are necessary for cell proliferation [60]. In addition, heparin decreases fibroblasts proliferation by binding to extracellular matrix components, thereby disrupting fibroblasts attachment, which is important for proliferation [61]. Heparin has also been reported to inhibit gel contraction by fibroblasts in a collagen gel [62].

Mast cells can also upregulate fibrosis through the release of several cytokines such as TGF-β, IL-4 and TNF-α, which are potent stimulators of collagen and fibronectin synthesis by fibroblasts. TNF-α was shown to stimulate fibroblast proliferation, chemotaxis and secretion of matrix metalloproteinases and other cytokines such as IL-6 [63–65]. Mast cells have also been shown to produce basic fibroblast growth factor (b-FGF) [66].

We have previously demonstrated that rat peritoneal mast cells co-cultured with 3T3 fibroblasts can increase the proliferation of these fibroblasts. Simulation of these mast cells resulted in a further increase of fibroblast proliferation, and an increase in collagen production [67]. It seems that mast cell activation in fibrosis is caused by the presence of constant endogenous stimuli, unlike mast cell activation in allergic diseases which is caused by a single or repetitive exposure to exogenous stimulus. We found that fibroblast proliferation in subconfluent cultures increased significantly over 4–5 days when mast cells were repeatedly activated, but not when they underwent single activation. Repeated activation of mast cells also caused a twofold increase in fibroblast collagen production in confluent cultures [67]. We have recently shown that mast cell sonicates added to dermal fibroblasts seeded in three-dimensional collagen lattices, increased fibroblast proliferation and collagen deposition, even at low mast cell concentrations [68]. However, there was a decrease in the speed and intensity of the gel contraction, which was partially attributed to heparin [68].

Effects of Mast Cells on Angiogenesis

Angiogenesis is an essential step in tissue repair and mast cells have been linked for almost two decades to both these processes. Several lines of histological evidence have implicated mast cells in the regulation of pathological or physiological examples of angiogenesis including hemangiomas [66], neoplasms [69, 70], rheumatoid arthritis [71], nasal polyps [72], wound healing [73] and ovulation [74]. Recently some research has focused on the production and secretion of angiogenic factors from mast cells.

Mast cells from human tissues with chronic inflammation [75, 76] and rat/ mouse tissues with anaphylaxis were shown to possess b-FGF in their cytoplasmic granules that can be released through degranulation [76].

Boesiger et al. [77] showed that murine or human cord blood derived mast cells release VPF/VEGF upon stimulation through FcεRI or c-Kit or after challenge with phorbol myristate acetate, or calcium ionophore. Such mast cells can rapidly release VPF/VEGF apparently from a preformed pool, and can then sustain release by secreting newly synthesized protein.

In addition, the human mast cell leukemic cell line HMC-1 can constitutively express and secrete three isoforms of VPF/VEGF [78].

Mast cells can contribute to various aspects of angiogenesis not only through the production of VEGF and b-FGF but also of other preformed mediators or cytokines. Heparin, contained in large amounts in mast cell secretory granules, is important in angiogenesis. In fact, it stimulates endothelial cell chemotaxis [79] and proliferation [80] and, by binding b-FGF, it renders it biologically active and protected from proteoloysis. Histamine and more recently tryptase have been shown to be angiogenic factors [81, 82]. In addition, TGF-β, TNF-α, IL-8 and other cytokines produced by mast cells might contribute to the angiogenic process [7, 83]. Also, the production of collagen type VIII by human mast cells in vivo may influence angiogenesis since this collagen is believed to facilitate the assembly of endothelial cords and tubes and its synthesis precedes that of pro-collagen type I [84].

Interestingly, angiogenic factors are not only produced by mast cells but they have also been shown to stimulate mast cell migration at sites of angiogenesis [85].

Recently, a direct role of mast cell in angiogenesis was demonstrated in an in vivo model [86] when degranulated mast cells and their secretory granules induced an angiogenic response. The addition of anti-FGF-2 (b-FGF) or anti-VEGF antibodies significantly reduces the angiogenic response, indicating that these two factors are primarily responsible for the mast cell vasoproliferative activity.

Conclusions

Mast cells play a major role in the onset and perpetuation of allergic inflammation, but also have major roles in the modulation of the subsequent tissue repair or fibrosis and angiogenesis. The network of interactions between mast cells and eosinophils creates mechanisms of dual stimulation, where mediators secreted from one cell type are activating the other, to release mediators that continue to activate the former. Some of these mediators are produced by both cell types, and can influence both of them. Moreover, some mediators can act in an autocrine fashion, thereby augmenting the allergic response. In addition to interacting with eosinophils, mast cells can interact with fibroblasts and with endothelial cells, and are therefore responsible for fibrogenic and angiogenetic responses.

In conclusion, we have shown that mast cells are not only responsible for the initiation of the allergic response, but also play a role as effector cells, secreting mediators that influence eosinophils and probably other inflammatory cells and tissue cells such as fibroblasts and endothelial cells. Consequently, they can be considered as target cells for drug intervention.

References

1. Kitamura Y, Shimada M, Hatanaka K, Miyano Y. Development of mast cells from grafted bone marrow cells in irradiated mice. Nature 268:442–443, 1977
2. Metcalfe DD, Baram D, Mekori YA. Mast cells. Physiol Rev 77:1033–1079, 1997
3. Stevens RL, Fox CC, Lichtenstein LM, Austen KF. Identification of chondroitin sulfate E proteoglycans and heparin proteoglycans in the secretory granules of human lung mast cells. Proc Natl Acad Sci USA 85:2284–2287, 1988
4. Gordon JR, Burd PR, Galli SJ. Mast cells as a source of multifunctional cytokines. Immunol Today 11:458–464, 1990
5. Schwartz L, Huff T. Biology of mast cells and basophils. In: Middlleton E Jr., Reed CE, Ellis EF, Adkinson FN, Yunginger JW, Busse WW, eds. Allergy. Principles and Practice. St. Louis, Missouri: Mosby 135–168, 1993
6. Coffman RL. T-helper heterogeneity and immune response patterns. Hosp Pract (Off Ed) 24:101–14, passim, 1989
7. Church MK, Levi-Schaffer F. The human mast cell. J Allergy Clin Immunol 99:155–160, 1997
8. Bradding P, Okayama Y, Howarth PH, Church MK, Holgate ST. Heterogeneity of human mast cells based on cytokine content. J Immuno 155:297–307, 1995
9. Okayama Y, Kobayashi H, Ashman LK, Dobashi K, Nakazawa T, Holgate ST, Church MK, Mori M. Human lung mast cells are enriched in the capacity to produce granulocyte-macrophage colony-stimulating factor in response to IgE-dependent stimulation. Eur J Immunol 28:708–715, 1998
10. Pincus SH, DiNapoli AM, Schooley WR. Superoxide production by eosinophils: activation by histamine. J Invest Dermatol 79:53–57, 1982

11. Gordon JR, Galli SJ. Mast cells as a source of both preformed and immunologically inducible TNF-alpha/cachectin. Nature 346:274–276, 1990

12. Bradding P, Roberts JA, Britten KM, Montefort S, Djukanvoic P, Mueller R, Heusser CH, Howarth PH, Holgate ST. IL-4, IL-5 and IL-6 and TNF-a in normal and asthmatic airways: evidence for the human mast cell as an important source of these cytokines. Am J Respir Cell Mol Biol 10:471–480, 1994

13. Casale TB, Costa JJ, Galli SJ. TNF alpha is important in human lung allergic reactions. Am J Respir Cell Mol Biol 15:35–44, 1996

14. Zeck-Kapp G, Czech W, Kapp A. TNF alpha-induced activation of eosinophil oxidative metabolism and morphology–comparison with IL-5. Exp Dermatol 3:176–188, 1994

15. Matsuyama G, Ochiai K, Ishihara C, Kagami M, Tomioka H, Koya N. Heterogeneous expression of tumor necrosis factor-alpha receptors I and II on human peripheral eosinophils. Int Arch Allergy Immunol 117 Suppl 1:28–33, 1998

16. Horie S, Gleich GJ, Kita H. Cytokines directly induce degranulation and superoxide production from human eosinophils. J Allergy Clin Immunol 98:371–381, 1996

17. Schwingshackl A, Duszyk M, Brown N, Moqbel R. Human eosinophils release matrix metalloproteinase-9 on stimulation with TNF-alpha. J Allergy Clin Immunol 104:983–989, 1999

18. Grewe M, Czech W, Morita A, Werfel T, Klammer M, Kapp A, Ruzicka T, Schopf E, Krutmann J. Human eosinophils produce biologically active IL-12: implications for control of T cell responses. J Immunol 161:415–420, 1998

19. Nakajima H, Gleich GJ, Kita H. Constitutive production of IL-4 and IL-10 and stimulated production of IL-8 by normal peripheral blood eosinophils. J Immunol 156:4859–4866, 1996

20. Han SJ, Kim JH, Noh YJ, Chang HS, Kim CS, Kim KS, Ki SY, Park CS, Chung IY. Interleukin (IL)-5 downregulates tumor necrosis factor (TNF)-induced eotaxin messenger RNA (mRNA) expression in eosinophils. Induction of eotaxin mRNA by TNF and IL-5 in eosinophils. Am J Respir Cell Mol Biol 21:303–310, 1999

21. Levi-Schaffer F, Temkin V, Malamud V, Feld S, Zilberman Y. Mast cells enhance eosinophil survival in vitro: Role of TNF-a and Granulocyte-Macrophage Colony-Stimulating Factor. J Immunol 160:5554–5562, 1998

22. Levi-Schaffer F, Smith SJ, Brown G, Fattah D, Ray K, Uings I. The effects of dexamethasone on eosinophils activated by Tumor Necrosis Factor-alpha (TNF-a): A comparison with GM-CSF. (Submitted). 2000.

23. Czech W, Krutmann J, Budnik A, Schopf E, Kapp A. Induction of intercellular adhesion molecule 1 (ICAM-1) expression in normal human eosinophils by inflammatory cytokines. J Invest Dermatol 100:417–423, 1993

24. Raible D, Schuman E, Dinuso J, Cardilo R, Post T. Mast cell mediators prostaglandin D$_2$ and histamine activate human eosinophils. J Immunol 148:3536–3542, 1992

25. Takafuji S, Tadokoro K, Ito K, Nakagawa T. Release of granule proteins from human eosinophils stimulated with mast-cell mediators. Allergy 53:951–956, 1998

26. Okayama Y, Kobayashi H, Ashman LK, Holgate ST, Church MK, Masatomo M. Activation of eosinophils with cytokines produced by lung mast cells. Int Arch Allergy Appl Immunol 114:75–77, 1997

27. Bonini S, Lambiase A, Bonini S, Levi-Schaffer F, Aloe L. Nerve growth factor: an important molecule in allergic inflammation and tissue remodelling. Int Arch Allergy Immunol 118:159–162, 1999

28. Nilsson G, Forsberg-Nilsson K, Xiang Z, Hallbook F, Nilsson K, Metcalfe DD. Human mast cells express functional TrkA and are a source of nerve growth factor. Eur J Immunol 27:2295–2301, 1997

29. Solomon A, Aloe L, Pe'er J, Frucht-Pery J, Bonini S, Bonini S, Levi-Schaffer F. Nerve growth factor is preformed in and activates human peripheral blood eosinophils. J Allergy Clin Immunol 102:454–460, 1998

30. Takafuji S, Bischoff SC, De Weck AL, Dahinden CA. Opposing effects of tumor necrosis factor-alpha and nerve growth factor upon leukotriene C4 production by human eosinophils triggered with N- formyl-methionyl-leucyl-phenylalanine. Eur J Immunol 22:969–974, 1992

31. Zhang S, Anderson DF, Bradding P, Coward WR, Baddeley SM, MacLeod JD, McGill JI, Church MK, Holgate ST, Roche WR. Human mast cells express stem cell factor. J Pathol 186:59–66, 1998

32. Yuan Q, Austen KF, Friend DS, Heidtman M, Boyce JA. Human peripheral blood eosinophils express a functional c-kit receptor for stem cell factor that stimulates very late antigen 4 (VLA-4)- mediated cell adhesion to fibronectin and vascular cell adhesion molecule 1 (VCAM-1). J Exp Med 186:313–323, 1997

33. Patella V, de Crescenzo G, Marino I, Genovese A, Adt M, Gleich GJ, Marone G. Eosinophil granule proteins activate human heart mast cells. J Immunol 157:1219–1225, 1996

34. Zheutlin LM, Ackerman SJ, Gleich GJ, Thomas LL. Stimulation of basophil and rat mast cell histamine release by eosinophil granule-derived cationic proteins. J Immunol 133:2180–2185, 1984

35. Okayama Y, el Lati SG, Leiferman KM, Church MK. Eosinophil granule proteins inhibit substance P-induced histamine release from human skin mast cells. J Allergy Clin Immunol 93:900–909, 1994

36. el Lati SG, Dahinden CA, Church MK. Complement peptides C3a- and C5a-induced mediator release from dissociated human skin mast cells. J Invest Dermatol 102:803–806, 1994

37. Yanagida M, Fukamachi H, Ohgami K, Kuwaki T, Ishii H, Uzumaki H, Amano K, Tokiwa T, Mitsui H, Saito H. Effects of T-helper 2-type cytokines, interleukin-3 (IL-3), IL-4, IL-5, and IL-6 on the survival of cultured human mast cells. Blood 86:3705–3714, 1995

38. Ochi H, De Jesus NH, Hsieh FH, Austen KF, Boyce JA. IL-4 and –5 prime human mast cells for different profiles of IgE- dependent cytokine production. Proc Natl Acad Sci USA 97:10509–10513, 2000

39. Hartman M-L, Piliponsky A, Temkin V, Levi-Schaffer F. Human peripheral blood eosinophils express stem cell factor. Blood (in press).

40. Tsai M, Takeishi T, Thompson H, Langley KE, Zsebo KM, Metcalfe DD, Geissler EN, Galli SJ. Induction of mast cell proliferation, maturation, and heparin synthesis by the rat c-kit ligand, stem cell factor. Proc Natl Acad Sci USA 88:6382–6386, 1991

41. Mitsui H, Furitsu T, Dvorak AM, Irani AM, Schwartz LB, Inagaki N, Takei M, Ishizaka K, Zsebo KM, Gillis S. Development of human mast cells from umbilical cord blood cells by recombinant human and murine c-kit ligand. Proc Natl Acad Sci USA 90:735–739, 1993

42. Meininger CJ, Yano H, Rottapel R, Bernstein A, Zsebo KM, Zetter BR. The c-kit receptor ligand functions as a mast cell chemoattractant. Blood 79:958–963, 1992

43. Dastych J, Metcalfe DD. Stem cell factor induces mast cell adhesion to fibronectin. J Immunol 152:213–219, 1994

44. Bischoff SC, Dahinden CA. c-kit ligand: a unique potentiator of mediator release by human lung mast cells. J Exp Med 175:237–244, 1992

45. Columbo M, Horowitz EM, Botana LM, MacGlashan DW, Jr., Bochner BS, Gillis S, Zsebo KM, Galli SJ, Lichtenstein LM. The human recombinant c-kit receptor ligand, rhSCF, induces mediator release from human cutaneous mast cells and enhances IgE-dependent mediator release from both skin mast cells and peripheral blood basophils. J Immunol 149:599–608, 1992

46. Matsuda H, Coughlin MD, Bienenstock J, Denburg JA. Nerve growth factor promotes human hemopoietic colony growth and differentiation. Proc Natl Acad Sci USA 85:6508–6512, 1988

47. Marshall JS, Gomi K, Blennerhassett MG, Bienenstock J. Nerve growth factor modifies the expression of inflammatory cytokines by mast cells via a prostanoid-dependent mechanism. J Immunol 162:4271–4276, 1999

48. Piliponsky AM, Pickholtz D, Gleich GJ, Levi-Schaffer F. Eosinophils activate mast cells to release histamine. Int Arch Allergy Immunol 118:202–203, 1999

49. Levi-Schaffer F, Riesel-Yaron N. Effects of prolonged incubation of rat peritoneal mast cells with compound 48/80. Eur J Immunol 20:2609–2613, 1990

50. Yoshikawa H, Nakajima Y, Tasaka K. Glucocorticoid suppresses autocrine survival of mast cells by inhibiting IL-4 production and ICAM-1 expression. J Immunol 162:6162–6170, 1999

51. Hawkins RA, Claman HN, Clark RA, Steigerwald JC. Increased dermal mast cell populations in progressive systemic sclerosis: a link in chronic fibrosis? Ann Intern Med 102:182–186, 1985

52. Wichman BE. The mast cell count during the process of wound healing: an experimental investigation in rats. Acat Pathol Microbiol Scand 108:1–35, 1955

53. Jordana M, Befus AD, Newhouse MT, Bienenstock J, Gauldie J. Effect of histamine on proliferation of normal human adult lung fibroblasts. Thorax. 43:552–558, 1988

54. Hatamochi A, Fujiwara K, Ueki H. Effects of histamine on collagen synthesis by cultured fibroblasts derived from guinea pig skin. Arch Dermatol Res 277:60–64, 1985
55. Kupietzky A, Levi-Schaffer F. The role of mast cell-derived histamine in the closure of an in vitro wound. Inflamm Res 45:176–180, 1996
56. Kanbe N, Tanaka A, Kanbe M, Itakura A, Kurosawa M, Matsuda H. Human mast cells produce matrix metalloproteinase 9. Eur J Immunol 29:2645–2649, 1999
57. Gruber BL, Kew RR, Jelaska A, Marchese MJ, Garlick J, Ren S, Schwartz LB, Korn JH. Human mast cells activate fibroblasts: tryptase is a fibrogenic factor stimulating collagen messenger ribonucleic acid synthesis and fibroblast chemotaxis. J Immunol 158 :2310–2317, 1997
58. Abe M, Kurosawa M, Ishikawa O, Miyachi Y, Kido H. Mast cell tryptase stimulates both human dermal fibroblast proliferation and type I collagen production. Clin Exp Allergy 28:1509–1517, 1998
59. Cairns JA, Walls AF. Mast cell tryptase stimulates the synthesis of type I collagen in human lung fibroblasts. J Clin Invest 99:1313–1321, 1997
60. Wright TC, Jr., Pukac LA, Castellot JJ, Jr., Karnovsky MJ, Levine RA, Kim-Park HY, Campisi J. Heparin suppresses the induction of c-fos and c-myc mRNA in murine fibroblasts by selective inhibition of a protein kinase C-dependent pathway. Proc Natl Acad Sci USA 86:3199–3203, 1989
61. Del Vecchio PJ, Bizios R, Holleran LA, Judge TK, Pinto GL. Inhibition of human scleral fibroblast proliferation with heparin. Invest Ophthalmol Vis Sci 29:1272–1276, 1988
62. Guidry C, Grinnell F. Heparin modulates the organization of hydrated collagen gels and inhibits gel contraction by fibroblasts. J Cell Biol 104:1097–1103, 1987
63. Dayer JM, Beutler B, Cerami A. Cachectin/tumor necrosis factor stimulates collagenase and prostaglandin E2 production by human synovial cells and dermal fibroblasts. J Exp Med 162:2163–2168, 1985
64. Kendall JC, Li XH, Galli SJ, Gordon JR. Promotion of mouse fibroblast proliferation by IgE-dependent activation of mouse mast cells: role for mast cell tumor necrosis factor-alpha and transforming growth factor-beta 1. J Allergy Clin Immunol 99:113–123, 1997
65. Postlethwaite AE, Seyer JM. Stimulation of fibroblast chemotaxis by human recombinant tumor necrosis factor alpha (TNF-alpha) and a synthetic TNF-alpha 31–68 peptide. J Exp Med 172:1749–1756, 1990
66. Qu Z, Liebler JM, Powers MR, Galey T, Ahmadi P, Huang XN, Ansel JC, Butterfield JH, Planck SR, Rosenbaum JT. Mast cells are a major source of basic fibroblast growth factor in chronic inflammation and cutaneous hemangioma. Am J Pathol 147:564–573, 1995
67. Levi-Schaffer F, Rubinchik E. Activated mast cells are fibrogenic for 3T3 fibroblasts. J Invest Dermatol 104:999–1003, 1995
68. Berton A, Levi-Schaffer F, Emonard H, Garbuzenko E, Gillery P, Maquart FX. Activation of fibroblasts in collagen lattices by mast cell extract: a model of fibrosis. Clin Exp Allergy 30:485–492, 2000
69. Imada A, Shijubo N, Kojima H, Abe S. Mast cells correlate with angiogenesis and poor outcome in stage I lung adenocarcinoma. Eur Respir J 15:1087–1093, 2000
70. Sawatsubashi M, Yamada T, Fukushima N, Mizokami H, Tokunaga O, Shin T. Association of vascular endothelial growth factor and mast cells with angiogenesis in laryngeal squamous cell carcinoma. Virchows Arch 436:243–248, 2000
71. Yamada T, Sawatsubashi M, Yakushiji H, Itoh Y, Edakuni G, Mori M, Robert L, Miyazaki K. Localization of vascular endothelial growth factor in synovial membrane mast cells: examination with „multi-labelling subtraction immunostaining". Virchows Arch 433:567–570, 1998
72. Vento SI, Wolff CH, Salven PJ, Hytonen ML, Ertama LO, Malmberg CH. Vascular permeability factor/vascular endothelial growth factor in nasal polyps. Acta Otolaryngol Suppl 543:170–174, 2000
73. Trabucchi E, Radaelli E, Marazzi M, Foschi D, Musazzi M, Veronesi AM, Montorsi W. The role of mast cells in wound healing. Int J Tissue React 10:367–372, 1988
74. Krishna A, Beesley K, Terranova PF. Histamine, mast cells and ovarian function. J Endocrinol 120:363–371, 1989
75. Qu Z, Huang X, Ahmadi P, Stenberg P, Liebler JM, Le AC, Planck SR, Rosenbaum JT. Synthesis of basic fibroblast growth factor by murine mast cells. Regulation by transforming growth

factor beta, tumor necrosis factor alpha, and stem cell factor. Int Arch Allergy Immunol 115:47–54, 1998

76. Qu Z, Kayton RJ, Ahmadi P, Liebler JM, Powers MR, Planck SR, Rosenbaum JT. Ultrastructural immunolocalization of basic fibroblast growth factor in mast cell secretory granules. Morphological evidence for bFGFf release through degranulation. J Histochem Cytochem 46:1119–1128, 1998

77. Boesiger J, Tsai M, Maurer M, Yamaguchi M, Brown LF, Claffey KP, Dvorak HF, Galli SJ. Mast cells can secrete vascular permeability factor/ vascular endothelial cell growth factor and exhibit enhanced release after immunoglobulin E-dependent upregulation of fc epsilon receptor I expression. J Exp Med 188:1135–1145, 1998

78. Grutzkau A, Kruger-Krasagakes S, Baumeister H, Schwarz C, Kogel H, Welker P, Lippert U, Henz BM, Moller A. Synthesis, storage, and release of vascular endothelial growth factor/vascular permeability factor (VEGF/VPF) by human mast cells: implications for the biological significance of VEGF206. Mol Biol Cell 9:875–884, 1998

79. Azizkhan RG, Azizkhan JC, Zetter BR, Folkman J. Mast cell heparin stimulates migration of capillary endothelial cells in vitro. J Exp Med 152:931–944, 1980

80. Folkman J. Regulation of angiogenesis: a new function of heparin. Biochem Pharmacol 34:905–909, 1985

81. Sorbo J, Jakobsson A, Norrby K. Mast-cell histamine is angiogenic through receptors for histamine1 and histamine2. Int J Exp Pathol 75:43–50, 1994

82. Blair RJ, Meng H, Marchese MJ, Ren S, Schwartz LB, Tonnesen MG, Gruber BL. Human mast cells stimulate vascular tube formation. Tryptase is a novel, potent angiogenic factor. J Clin Invest 99:2691–2700, 1997

83. Norrby K. Mast cells and de novo angiogenesis: angiogenic capability of individual mast-cell mediators such as histamine, TNF, IL-8 and bFGF. Inflamm Res 46 Suppl 1:S7-S8, 1997

84. Ruger B, Dunbar PR, Hasan Q, Sawada H, Kittelberger R, Greenhill N, Neale TJ. Human mast cells produce type VIII collagen in vivo. Int J Exp Pathol 75:397–404, 1994

85. Gruber BL, Marchese MJ, Kew R. Angiogenic factors stimulate mast-cell migration. Blood 86:2488–2493, 1995

86. Ribatti D, Crivellato E, Candussio L, Nico B, Vacca A, Roncali L, Dammacco F. Mast cells and their secretory granules are angiogenic in the chick embryo chorioallantioc membrane. Clin Exp Allergy 2000 (in press)

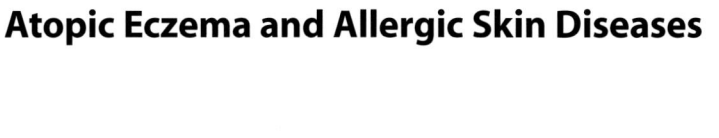

Atopic Eczema and Allergic Skin Diseases

15 Modulation of Skin Barrier Function

W. Wohlrab, C. Huschka, D. Fröde, J.-M. Schneider

Clinical unaffected skin of patients suffering from atopic eczema is characterized by a high degree of disturbances of structural and functional properties of
the stratum corneum [16, 19]. The aim of skin care during a clinical unaffected
interval is the reconstruction of disturbed barrier function by substitution of
moisturizing substances and lipids. The reconstruction of the barrier function
of the skin is possible both by substitution of reduced lipid components and by
stimulation of the epidermal lipid synthesis. Among the lipids fatty acids (FA)
play an important role in the synthesis of epidermal lipids [5, 6, 13]. As linked to
specific epidermal ceramides, they are involved in forming and maintaining the
barrier function of the skin.

Penetration of FA into Human Skin

The efficiency of topically applied FA containing vehicles with drugs or skin care
products largely depends on the penetrated FA amount in the different skin layers. Equally, the influence on keratinocyte proliferation is dependent on the type
and the penetrated concentration of FA. According to the FA content of human
epidermis (EP) [3, 4, 21], we examined a number of saturated and unsaturated
middle chain FA and middle chain methylbranched FA as well (Fig. 1)

The investigations of the FA penetration into different skin layers yielded differences in FA penetration. We could find unsaturated FA (e.g. oleic acid) in the

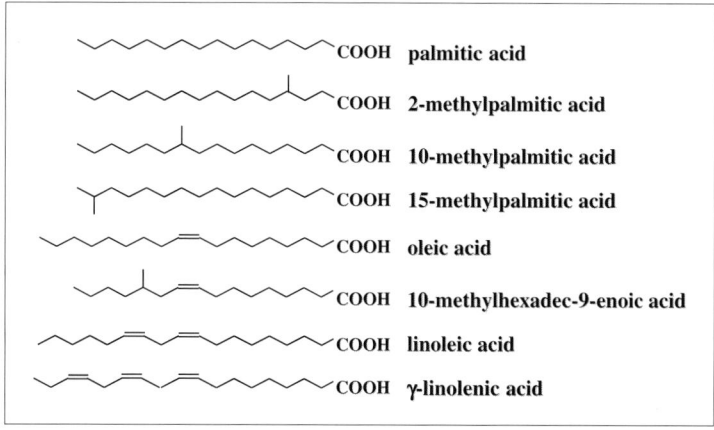

Fig. 1. Structures of fatty acids

New Trends in Allergy V
J. Ring, H. Behrendt (Eds.)
© Springer-Verlag Berlin, Heidelberg 2002

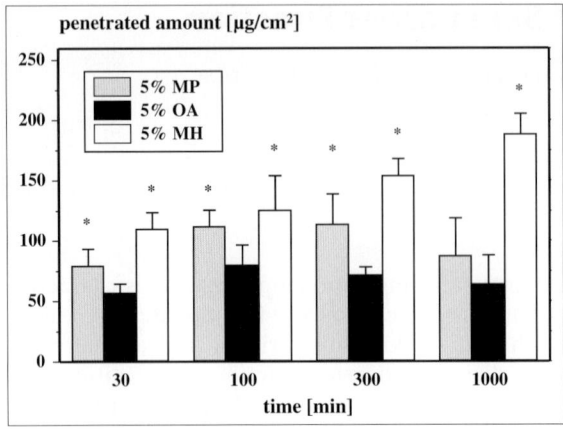

Fig. 2. Fatty acid penetration into human stratum corneum ex vivo ($n=3$; *significant to the control, $p=0.05$). *MP*, 2-methylpalmitic acid; *OA*, oleic acid; *MH*, 10-methylhexadec-9-enoic acid

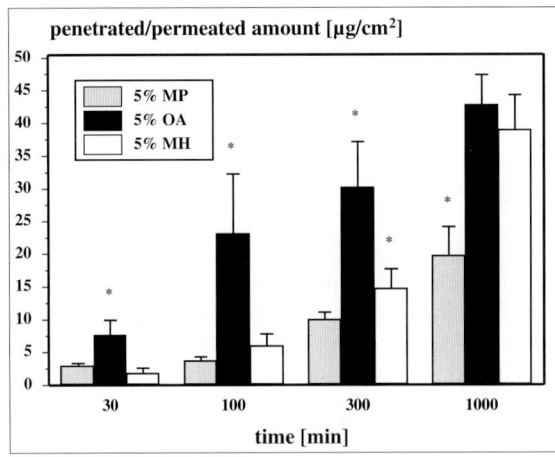

Fig. 3. Fatty acid penetration into viable epidermis and dermis and permeation into the acceptor ($n=3$; *significant to the control, $p=0.05$). *MP*, 2-methylpalmitic acid; *OA*, oleic acid; *MH*, 10-methylhexadec-9-enoic acid

stratum corneum also after longer penetration time only in a very low concentration but the methylbranched type (e.g. of oleic acid) in higher concentrations (Fig. 2). We saw other results in the living part of EP (Fig. 3). In this skin layer, the highest concentration was reached by the application of unbranched unsaturated FA, for example oleic acid.

Summarizing, it may be said that the penetration of FA into different skin layers is not only dependent on concentration applied and application time but also on the molecular structure of FA [23, 27, 28].

Modulation of Epidermal Proliferation

Hence, differences in keratinocyte (KC) reactions also resulted from different types of FA. After incubation with low linoleic acid concentrations, an increase in tritium thymidine incorporation could be measured, while a decrease in pro-

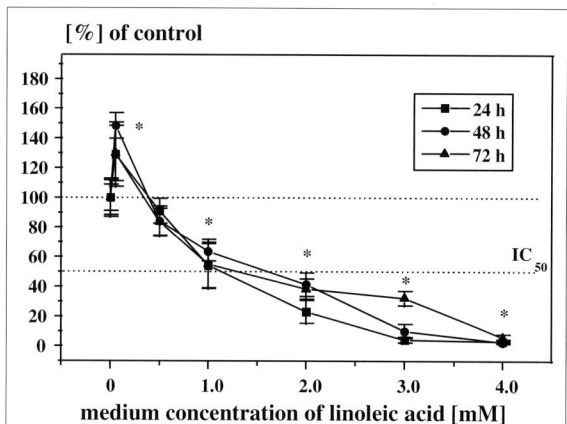

Fig. 4. Influence of linoleic acid on the proliferation of human keratinocytes. (*Significant to the control, $p=0.05$)

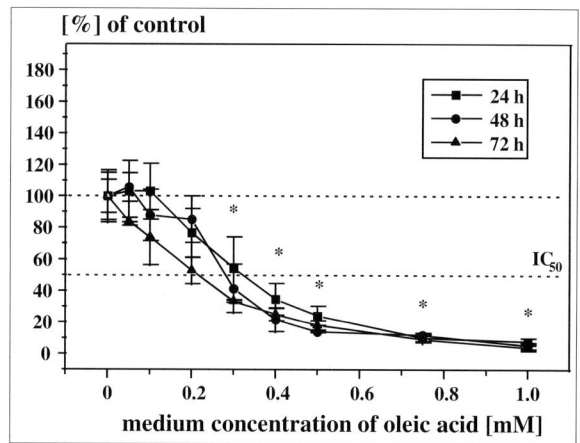

Fig. 5. Influence of oleic acid on the proliferation of human keratinocytes. (*Significant to the control, $p=0.05$)

liferation was observed with higher linoleic acid concentrations (Fig. 4). On the other hand, a drastic reduction in tritium thymidine incorporation was observed by oleic acid already at a low concentration (Fig. 5).

The mechanism of this reduced KC proliferation is primarily not a toxic effect. With different methods, we could demonstrate that apoptosis of KC occurred after contact with FA [2]. Examples with linoleic acid (Fig. 6) and γ-linolenic acid (Fig. 7) showed a reduced number of intact KC in dependence on increased FA concentration. At the same time, the number of apoptotic cells was increased while the necrotic cell proportion remained unchanged. Annexin-V-FITC, Cell Death Detection Elisa Test and DNA-Fragmentation Test were used to detect apoptosis (Figs. 8, 9).

The induction of KC apoptosis is dependent on the type as well as the concentration of FA. In connection with these processes, changes in the free intracellular $[Ca^{2+}]_i$-content, p53 and bcl2/bax expression could be demonstrated [14]. High concentrations of free FA (e.g. linoleic acid; γ-linolenic acid) led within

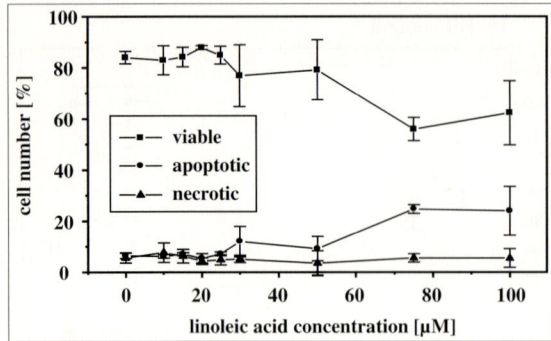

Fig. 6. Apoptosis in human keratinocytes after 24 h incubation with linoleic acid. (Method: Annexin-V-FLUOS)

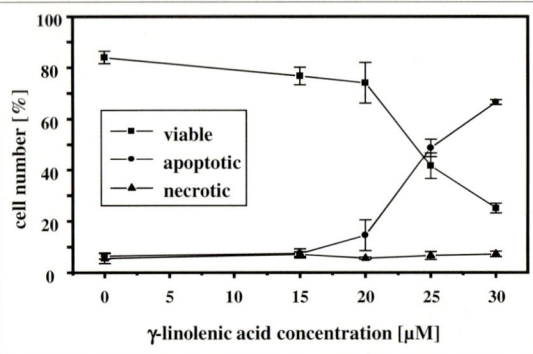

Fig. 7. Apoptosis in human keratinocytes after 24 h incubation with γ-linolenic acid. (Method: Annexin-V-FLUOS)

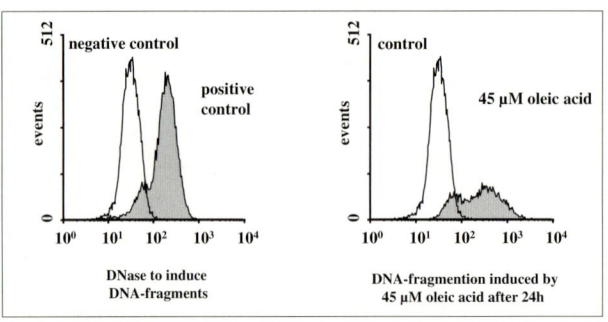

Fig. 8. Detection of late apoptosis in human keratinocytes induced by oleic acid

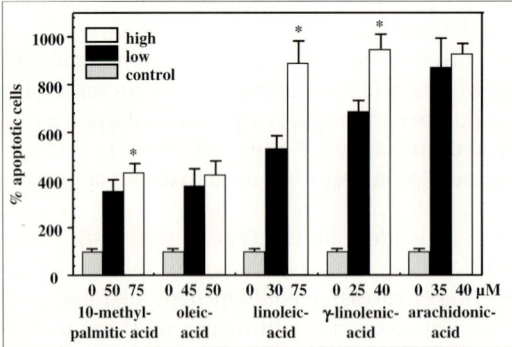

Fig. 9. Influence of fatty acids on apoptosis of human keratinocytes. (Method: Cell Death Detection ELISAPLUS; incubation time 24 h)

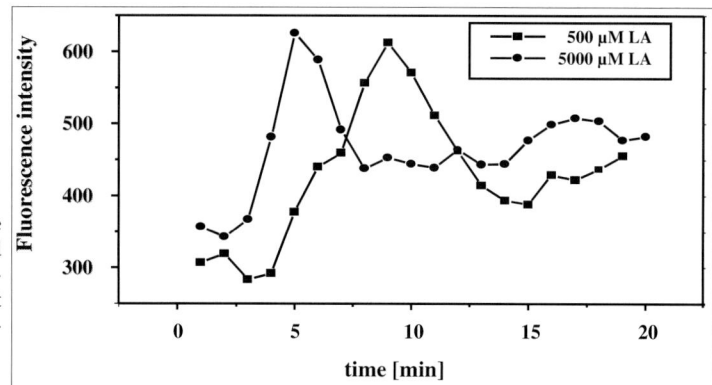

Fig. 10. Influence of linoleic acid on the intracellular Ca²⁺-content of human keratinocytes

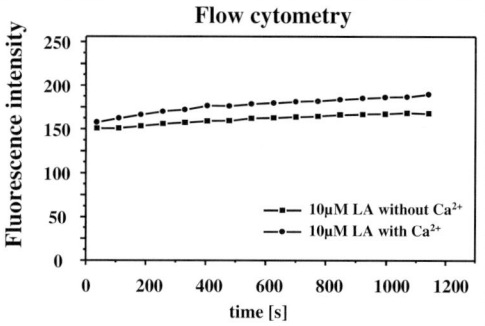

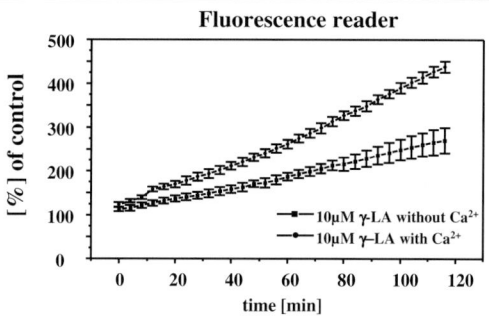

Fig. 11. Influence of free fatty acids on the intracellular Ca²⁺-concentration in human keratinocytes. *LA*, linoleic acid; *γ-LA*, γ-linolenic acid

minutes to a distinct rise in the free intracellular $[Ca^{2+}]_i$-concentration for a short time (Fig. 10). Low concentrations of free FA led to a continuous increase in free intracellular $[Ca^{2+}]_i$–content over several minutes (Fig. 11). The result that apoptosis occurred after adding fatty acids is probably related to these findings.

At the same conditions changes of p53 (Fig. 12) and bcl2/bax (Fig. 13) expression could be demonstrated.

Altogether, it may be said that the knowledge of the KC reaction after contact with FA plays an important role for the substitution of reduced lipids to reconstruct skin barrier function [23, 26, 27].

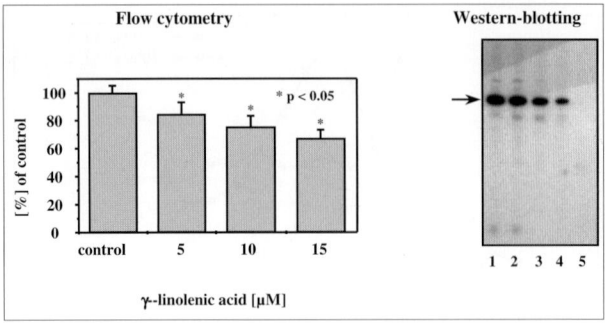

Fig. 12. Effect of γ-linolenic acid on p53 expression in human keratinocytes. Western blotting lanes: *1*, control with 0.2% ethanol; *2*, 15 μM γ-linolenic acid; *3*, 20 μM γ-linolenic acid; *4*, 25 μM γ-linolenic acid; *5*, buffer

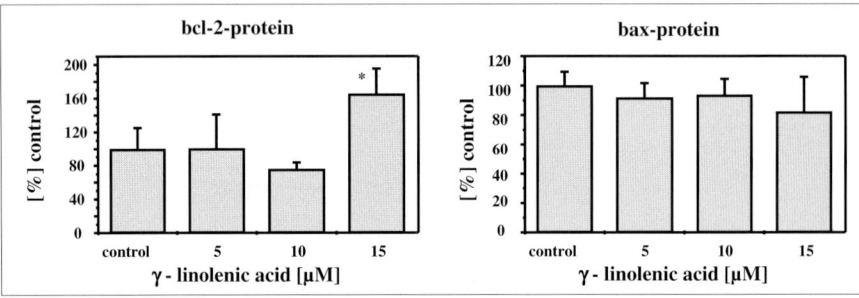

Fig. 13. Expression of apoptosis associated proteins in human keratinocytes (after incubation with γ-linolenic acid; incubation time 24 h)

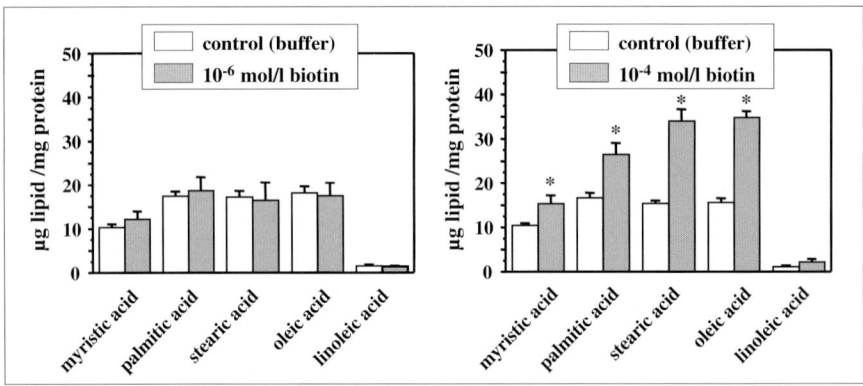

Fig. 14. Influence of biotin on the fatty acid content of human keratinocytes. (Mean±SD; *significant to the control, $p \leq 0.05$; $n=6$)

FA Synthesis in Human Keratinocytes

From this point of view, we should return to the importance of FA content for the formation of the barrier function of the skin. It is well known that human KC have the capacity to synthesize FA and the FA synthesis does not occur in the

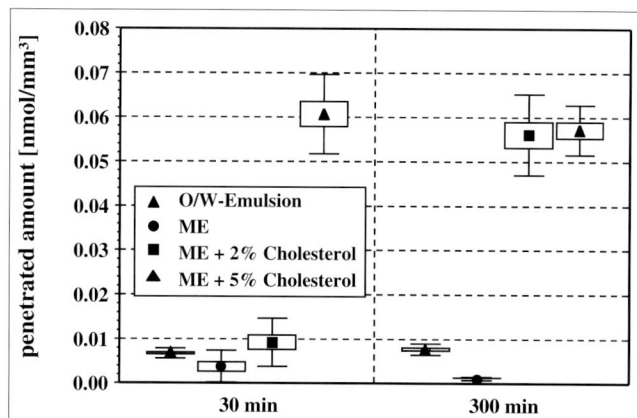

Fig. 15. Penetration of biotin from microemulsions (*ME*) compared with an oil in water emulsion into human skin ex vivo – epidermis (*p*≤0.05; *n*=9)

dermis [15, 17, 18, 20, 22]. On the other hand, several observations indicate that KC recycle FA derived from the extracellular degradation of precursor lipids [19, 26, 28]. Under the influence of biotin [1, 7], we could demonstrate an increased content of FA in human KC (Fig. 14) [10].

At the same conditions changes of intracellular $[Ca^{2+}]_i$–concentrations, involucrin or KI67 expression could not be detected [8, 12]. On the other hand, to increase FA synthesis in human KC, an epidermal biotin concentration of at least 10^{-5} mol is necessary. We observed the biotin penetration into human skin from different vehicles and commercial formulations (Fig. 15). In none of the tested formulations could we find a sufficient therapeutic effective drug concentration in the viable part of the epidermis. Only a specific microemulsion led to a therapeutically effective drug concentration [9, 11, 24, 25].

More recent investigations have shown in all probability a modified ceramide synthesis in KC under the influence of biotin.

Summarizing we conclude that the action of FA and the stimulation of epidermal lipid synthesis could lead to an improvement and to a reconstruction of the barrier function of human skin.

References

1. Bitsch, R.; Bartel, K.: Biotin. Stuttgart: Wissenschaftliche Verlagsgesellschaft mbH, 1994
2. Darzynkiewicz, Z.; Juan, G.; Li, X.; Gorczyca, W.; Murakami, T.; Traganos, F.: Cytometry in cell necrobiology: analysis of apoptosis and accidental cell death (necrosis). Cytometry 27 (1997), 1–20
3. Elias, P.M.: Epidermal lipids, barrier function, and desquamation. J Invest Dermatol 80 Suppl.6 (1983), 44–49
4. Elias, P.M.: Epidermal barrier function : intercellular lamellar lipid structures, origin, composition and metabolism. J Contr Rel 15 (1991), 199–208
5. Elias, P.M.: Stratum corneum architecture, metabolic activity and interactivity with subjacent cell layers. Exp Dermatol 5 (1996), 191–201
6. Elias, P.M.; Brown, B. E.; Ziboh, V. A.: The permeability barrier in essential fatty acid deficiency: Evidence for direct role for linoleic acid in barrier function. J Invest Dermatol 74 (1980), 230–233

7. Friedrich, W.: Vitamins. Berlin: De Gruyter, 1988
8. Fritsche, A.; Mathis, G.A.; Althaus, F.R.: Pharmakologische Wirkungen von Biotin auf Epidermiszellen. Schweiz Arch Tierheilk 133 (1991), 277–283
9. Göbel, S.; Schmalfuß, U.; Neubert, R.; Wohlrab, W.: Penetration of biotin from a microemulsion into human skin. Skin Pharmacol 9 (1996), 82
10. Huschka, Chr.; Wohlrab, W.; Neubert, R.: Stimulation of fatty acid sythesis in keratinocytes. J Invest Dermatol 110 (1998), 559
11. Huschka, Chr.; Wohlrab, W.; Neubert, R.; Motitschke, L.: Die Penetration von Biotin in humane Haut ex vivo aus verschiedenen Vehikeln. Kosmet Med 18 (1997), 214–217
12. Limat, A.; Suorrmala, T.; Hunziker, T.; Waelti, E.R.; Braathen, L.R.; Baumgartner, R.: Proliferation and differentiation of cultured human follicular keratinocytes are not influenced by biotin. Arch Dermatol Res 288 (1995), 31–38
13. Mauro, T.; Grayson, S.; Gao, W.N.; Man, M-Q.; Kriehuber, E.; Behne, M.; Feingold, K.R.; Elias, P.M.: Barrier recovery is impeded at neutral pH, independent of ionic effects: implications for extracellular lipid processing. Arch Dermatol Res 290 (1998), 215–222
14. McGovern, U.B.; Jones, K.T.; Sharpe, G.R.: Intracellular calcium as a second messenger following growth stimulation of human keratinocytes. Br J Dermatol 132 (1995), 892–896
15. Ottey, K.A.; Wood, L.C.; C.Gunfeld; Elias, P.M.; Feingold, K.R.: Cutaneous permeability barrier disruption increasa fatty acid synthetic enzyme activity in the epidermis of hairless mice. J Invest Dermatol 104 (1995), 401–404
16. Plewig, G.; Jansen, T.; Schürer, N.Y.: Das Stratum corneum. Hautarzt 48 (1997), 510–521
17. Proksch, E.; Holleran, W.M.; Menon, G.K.; Elias, P.M.; Feingold, K.R.: Barrier function regulates epidermal lipid and DNA synthesis. Br J Dermatol 128 (1993), 473–482
18. Proud, V.K.; Rizzo, W.B.; Patterson, J.W.; Heard, G.S.; Wolf, B.: Fatty acid alterations and carboxylase deficientcies in the skin of biotin-deficient rats. Am J Clin Nutr 51 (1990), 853–858
19. Schaefer, H.; Redelmeier, T.E.: Skin barrier. Principles of percutaneous absorption Basel: Karger Verlag, 1996
20. Schürer, N.Y.; Köhne, A.; Schliep, V.; Barlag, K.; Goerz, G.: Lipid composition and synthesis of HaCaT cells, an immortalized human keratinocyte line, in comparison with normal human adult keratinocytes. Exp Dermatol 2 (1993), 179–185
21. Schürer, N.Y.; Plewig, G.; Elias, P. M.: Stratum corneum lipid function. Dermatologica 183 (1991), 77–94
22. Schürer, N.Y.; Stremmel, W.; Grundmann, J.-U.; Schliep, V.; Kleinert, H.; Bass, N.M.; Williams, M.L.: Evidence for a novel keratinocyte fatty acid uptake mechanism with preference for linoleic acid: Comparison of oleic and linoleic acid uptake by cultured human keratinocytes, fibroblasts and a human hepatoma cell line. Biochim Biophys Acta 1211 (1994), 51–60
23. Siegenthaler, G.; Hotz, R.; Chatellard-Gruaz, D.; Diderjean, L.; Hellmann, U.; Saurat, J.H.: Purification and characterization of the human epidermal fatty acid – binding protein: localization during epidermal cell differentiation in vivo and in vitro. Biochem J 302 (1994), 363–371
24. Wagner, C.; Göbel, S.; Wohlrab, W.; Neubert, R.: Vehicle dependent liberation and penetration of biotin into human skin. Skin Pharmacol 10 (1997), 34–39
25. Wolf, R.; Huschka, Chr.; Raith, K.; Wohlrab, W.; Neubert, R.: Rapid quantification of biotin in human skin extracts after dermal application using HPLC-ESI-MS. Analytical Communications 34 (1997), 335–337
26. Yang, L.; Mao-Qiang, M.; M.Taljebini; Elias, P.M.; Feingold, K.R.: Topical stratum corneum lipids accelerate barrier repair after tape stripping, solvent treatment and some but not all types of detergent treatment. Br J Dermatol 133 (1995), 679–685
27. Zakim, D.: Fatty acids enter cells by simple diffusion. Proc Soc Exp Biol Med 212 (1996), 5–14
28. Ziboh, V.A.; Chapkin, R.S.: Metabolism and function of skin lipids. Prog Lipid Res 27 (1988), 81–105

16 T Cells and Effector Mechanisms in Atopic Dermatitis

M. Akdis, A. Trautmann, S. Klunker, K. Blaser, C.A. Akdis

Summary

T cells constitute a large population of cellular infiltrate in atopic dermatitis (AD) and a dysregulated, cytokine mediated immune response appears to be an important pathogenetic factor. The great majority of T cells homing to skin express CD45RO$^+$ memory/effector phenotype and the skin-selective homing receptor, the cutaneous lymphocyte-associated antigen (CLA). Aeroallergens, food antigens, autoantigens and bacterial superantigens activate T cells in AD. Continuous stimulation of T cells in lymphatic organs and skin plays an important role in AD with induction of hyper IgE and eosinophilia. Activated T cells induce keratinocyte apoptosis as a key pathogenetic event in the formation of eczema. To mediate these effector functions after skin homing, activated T cells show continuous survival in the skin. Activation-induced cell death of T cells (AICD) is prevented by cytokines and extracellular matrix components in the eczematous skin.

Mechanisms of T Cell Activation in AD

Several studies pointed to the role of activated CD4$^+$ T cells in AD and other allergic inflammatory disease (reviewed in [1]). Increased numbers of activated CLA-bearing T cells in the circulation and increased levels of serum L-selectin, a marker for leukocyte activation correlating with disease severity demonstrate systemic T cell activation in AD [2–4]. Several stimuli leading to T cell activation in AD including aeroallergens, food allergens and superantigens have been emphasized. Aeroallergens can induce both immediate type and delayed type responses in the skin [5]. The frequency of aeroallergen-specific T cells was investigated in AD lesions and they were found to be less than 1% in non-challenged AD lesions [6]. The contribution of food allergens in the exacerbation of AD by T cell activation was also demonstrated [7]. Dermal cellular infiltrate in AD mainly consists of CD4$^+$ and CD8$^+$ T cells with a CD4/CD8 ratio similar to peripheral blood levels [8, 9]. In recent studies, CD8$^+$CLA$^+$ T cells were demonstrated to be as potent as CD4$^+$CLA$^+$ T cells in induction of IgE and prolonged of eosinophil survival [8, 9]. Normally allergen-specific T cell responses in food and aeroallergen allergy are confined to CD4$^+$ T cells. This, however, may not explain the activation and recruitment of CD8$^+$ T cells in AD skin lesions. It is known that bacterial superantigens can interact with certain Vβ elements of the TCR leading to activation, expansion, anergy or deletion of T cells. CD8$^+$ T cells [8]

New Trends in Allergy V
J. Ring, H. Behrendt (Eds.)
© Springer-Verlag Berlin, Heidelberg 2002

and even CD4⁻ CD8⁻ T cells can respond to superantigenic stimuli [10], which may explain the existence of activated CD8⁺ T cells in eczema lesions and their contribution to IgE production and eosinophil survival [8, 9].

From a number of studies it can be concluded that bacterial superantigens contribute to the pathogenesis and exacerbation of AD. Staphylococcal superantigens were isolated from AD skin [11]. Superantigen patch test elicits skin inflammation in AD patients [12] and in human severe combined immunodeficiency mouse model [13]. In addition, specific IgE antibodies to bacterial superantigens exist in AD [14]. It was also demonstrated that CD8⁺ T cells isolated from skin or CLA⁺ CD8⁺ T cells isolated from peripheral blood efficiently proliferate by superantigenic stimulation [8]. Furthermore, purified CD4⁺ or CD8⁺ T cells cultured from skin biopsies secrete high IL-5 and IL-13 by Staphylococcal enterotoxin B (SEB) stimulation [8]. Induction of CLA expression by superantigens on Th2 cells in addition to Th1 cells may play an important role in the pathogenesis of AD [15]. Staphylococcal superantigens secreted at the skin surface may penetrate through the inflamed skin and stimulate epidermal macrophages or Langerhans cells to produce IL-1, TNF and IL-12. Local production of IL-1 and TNF may induce E-selectin on vascular endothelium allowing an initial migration of CLA⁺ memory/effector cells [16].

Cytokine Profile of T Cells in AD

Elevated IgE levels and eosinophilia in AD suggest increased expression of Th2 type cytokines [17]. The majority of allergen-specific T cells derived from skin lesions that have been provoked in AD patients by epicutaneous allergen application or peripheral blood skin homing T cells, produce predominantly Th2 cytokines such as IL-4, IL-5 and IL-13 [2, 3, 8, 18]. Previously, such polarized Th2 cytokine pattern was regarded as a specific feature reflecting immune dysregulation in AD. However, current studies demonstrate that IFN-γ predominates over IL-4 in chronic skin lesions and older patch test reactions in AD, whereas, IL-5 and IL-13 still remain at high levels [6, 9, 19, 20]. A number of factors may be involved in increased IFN-γ in older skin lesions. IL-12 produced by Langerhans cells, eosinophils and keratinocytes appears to be a predominant mediator for the induction of IFN-γ in T cells after homing to skin [21–23]. Furthermore, IL-18 produced in the microenvironment of skin may act in parallel to IL-12 [24].

T Cell-Mediated Effector Mechanisms in Atopic Dermatitis

A Role for IL-5 and IL-13 in Atopic Dermatitis

Although most patients with AD show high concentrations of total and allergen-specific IgE in blood and skin, some of them express normal IgE levels and show no allergen-specific IgE antibodies. The diagnostic criteria of AD by Hanifin and Rajka [25] can be fulfilled also in the absence of elevated total IgE and allergen-specific IgE. This suggests that elevated IgE levels and IgE sensitization are not prerequisites in the pathogenesis of the disease. The subgroup of AD patients with normal IgE levels and without specific IgE sensitization has been termed the non-allergic form of AD (NAD) or intrinsic-type AD [9, 26]. Recent data suggest that T cells are likely involved in the pathogenesis of AD and NAD [27]. CD4$^+$ and CD8$^+$ subsets of skin infiltrating T cells as well as skin homing CLA$^+$ T cells from peripheral blood, equally respond to superantigen, SEB, and produce IL-2, IL-5, IL-13 and IFN-γ in both forms of the disease [8, 9]. Interestingly, skin T cells from „extrinsic AD" patients express higher IL-5 and IL-13 levels compared to NAD patients. Accordingly, T cells isolated from skin biopsies of extrinsic AD, but not from „intrinsic", induced high IgE production in cocultures with normal B cells, which is mediated by IL-13. In addition, B cell activation with high CD23 expression is observed in the peripheral blood of „extrinsic AD", but not „intrissic" patients [9]. These findings suggest a lack of IL-13-induced B cell activation and consequent IgE production in non-atopic eczema, although high numbers of T cells are present in lesional skin of both types [9]. More importantly, IL-4 and IL-13 neutralization in B cell cocultures with peripheral blood CLA$^+$ skin homing T cells or skin infiltrating T cells demonstrated that IL-13 represents the major cytokine for induction of IgE production in AD [3, 8, 9].

Cytokine determinations from peripheral blood CLA$^+$ T cells and skin biopsies of AD patients show increased IL-5 expression [8, 9, 18, 27]. Accordingly, supernatants from CLA$^+$ T cells of both CD4$^+$ and CD8$^+$ subsets extend the life span of freshly purified eosinophils in vitro, whereas supernatants of CLA$^-$ T cells do not influence eosinophil survival. Neutralization of cytokines demonstrated the predominant role of IL-5-secreted from CLA$^+$ T cells in prolonged eosinophil survival in AD [8].

Dysregulated T Cell Apoptosis in AD

Cell death by apoptosis is a tightly regulated process that enables removal of unnecessary, aged or damaged cells. During apoptosis a complex death program is initiated that ultimately leads to phagocytosis of the apoptotic cell. Although the death of certain cells can lead to functional deficiencies, prolonged survival of some effector cells can cause tissue injury and play a role in the pathogenesis of disease [28]. During the development of the immune response, T cells are stimulated by antigens presented by antigen-presenting cells that leads to T cell activation and clonal expansion. Some of the activated T cells die by activation-induced cell death (AICD) under certain conditions [29]. AICD is thought to play an important role in maintaining homeostasis of the immune response and prevention of excessive immune reactivity.

A difference in control of life span is observed between peripheral blood CLA$^+$ T cells and T cells infiltrating the eczema lesions. In peripheral blood of AD patients both CD4$^+$ and CD8$^+$ subsets of CLA$^+$ CD45RO$^+$ T cells express upregulated Fas and Fas ligand and undergo AICD. CLA$^-$ CD45RO$^+$ T cells are in a resting state, do not express Fas and Fas ligand and are resistant to anti-Fas mAb induced apoptosis [30]. In contrast, T cells infiltrating the skin of AD patients express both Fas and Fas ligand; however, they do not show any signs of apoptosis.

Inflammatory cells reside in a protein network in the tissues, the extracellular matrix (ECM), which exerts a profound control over them. The effects of ECM are primarily mediated by integrins, a family of cell surface receptors that attach cells to the matrix and mediate mechanical and chemical signals from it. Cell adhesion to the extracellular matrix has been implicated in protection from apoptosis in anchorage-dependent cell types [31]. Apparently, integrin signaling by ECM represents an important survival signal in T cells, although they do not require anchorage in the tissues. Apoptosis of CLA⁺ CD45RO⁺ T cells is inhibited by fibronectin, tenascin, laminin and collagen IV as Collagen IV as ECM proteins and transferrin demonstrating a multifactorial survival of skin infiltrating T cells in the tissue [30]. In addition to ECM proteins, IL-2, IL-4 and IL-15 also prevent T cell apoptosis [30]. The common γ-chain is an essential signaling component shared by IL-2, IL-4 and IL-15 receptors as well as all other known T cell growth factor receptors. Interleukin-15 shares many biological activities with IL-2 and signals through the IL-2 receptor beta and gamma chains [32]. Blocking the common γ-chain in mice inhibits T cell proliferation and induces T cell apoptosis that induces stable allograft survival [33].

Together, these results demonstrate the control of in vivo activated skin-homing T cell numbers in peripheral blood with increased apoptosis, in contrast, T cell apoptosis is prevented by cytokines and extracellular matrix components in the eczematous skin.

T Cell-Mediated Keratinocyte Apoptosis as an Essential Pathogenic Event in Eczema Formation

The histological hallmark of eczematous disorders is characterized by marked keratinocyte pathology. Spongiosis in the epidermis is identified by impairment or loss of cohesion between KC and the influx of fluid from dermis, sometimes progressing to vesicle formation. A recent study by Trautmann et al. delineated activated skin-infiltrating T cell-induced epidermal keratinocyte apoptosis as a key pathogenic event in eczematous disorders [34,35]. IFN-γ released from activated T cells upregulates Fas (CD95) on keratinocytes, which renders them susceptible to apoptosis. When the Fas number on keratinocytes reaches a threshold of approximately 40,000 Fas molecules per keratinocyte, the cells become susceptible to apoptosis. Keratinocytes exhibit a relatively low threshold for IFN-γ-induced Fas expression (0.1–1 ng/ml). This requirement is substantially achieved by low IFN-γ secreting T cells that also produce high amounts of IL-5 and IL-13 and thereby contribute to eosinophilia and IgE production [34]. The lethal hit is delivered to keratinocytes by Fas ligand expressed on the surface of T cells and soluble Fas ligand released from T cells. In these studies, the involvement of cytokines other than IFN-γ was eliminated by experiments with different cytokines and anti-cytokine neutralizing antibodies. In addition, apoptosis pathways other than the Fas-pathway were ruled out by blocking T cell-induced keratinocyte apoptosis with caspase inhibitors and soluble Fas-Fc protein. Keratinocyte apoptosis was demonstrated in situ in lesional eczematous skin and patch test lesions of both AD and allergic contact dermatitis. Exposure of normal human skin and cultured skin equivalents to activated T cells demonstrated that keratinocyte apoptosis caused by skin infiltrating T cells represent a key event in the pathogenesis of eczematous dermatitis [34].

Although allergic contact dermatitis and drug-induced skin rashes are not related to AD, the mechanism of epidermal injury should be mentioned because of histopathological similarities. Traidl et al. demonstrated that keratinocytes could be the target of multiple hapten-specific cytotoxic T cell responses, which play a role in epidermal injury during allergic contact dermatitis [36]. They found that both nickel-reactive CD4[+] and CD8[+] T cells were exclusively cytotoxic against resting keratinocytes and IFN-γ treatment rendered keratinocytes susceptible to Th1 cytotoxicity [36]. T cell mediated cytotoxicity against keratinocytes has also been studied in sulfamethoxazol-induced skin reactions [37]. Sulfamethoxazol-specific both CD4[+] and CD8[+] T cells expressed high perforin and again IFN-γ-pretreated-keratinocytes were predominantly killed by CD4[+] T cells [37].

These studies demonstrate that both CD4[+] and CD8[+] T cells may play a role in keratinocyte injury according to their activation status. A direct contact of T cell to keratinocyte is not always required and soluble Fas ligand released from activated T cells can also induce keratinocyte apoptosis. IFN-γ appears to be a decisive cytokine to render keratinocytes susceptible to apoptosis [34, 36, 37]. Recent mice studies also provide evidence for the role of IFN-γ in eczema formation. IFN-γ knockout mice show significantly decreased allergic eczema formation [38] and transgenic mice expressing IFN-γ in the epidermis spontaneously developed eczema [39].

Conclusion

Activation and skin-selective homing of peripheral-blood T cells, and effector functions in the skin represent sequential immunological events in the pathogenesis of AD (Fig. 1). The CLA molecule represents a homing receptor involved in selective migration of memory/effector T cells to the skin. CLA is expressed on Th1 cells during the differentiation process and can be induced on Th2 cells by stimulation with bacterial superantigen and/or IL-12. Both CD4[+] and CD8[+] T cells bearing CLA represent activated memory/effector T cell subsets in peripheral blood of AD patients. They induce IgE mainly by IL-13 and prolong eosinophil life span mainly by IL-5. Dysregulated apoptosis in skin-infiltrating T cells and epidermal keratinocytes contributes to the elicitation and progress of AD. Activation-induced T cell apoptosis plays a role in the control of circulating skin-homing memory/effector T cell numbers in peripheral blood. In contrast, T cell apoptosis is prevented by cytokines and extracellular matrix components in the eczematous skin to form dermal T cell infiltrates and mediate effector functions. These activated T cells induce keratinocyte apoptosis via the Fas dependent pathway representing a key pathogenetic factor in the formation of eczematous lesions. In this context, future studies for treatment of AD should be directed to T cells by inhibition of various modes of activation, inhibition of skin-homing and inhibition of certain cytokines/chemokines that play a role in the pathogenesis.

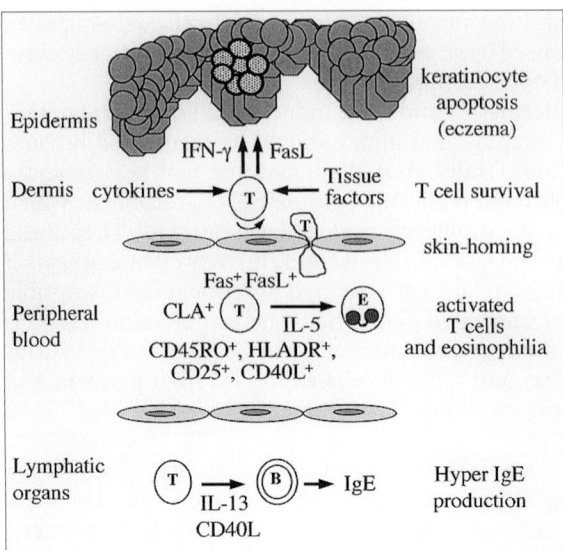

Fig. 1. Immune effector mechanisms in AD. In the peripheral blood of AD patients, both CD4$^+$ and CD8$^+$ subsets of CLA$^+$ CD45RO$^+$ T cells are in an activated state (CD25$^+$, CD40L$^+$, HLADR$^+$). They express Fas and Fas ligand (*FasL*) and undergo activation-induced apoptosis. In contrast, T cells infiltrating the skin of AD patients – despite expressing both Fas and FasL – do not show any apoptosis, because they are protected from apoptosis by cytokines and ECM proteins. These T cells secrete IFN-γ, which upregulates Fas on keratinocytes and renders them susceptible to apoptosis. Keratinocyte apoptosis is induced by FasL expressed on the surface of activated T cells or released to microenvironment. Both CD4$^+$ and CD8$^+$ T cells isolated from skin or CLA$^+$ CD45RO$^+$ T cells from peripheral blood secrete high levels of IL-5 and IL-13 and therefore are capable of prolonging eosinophil (*E*) life span and inducing IgE production by B cells

The knowledge of the molecular basis of dysregulated apoptosis is pivotal in understanding the pathology in AD and may lead to more focused therapeutic applications in the future.

Acknowledgements. The work of the authors is supported by the Swiss National Foundation (31.50590.97). Axel Trautmann is a recipient of a fellowship by the Deutsche Forschungsgemeinschaft (TR460/1.1).

References

1. CA Akdis, M Akdis, A Trautmann, K Blaser. Immune regulation in atopic dermatitis. Current Opin Immunol 12:641–646, 2000.
2. LF Santamaria Babi, LJ Picker, MT Perez Soler, K Drzimalla, P Flohr, K Blaser, C Hauser. Circulating allergen-reactive T cells from patients with atopic dermatitis and allergic contact dermatitis express the skin-selective homing receptor, the cutaneous lymphocyte-associated antigen. J Exp Med 181:1935–1940, 1995.
3. M Akdis, CA Akdis, L Weigl, R Disch, K Blaser. Skin-homing, CLA$^+$ memory T cells are activated in atopic dermatitis and regulate IgE by an IL-13-dominated cytokine pattern. IgG4 counter-regulation by CLA$^-$ memory T cells. J Immunol 159:4611–4619, 1997.
4. Y Shimada, S Sato, M Hasegawa, TF Tedder, K Takehara. Elevated serum L-selectin levels and abnormal regulation of L-selectin expression on leukocytes in atopic dermatitis: soluble L-selectin levels indicate disease severity. J Allergy Clin Immunol 104:163–168, 1999.
5. VA Varney, QA Hamid, M Gaga, S Ying, M Jacobson, AJ Frew, AB Kay, SR Durham. Influence of grass pollen immunotherapy on cellular infiltration and cytokine mRNA expression during allergen-induced late-phase cutaneous responses. J Clin Invest 92:644–651, 1993.

6. T Werfel, A Morita, M Grewe, H Renz, U Wahn, J Krutmann, A Kapp. Allergen-specificity of skin-infiltrating T-cells is not restricted to a type 2 cytokine pattern in chronic skin lesions of atopic dermatitis. J Invest Dermatol 107:871–876, 1996.

7. KJ Abernathy-Carver, HA Sampson, LJ Picker, DYM Leung. Milk-induced eczema is associated with the expansion of T cells expressing cutaneous lymphocyte antigen. J Clin Invest 95:913–918, 1995.

8. M Akdis, H-U Simon, L Weigl, O Kreyden, K Blaser, CA Akdis. Skin homing (Cutaneous Lymphocyte-Associated Antigen-positive) CD8$^+$ T cells respond to superantigen and contribute to eosinophilia and IgE production in atopic dermatitis. J Immunol 163:466–475, 1999.

9. CA Akdis, M Akdis, D Simon, B Dibbert, M Weber, S Gratzl, O Kreyden, R Disch, B Wüthrich, K Blaser, H-U Simon. T cells and T cell-derived cytokines as pathogenic factors in the non-allergic form of atopic dermatitis. J Invest Dermatol 113:628–634, 1999.

10. MC Chou, SC Lee, YS Lin, HY Lei. V b 8$^+$ CD4$^-$ CD8$^-$ subpopulation induced by staphylococcal enterotoxin B. Immunol Let 55:85–91, 1997.

11. JE Leyden, RR Marpies, AM Kligman. Staphylococcus aureus in the lesions of atopic dermatitis. Br J Dermatol 90:525–530, 1974.

12. P Strange, L Skov, S Lisby, PL Nielsen, O Baadsgaard. Staphylococcal enterotoxin B applied on intact normal and intact atopic skin induces dermatitis. Arch Dermatol 132:27–33, 1996.

13. U Herz, N Schnoy, S Borelli, L Weigl, U Käsbohrer, A Daser, U Wahn, R Köttgen, H Renz. A hu-SCID mouse model for allergic immune responses: Bacterial superantigen enhances skin inflammation and supresses IgE production. J Invest Dermatol 110:224–231, 1998.

14. DYM Leung, R Harbeck, P Bina, JM Hanifin, RF Reiser, HA Sampson. Presence of IgE antibodies to staphylococcal exotoxins in the skin of patients with atopic dermatitis: evidence for a new group of allergens. J Clin Invest 92:1374–1380, 1993.

15. M Akdis, S Klunker, M Schliz, K Blaser, CA Akdis. Expression of cutaneous lymphocyte-associated antigen on human CD4$^+$ and CD8$^+$ Th2 cells. Eur J Immunol 30:3533–3541, 2000.

16. DYM Leung, RS Cotran, JS Pober. Expression of an endothelial leukocyte adhesion molecule (ELAM-1) in elicited late phase allergic skin reactions. J Clin Invest 87:1805–1810, 1991.

17. DYM Leung. Atopic dermatitis: new insights and opportunities for therapeutic intervention. J Allergy Clin Immunol 105:860–876, 2000.

18. Q Hamid, M Boguniewicz, DYM Leung. Differential in situ cytokine gene expression in acute versus chronic atopic dermatitis. J Clin Invest 94:870–876, 1994.

19. M Grewe, CAFM Bruijnzeel-Koomen, E Schöpf, T Thepen, AG Langeveld-Wildschut, T Ruzicka, J Krutmann. A role for Th1 and Th2 cells in the immunopathogenesis of atopic dermatitis. Immunol Today 19:359–361, 1998.

20. T Thepen, EG Langeveld-Wildschut, IC Bihari, DF van Wichen, FC Van Reijsen, GC Mudde, CAFM Bruijnzeel-Koomen. Biphasic response against aeroallergen in atopic dermatitis showing a switch from an initial Th2 response to a Th1 response in situ: An immunochemical study. J Allergy Clin Immunol 97:828–837, 1996.

21. M Grewe, W Czech, A Morita, T Werfel, M Klammer, A Kapp, T Ruzicka, E Schöpf, J Krutmann. Human eosinophils produce biologically active IL-12: implications for control of T cell responses. J Immunol 161:415–420, 1998.

22. K Kang, M Kubin, KD Cooper, SR Lessin, G Trinchieri, AH Rook. IL-12 synthesis by human Langerhans cells. J Immunol 156:1402–1407, 1996.

23. G Müller, J Saloga, T Germann, I Bellinghausen, M Mohamadzadeh, J Knop, AH Enk. Identification and induction of human keratinocyte-derived IL-12. J Clin Invest 94:1799–1805, 1994.

24. S Stoll, H Jonuleit, E Schmitt, G Müller, H Yamauchi, M Kurimoto, J Knop, AH Enk. Production of functional IL-18 by different subtypes of murine and human dendritic cells (DC): DC-derived IL-18 enhances IL-12-dependent Th1 development. Eur J Immunol 28:3231–3239, 1998.

25. JM Hanifin, G Rajka. Diagnostic features of atopic dermatitis. Acta Derm Venerol 92:44–47, 1980.

26. B Wüthrich. Serum IgE in atopic dermatitis. Clin Allergy 8:241–248, 1978.

27. M Akdis, A Trautmann, S Klunker, H-U Simon, D Simon, R Disch, K Blaser, CA Akdis. Regulation of allergic inflammation by T cells and cytokines in atopic dermatitis. Int Arch Allergy Immunol 124:296–298, 2001.

28. H-U Simon, K Blaser. Inhibition of programmed eosinophil death: A key pathogenic event for eosinophilia. Immunol Today 16:53–55, 1995.

29. DR Green, DW Scott. Activation-induced apoptosis in lymphocytes. Curr Opin Immunol 6:476–487, 1994.

30. M Akdis, A Trautmann, K Blaser, CA Akdis. Life span of skin homing T cells in atopic dermatitis: survival in skin, activation induced apoptosis in peripheral blood. J Allergy Clin Immunol 105:167, 2000.

31. EA Clöark, SJ Brugge. Integrins and signal transduction pathways: The road taken. Science 268:233–238, 1995.

32. JG Giri, S Kumaki, M Ahdieh, DJ Friend, A Loomis, K Shanebeck, R Dubose, D Cosman, LS Park, DM Anderson. Identification and cloning of a novel IL-15 binding protein that is structurally related to the a chain of the IL-2 receptor. EMBO J 14:3654–3663, 1995.

33. WC Li, A Ima, Y Li, XX Zheng, TR Malek, TB Strom. Blocking the common g-chain of cytokine receptors induces T cell apoptosis and long term islet allograft survival. J Immunol 164:1193–1199, 2000.

34. A Trautmann, M Akdis, D Kleeman, F Altznauer, H-U Simon, T Graeve, M Noll, K Blaser, CA Akdis. T cell-mediated Fas-induced keratinocyte apoptosis plays a key pathogenetic role in eczematous dermatitis. J Clin Invest 106:25–35, 2000.

35. A Trautmann, M Akdis, K Blaser, CA Akdis. Role of dysregulated apoptosis in atopic dermatitis. Apoptosis 5:425–429, 2001.

36. C Traidl, S Sebastiani, C Albanesi, HF Merk, P Puddu, G Girolomoni, A Cavani. Disparate cytotoxic activity of nickel-specific CD8+ and CD4+ T cell subsets against keratinocytes. J Immunol 165:3058–3064, 2000.

37. B Schnyder, K Frutig, D Mauri-Hellweg, A Limat, N Yawalkar, WJ Pichler. T-cell mediated cytotoxicity against keratinocytes in sulfamethoxazol-induced skin reactions. Clin Exp Allergy 28:1412–1417, 1998.

38. JM Spergel, E Mizoguchi, H Oettgen, AK Bhan, RS Geha. Roles of Th1 and Th2 cytokines in a murine model of allergic dermatitis. J Clin Invest 103:1103–1111, 1999.

39. JM Carroll, T Crompton, JP Seery, FM Watt. Transgenic mice expressing IFN-g in the epidermis have eczema, hair hypopigmentation and hair loss. J Invest Dermatol 108:412–422, 1997.

17 Material-Odor Analysis as a Prerequisite for the Allergological Evaluation of Outgassing Odoractive Volatile Compounds

K. Breuer, F. Mayer, E. Mayer

Abstract

The evaluation of material odors is an important device of product optimization and consumer information. As a prerequisite for it, by means of gas chromatography-olfactometry of headspace samples (GCOH), using the human nose as an odor sensitive detector at the end of the capillary of a gas chromatograph, the odoractive volatiles emitted by certain materials were analyzed. By reducing the analyzed headspace volume step by step, finally only the most odoractive compounds emitted by the material are perceived. Subsequently, these odorants are identified by comparing their smell, their retention indices on two gas chromatography capillaries of different polarity and, when available, their mass spectra with authentic reference compounds. With this method the volatiles mainly causing the odor of a waxed and oiled parquet floor, of a varnished parquet floor and of a polymerous insulation material were identified.

Introduction

Indoor-air odors and odoractive substances are present in almost every room. If certain perceptions of odors cannot be clearly attributed to common activities usually performed in (living) rooms, such as cleaning or preparing food, but are emanating from various materials like building products, indoor materials or domestic appliances, odors may often cause fears concerning disturbances of health due to emissions from materials, or they have to serve as an alleged reason for feelings of ill-health. Possible interrelations between odor perceptions, annoyance or nuisance caused by odors, individual associations and other phenomena (such as the Sick Building Syndrome or Multiple Chemical Sensitivity, for instance) are being discussed [1]. Recently, this situation has induced both researchers and industrial manufacturers to join their efforts with the aim of examining and evaluating materials regarding their odor properties [2–4]. Two important objectives were given priority in doing so, namely to develop reproducible methods to evaluate material odors in order to be able to identify products that are „peculiar" in terms of odor [5] and, secondly, to improve the quality of products by reducing their TVOC (Total Volatile Organic Compounds) emissions (e.g. solvents) during their useful life.

Quite often, there is no direct correlation between the emission properties of odoractive substances and the TVOC emission [6]. This means that a TVOC reduction will not necessarily lead to improve a material's odor quality. So far, it

New Trends in Allergy V
J. Ring, H. Behrendt (Eds.)
© Springer-Verlag Berlin, Heidelberg 2002

can be stated that material odors still are a more or less random side effect occurring in the industrial manufacturing process of building products, interior decoration materials or domestic appliances, and that the reasons for this are to be found presumably in formulation ingredients or the production process itself.

Up to now, statements on material-inherent causes, i.e. concerning the chemical nature of the odoractive substances characterizing a specific material's odor, were possible to a very limited extent only. It is, however, precisely the knowledge of these odoractive substances as a prerequisite for the allergological evaluation and thus for improving both product and consumer information.

Gas chromatography-olfactometry (GC-O) [7] is a method that allows the differentiation of odoractive compounds from odorless substances within a complex mixture of volatiles. It has been successfully applied for several years now to investigate aroma compounds of foods [8]. For this purpose, the whole mixture of volatile compounds either in a purified organic solvent extract or in a defined headspace volume is separated into its different components by means of gas chromatography, the effluent gas flow at the end of the gas chromatography capillary column then being split between a flame ionization detector and a test person's nose. By sniffing the column effluent, using the human nose as a sensitive detector, it is possible to perceive odoractive substances contained in a complex mixture and to mark the corresponding spot in the flame-ionization detector chromatogram. Further, a stepwise dilution of the investigated mixture of volatile compounds allows to identify the odorants that are mostly contributing to the sample odor [9–11], namely those odorants still to be detected at maximum dilution. The evaluation of the most important odorous substances in materials by means of gas chromatography-olfactometry is explained using three different building products as examples.

Materials and Methods

Parquet floors from beech (2×2 slabs, 123×54×1.3 cm³ each) put together back to back and the edges sealed with solvent free aluminum foil were packed in an aroma sealing non-airtight foil (124×55×6 cm³). The surface of the parquet was either sealed with wax and oil or with varnish. A polymerous insulation material (butadiene-styrene-rubber), 50×200×2 cm³, freshly produced was stored in contact with air for 6 h. Afterwards a piece of the material (50×20×2 cm³) was cut in small pieces (5×1×2 cm³) and put in a glass vessel (2 l) sealed with a septum and a carbon filter for air pressure equalization. The rest of the material was stored in an aroma sealing foil. The chemicals referred to in the Tables 1 and 2 and in the text were obtained commercially, apart from 1-octene-one, which was a gift from the Deutsche Forschungsanstalt für Lebensmittelchemie (German Research Institute for Food Chemistry). Gas chromatography-olfactometry of headspace samples was performed on a gas chromatograph with a carbon dioxide oven cooling system and a purge-and-trap injection system. The empty glass liner in the desorption unit of the purge-and-trap system was deactivated by treatment with a mixture of 1,3-diphenyltetramethyldisilazan/hexamethyldisilazan/pentane (1/

1/2, v/v/v) [12]. The capillaries used for gas chromatography were a HP-5 (50 m×0.32 mm, film thickness 1.05 μm) and a DB-1701 (30 m×0.32 mm, film thickness 1 μm). At the end of the capillary the effluent was split 1:6 between a flame ionization detector and a sniffing port using deactivated fused silica capillaries (40 cm×0.18 mm and 70 cm×0.32 mm, respectively). The flame ionization detector and the sniffing port were held at a temperature of 300°C. The flow of the carrier gas helium was 2.5 ml/min, the split gas helium had a flow of 1.6 ml/min, the auxiliary gas of the flame ionization detector was also helium with a flow of 30 ml/min. For sample collection defined volumes of the headspace were either collected on a Tenax-trap (16×0.4 cm) with a flow of 100 ml/min (400–100 ml) and the trap installed into the desorption heating block of the purge-and-trap system or small volumes of the headspace (3–50 ml) were drawn by a gas-tight syringe and injected into the purge-and-trap system with a velocity of 10 ml/min. The volatiles in the sample were desorbed by heating the desorption block up to 250°C for 10 min. During this time the carrier gas helium (20 ml/min) flushed the sample into a trap-capillary (20 cm×0.53 mm, coated with CP-Sil 8, film thickness 5 μm) cooled with liquid nitrogen down to −100°C, where the volatiles were cryofocussed. For injection the cooling trap was rapidly heated up to 250°C, the temperature held for 1 min and the sample flushed by the carrier gas helium onto the gas chromatography capillary. The initial temperature of the oven of 20°C was held for 5 min, then raised by 6°C/min to 250°C and finally held for 10 min. The retention indices of the odorants were determined by co-chromatography with a solution of *n*-alkanes (hexane to hexadecane, 0.05%) in pentane. The retention index of each alkane results by multiplication of the number of carbon atoms by 100 and the retention index of a compound by linear interpolation according to van den Dool and Kratz [13]. Gas chromatography-mass spectrometry of headspace samples was performed on a gas chromatograph with a carbon dioxide oven cooling system and a mass selective detector. As gas chromatography capillary a HP-5 (50 m×0.32 mm, film thickness 1.05 μm) was used. The headspace sample (100–500 ml) was drawn on a Tenax trap (9×0.6 cm) with a velocity of 100 ml/min and the trap installed into an automatic desorption sys-

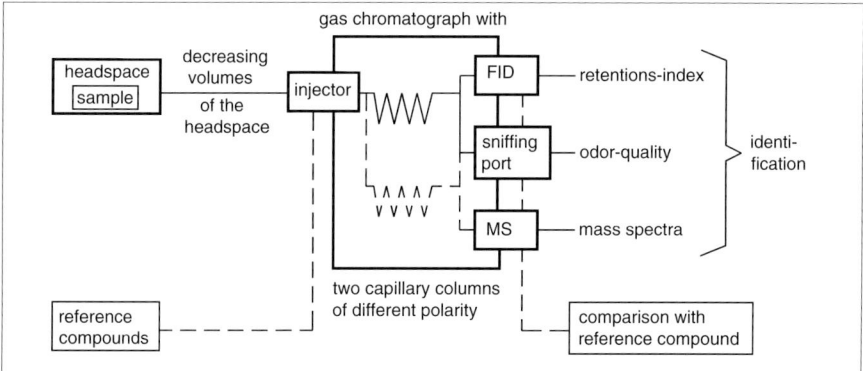

Fig. 1. Principle of the combination of gas chromatography–olfactometry and gas chromatography–mass spectrometry

tem. The sample was desorbed from the trap by heating it up to 360°C in a stream of helium (33 ml/min) for 10 min. The volatiles were cryofocussed in a cold trap, piezo-electrically cooled down to 5°C. For injection the trap was heated up to 350°C for 3 min and the volatiles were flushed in a stream of helium onto the gas chromatography column. The temperature program was the same as for gas chromatography-olfactometry. Mass spectra were generated at 70 eV by electrical ionization.

Figure 1 shows the principle of gas chromatography-olfactometry in combination with gas chromatography-mass spectrometry.

Results and Discussion

The odorants emitted by building materials were analyzed by gas chromatography-olfactometry of headspace samples (GCOH) using the human nose at the end of a gas chromatography capillary as a sensitive detector for odoractive compounds. By reducing the analyzed headspace volume step by step always less odorants were perceived until in the smallest volume only the most important odoractive compounds can be detected. The results were verified by repeating this procedure on another gas chromatography column of different polarity. The substances causing the odors were finally identified by comparing the perceived smell at the end of the gas chromatography capillaries and their retention indices on the two different capillaries with authentic reference compounds. By analyzing the samples also by gas chromatography-mass spectrometry the identification of the odorants was confirmed by mass spectra data, although sometimes the concentration of an odorant was high enough for the detection by the sensitive human nose but not high enough for obtaining a clear mass spectra.

With this method the important odorants of two different types of parquet floor either sealed with wax and oil or with varnish and a polymerous synthetic butadiene-styrene-rubber were determined.

The volatile compounds that are mostly responsible for the odor of a waxed and oiled parquet floor, perceptible in a headspace volume of 10 ml, are pentanal, hexanal, α-pinene, β-pinene, 1-octene-3-one, octanal, Z-2-nonenal and E-2-nonenal (Table 1). Of those β-pinene and octanal could still be detected in a headspace volume of 3 ml. Some of the odorants completing the overall odor are acetaldehyde, methylpropanal, 3-methylbutanal, heptanal, 1-nonene-3-one and nonanal which were additionally smelled in a volume of 30 ml.

In contrast, the most important odorants of a varnished parquet floor are pentanal, hexanal, α-pinene, β-pinene, 1-octene-3-one and benzaldehyde (Table 1). These compounds were perceptible in a headspace volume of 30 ml. The odor is completed among others by acetophenone, 3-methylbutanal, butanal and acetaldehyde, which were additionally detected in a headspace volume of 100 ml. The number of odorants found in the same sample volume was smaller in the headspace of the varnished parquet floor than in the waxed and oiled parquet floor. A comparable number of odorants was perceived in the headspace of 30 ml of the varnished and in 10 ml of the waxed and oiled parquet, indicating that the concentration of odorants in the headspace above the waxed and oiled parquet

Table 1. Most important odorants of parquet floors sealed with wax and oil or with varnish

Odor quality	Retention index		Smallest headspace volume of a parquet floor for detection (ml)		Compound
	HP-5	DB-1701	Waxed/oiled	Varnished	
Fruity	<600	<600	30	100	Acetaldehyde[a]
Malty	<600	640	30	>300	Methylpropanal[a)]
Sweet	<600	680	100	100	Butanal[a]
Malty	653	741	30	100	3-Methylbutanal[a]
Green	700	784	10	30	Pentanal[a]
Green	800	889	10	30	Hexanal[a]
Citrus-like	899	995	30	>300	Heptanal[a]
Terpeny	950	953	10	30	α-Pinene[a,b]
Marzipan-like	967	1,104	>300	30	Benzaldehyde[a]
Mushroom-like	980	1,074	10	30	1-Octene-3-one[c]
Terpeny/wooden	998	1,009	3	30	β-Pinene[a,b]
Citrus-like	1,005	10,97	3	>300	Octanal[a]
Pungent	1,077	1,193	>300	100	Acetophenone[a]
Mushroom-like	1,080	1,175	30	>300	1-Nonene-3-one[c]
Citrus-like	1,107	1,202	30	>300	Nonanal[a]
Fatty	1,148	1,253	10	>300	Z-2-nonenal[c]
Fatty	1,162	1,274	10	>300	E-2-nonenal[c]

[a] The compound was identified in accordance with the reference compound because of its odor, its retention indices on the two capillaries of different polarity and because of its mass spectra.
[b] Distribution of the enantiomeres not investigated.
[c] The compound was identified in accordance with the reference compound because of its odor and its retention indices on the two capillaries of different polarity.

floor is higher than above the varnished parquet floor. The varnish prevents the release of the odorants from the wooden parts of the parquet more than wax and oil. Consequently the overall odor of the varnished parquet is less intense than of the waxed and oiled parquet. Apart from the difference in the odor intensity also their odor quality is different. Both types of parquet floor contain short chained green smelling aldehydes and wooden smelling terpenes, but in the waxed and oiled parquet the long chained citrus-like smelling aldehydes and some fatty smelling compounds, presumably resulting from the sealing, contribute to the odor, while in the varnished parquet, benzaldehyde and acetophenone, originating from the varnish, were important odorants and higher aldehydes and fatty compounds were missing (Table 1).

As third product a polymerous synthetic insulation material, a butadiene-styrene-rubber, was analyzed. The first impression of the odor of this freshly produced material was sulfurous-rotten, caused by dimethyl sulfide and related compounds. First of all it was stored in the presence of air for 6 h to loose parts of the disgusting smelling high volatile compounds, which had nothing to do with the well known usual odor of the product. Then it was subject to analysis. The most important odorants of the polymerous rubber, perceptible in a headspace volume of 25 ml, are dimethyl disulfide, ethyl methylpropanoat, ethyl 2-methylbutanoat, 4-vinyl cyclohexene, m- and p-cresol (Table 2).

Table 2. Most important odorants of a polymerous butadiene-styrene rubber, perceived in a headspace volume of 25 ml

Odor quality	Retention index		Compound
	HP-5	DB-1701	
Cabbage-like	740	794	Dimethyl disulfide[a]
Fruity	755	816	Ethyl methylpropanoate[b]
Rubber-like	840	862	4-Vinyl cyclohexene[b]
Fruity	850	907	Ethyl 2-methylbutanoate[b]
Fruity/currant-like	900	969	Unknown
Rubber-like	1,083	1,301	p-Cresol
Rubber-like	1,090	1,304	m-Cresol

[a] The compound was identified in accordance with the reference compound because of its odor and its retention indices on the two capillaries of different polarity.
[b] The compound was identified in accordance with the reference compound because of its odor, its retention indices on the two capillaries of different polarity and because of its mass spectra.

Additionally one fruity, currant-like smelling compound has been detected, but could not be identified so far. The odor of this compound and the retention indices on two gas chromatography capillaries of different polarity supplied not enough information for identification and besides, no mass spectra for the unknown substance could be obtained. One approach to isolate higher amounts of unknown odorants for identification would be solvent extraction of the material.

Conclusion

The present method which was developed in order to identify odors emitted from building products provides an instrument to characterize the random side effect of „material odors" with respect to the substances involved. Precise knowledge of the relevant odoractive substances is the basis for any causality research. Consequently, it will become possible to attribute specified odoractive substances (and thus specific problematic odors) to certain ingredients or processing steps, respectively.

As material odors are probably inevitable in some cases, the present method might also open up new ways of consumer information. For instance, it is conceivable that concentrations of odoractive substances which are the cause of definite material odors (e.g. trace concentrations of odoractive substances being perceived by the sensitive detector human nose) will also be evaluated with regard to aspects of allergy.

Acknowledgements. This research project was supported by the Gips-Schüle-Foundation, Stuttgart (Germany).

References

1. Fanger, P. O. 1987. A Solution to the Sick Building Mystery. Proceedings of the 4th International Conference on Indoor Air Quality and Climate in Berlin, Vol. 4, pp 49–55.
2. Breuer, K., Mayer, E.1998. Kann man die Gesundheitsverträglichkeit von Bauprodukten ermitteln ? Bauphysik 20, Vol. 6, pp 226–232.
3. Breuer, K., Mayer, E.1999. Bewertung der Gesundheitsverträglichkeit von Bauprodukten auf der Basis von Prüfkammerexperimenten. Tagungsband Reihe T/2, Gemeinschaftstagung DIBt/IBP, Berlin, 17.11.1999.
4. Schwab, R., Mair, S., Mayer, E. 1998. Geruchsbewertung von Baustoffen und Büroräumen. VDI-Berichte 1373 Kommission Reinhaltung der Luft im VDI und DIN „Gerüche in der Umwelt" Innenraum- und Außenluft, pp 145–153.
5. Fraunhofer-Institut für Bauphysik. 1999. Verbundvorhaben „Gesundheits- und umweltverträgliche Bauprodukte (GUB)", 3. Sachstandsbericht RKB-1/1999.
6. Mayer, F., Breuer, K. 2000. Geruchsstoffe von Bauprodukten in Innenräumen – Gaschromatographisch-olfaktometrische Untersuchung des Materialgeruchs eines Parkettboden. Bauphysik 22, Vol. 2, pp 96–100.
7. Fuller, G. H., Steltenkamp, R., Tisserand, G. A. 1964. The gas chromatograph with human sensor. Ann. NY Acad. Sci., Vol. 116, pp 711–724.
8. Grosch, W. 1993. Detection of potent odorants in food by aroma extract dilution analysis. Trends in Food Science and Technology, Vol. 4, pp 68–73.
9. Ullrich, F., Grosch, W. 1987. Identification of the most intense volatile flavour compounds formed during autoxidation of linoleic acid. Z. Lebensm. Unters. Forsch., Vol. 184, pp 277–282
10. Holscher, W., Steinhart, H. 1992. Investigation of roasted coffee freshness with an improved headspace technique. Z. Lebensm. Unters. Forsch., Vol. 195, pp 33–.
11. Acree, T. E., Barnard, J., Cunningham, D. G. 1984. A procedure for the sensory analysis of gas chromatographic effluents. Food Chem., Vol. 14, pp 273–286.
12. Guth, H., Stein, J.1994,1999. Deutsche Forschungsanstalt für Lebensmittelchemie (German Research Institute for Food Chemistry), personal communication
13. van den Dool, H., Kratz, P. D. 1963. A generalization of the retention index system including linear temperature programmed gas-liquid partition chromatography. J. Chromatog., Vol. 11, pp 463–.

18 The Atopy Patch Test: Use and Perspectives

U. Darsow, J. Ring

Summary

Among the trigger factors of atopic eczema (AE), aeroallergens like house dust mite, animal dander or pollen are often clinically important. The atopy patch test (APT) is an epicutaneous patch test with allergens known to elicit IgE-mediated reactions, and the evaluation of eczematous skin lesions. It can be used for the diagnosis in atopic eczema patients with suspected allergy to aeroallergens. With regard to clinical history, the atopy patch test gave more specific results than skin prick test or radioallergosorbent test.

Introduction

Atopic eczema (AE, atopic dermatitis) is a clinically defined inflammatory, chronically relapsing skin disease with a prevalence of 2–5% (in children and young adults about 10%) [22, 23, 29]. AE is a multifactorial disease with a large number of individually different trigger factors [33, 37, 55, 60]. Different names like „prurigo Besnier", „neurodermatitis", „endogenous eczema", „neurodermitis constitutionalis siva atopica" are influenced by different concepts of pathophysiology of AE. Atopy is a very common finding in patients with AE and their families [25, 29, 38]. Atopy is defined as familial tendency towards the development of certain diseases (extrinsic bronchial asthma, allergic rhinoconjunctivitis, and/or atopic eczema) based on a hypersensitivity of skin and mucous membranes against environmental substances. This is associated with elevated IgE-production and/or altered unspecific reactivity [46, 47]. The clinical definition of AE also includes a typically age-related distribution and morphology [22, 25, 67].

High IgE production in patients with AE is explained by an impaired balance of the CD4-positive T helper cell populations TH1 and TH2 with a predominance of Interleukin-4 and Interleukin-13 producing TH2-cells [21, 28, 35, 42, 56]. The inflammatory infiltrate of AE lesions consists to a large proportion of TH cells. Interleukin-4 induces IgE production [42, 63]. Some patients with AE report exacerbations of their skin lesions after contact with certain immediate-type (IgE-inducing) allergens like house dust mite, pollen or animal dander. Appropriate avoidance strategies, on the other hand, often improve the course of AE [3, 19, 44, 50, 57, 59]. Due to the epidermal barrier function disturbance that was described in AE [51], aeroallergens are obviously able to penetrate the skin barrier and to come in direct contact with antigen-presenting Langerhans cells [30]. The role of IgE in antigen presentation could recently be shown by the group of G. Stingl

New Trends in Allergy V
J. Ring, H. Behrendt (Eds.)
© Springer-Verlag Berlin, Heidelberg 2002

[31]. This mechanism involves IgE and IgE-binding structures on the surface of epidermal Langerhans cells [4, 5, 6, 8].

Diagnosis of Aeroallergen-Triggered Atopic Eczema

From a practical point of view, the identification of an aeroallergen causing an eczema flare in this way is of high importance for the patient. Moreover, the relevant allergen has to be identified for a successful allergen avoidance strategy. A diagnostic tool for aeroallergen-triggered AE is needed. IgE-mediated sensitizations are usually diagnosed by determination of specific serum IgE and skin prick tests or intracutaneous injections of allergen solutions [10, 46]. This reveals mostly multiple sensitizations in AE, but often without clinical relevance. Also, the skin test reactions wheal and flare are neither intended to simulate the clinical picture of eczema nor do they represent the appropriate dimension of the skin immune system. In 1937, Rostenberg und Sulzberger [48] described a total of 12,000 patch tests with a wide variety of allergens, including aeroallergens in different patient groups. However, the first patch test with aeroallergens especially in patients with AE was published 1982 by Mitchell et al. [32]. Other groups also succeeded in eliciting eczematous reactions with different methodological approaches and allergen concentrations [1, 9, 24, 36, 40, 41, 52–54, 65]. Studies on aeroallergen patch testing on untreated, nonabraded skin were an exception [64], whereas stratum corneum abrasion [20, 32, 34] or tape stripping [7, 26, 62] and addition of sodiumlaurylsulfate [58] were used to enhance allergen penetration. The number and definition of positive reactions in these experimental systems varied (15–100%). No clear correlation with history was obtained in larger groups of patients. In 1989, the term „atopy patch test" was proposed with the following definition: an epicutaneous patch test with allergens known to elicit IgE-mediated reactions, and the evaluation of eczematous skin lesions [43, 45]. We investigated methodological aspects and clinical covariates of the APT in order to obtain a method for clinical routine that gives positive results only in patients with AE. The results of the studies that led to an APT technique applicable on unabraded, uninvolved back skin were already reviewed in *New Trends in Allergy IV* [14, 15]. The use of lipophilic petrolatum vehicles, initially not expected to give better results, is now widely accepted for APT and has since been standard in our further investigations.

Allergen Preparations for the APT

All APT studies were performed after discontinuance of antihistamines, systemic and topical (test area) steroids for at least 7 days. The effect of antihistamines on APT is not known to date. We performed APT studies with allergen lyophilisates from house dust mite *Dermatophagoides pteronyssinus*, cat dander and grass pollen. In a lower number of patients, birch and mugwort pollen were also included. The test substances were applied in large Finn chambers (12 mm diameter) on clinically uninvolved, non-abraded and untreated back skin. In control areas, vehicles without allergens were tested. Results were evaluated after 48 and 72 h.

Table 1. Clinical covariates of the APT in a randomized, double-blind multicenter trial; *n*=253 adults and 30 children with atopic eczema (data from [13] and [16])

	Skin prick		slgE		APT		History	
	C	A	C	A	C	A	C	A
D. pteronyssinus	67%	59%	40%	56%	41%	34%	30%	52%
Cat dander	43%	54%	43%	49%	17%	12%	23%	23%
Grass pollen	57%	65%	57%	75%	15%	18%	20%	33%

A, adults 15–63 years, *n*=253, 3000–10000 PNU/g; C, children 5–14 years, *n*=30, 300–5000 PNU/g.

Grading of positive APT reactions was similar to the criteria used in conventional contact allergy patch testing (ICDRG rules, [2, 18]), only clear-cut positive reactions (with infiltration, not only erythematous) were statistically evaluated.

A dose-response double-blind multicenter study involved 253 adult patients and 30 children with atopic eczema ([16]; Table 1). This study investigated the allergen concentration range from 5,000 to 10,000 protein nitrogen units (PNU)/ g (adults). The allergen dose with the most clear-cut results (positive or negative) could be determined for house dust mite, cat dander and grass pollen between 5,000 and 7,000 PNU/g. In children, lower allergen doses seem possible [13]. In another clinical trial comparing different allergen standardization systems, the allergen doses of 7,000 PNU/g and 200 IR/g (biological unit) were intraindividually compared in 50 patients with AE. Both systems showed comparable concordance with the patients clinical history: 71–73% of APT were corroborated by a corresponding positive or negative history of AE flares after contact with the specific allergen (submitted). A typical picture of a positive APT reaction is given in Figure 1.

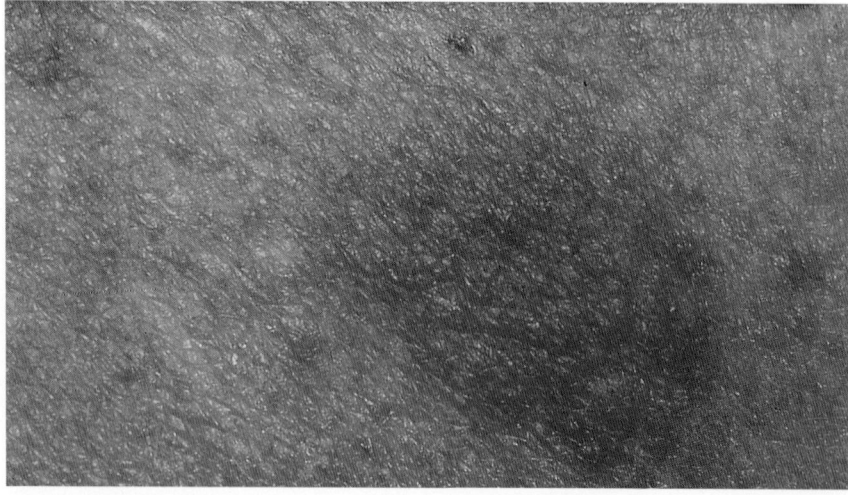

Fig. 1. APT with house dust mite *D. pteronyssinus* in a patient with atopic eczema. Eczematous reaction after 48 h

APT and Specific IgE

The frequency of positive APT was reproducibly lower than the numbers of positive skin prick tests or radioallergosorbent tests to the same allergen. The individually positive APT allergen pattern of the patients varied with their skin prick test and specific IgE results. The percentages of positive reactions in the German multicenter study are shown in Table 1 (calculated with regard to n, which included patients with questionable results and 10 dropouts). Birch pollen (data not shown) elicited positive APT reactions in 11% of patients. Cross-table analysis and logistic regression (Tables 2 and 3) revealed significant concordances of APT results with history, skin prick test, and specific corresponding IgE for *D. pteronyssinus*, cat dander and grass pollen ($p<0.001$). However, the results also showed that high allergen-specific IgE in serum is not mandatory for a positive atopy patch test, same holds true for the correlation with skin prick tests. An example is given in Table 3 (very similar results were obtained for specific IgE). One may conclude that the APT may give further diagnostic information in addition to patient's history and classical tests of IgE-mediated hypersensitivity. On one hand a role for IgE in the reaction mechanism of APT is suggested, since in most APT-positive patients elevated specific IgE was found compared to those with negative APT. On the other hand, a cellular mechanism without direct involvement of IgE may be hypothesized to explain the clear-cut positive APT reactions in a subgroup of AE patients.

Table 2. APT multicenter study: significant predictors of a positive APT in a logistic regression model. The lower three covariates were only significant ($p<0.05$) when the upper three covariates were excluded

Positive reactions are associated with:
   Increased specific serum IgE
   Positive skin prick test reaction
   Allergen-specific corresponding history
   Increased total IgE
   Long eczema duration
   Rhinoconjunctivitis (grass pollen)

Table 3. APT and skin prick test results in a multicenter study (data from [16])

	SP neg+/–	SP pos	Total
APT neg.	61	44	105
APT pos.	13	70	83
Total	74	114	188

SP, skin prick test; 48 h results in adult patients; house dust mite *D. pteronyssinus*. Fisher's exact test $p<0.00001$.

Clinical Relevance of the APT

A „golden standard" for the diagnosis of aeroallergen-induced AE is not available. Like in conventional, classic patch testing for contact allergy, the prospectively obtained history of allergen-induced eczema exacerbation can be used as proof of clinical relevance of an APT result. In the German multicenter study, up to 52% of the 253 adult patients reported previous eczema flares after contact with specific allergen (Table 1). APT results of *D. pteronyssinus*, cat dander and grass pollen were statistically significantly associated with clinical history ($p < 0.001$, Chi^2- and logistic regression; birch pollen $p = 0.1$). The association of clinical history and APT was used to calculate sensitivity and specificity of the classical and new tests in comparison. The APT showed a higher specificity (depending on allergen) with regard to clinical relevance of an allergen as compared to skin prick test and specific IgE, but also in most allergens a lower sensitivity (Table 4).

The association of eczema flares and allergen exposure can be investigated more easily in a seasonal aeroallergen. One third of AE patients report on eczema flares during spring and summer, the pollen seasons of birch and grass (summer eruption) [38]. Also, according to our results, one third of patients with specific IgE to grass pollen develop a positive APT result to this allergen [16]. In a study on the influence of grass pollen on AE, 79 patients were tested with an APT with 10,000 PNU/g grass pollen allergen mixture of 6 species in petrolatum and simultaneously with 10 mg dry unprocessed pollen of *Dactylis glomerata* grass [12]. Again, the APT results were compared with history, skin prick tests, specific corresponding IgE and the clinical eczema pattern of „air-exposed eczema". Indeed, significantly higher frequencies of positive APT were seen in patients with corresponding history of exacerbation of their eczema in the summer months of the previous year and/or in direct contact with grass (12 of 79 patients, 75% had positive APT) compared to patients without this history (67 of 79, 16% had positive APT; $p < 0.001$). Sensitivity and specificity of the different diagnostic methods are shown in Table 4. The standardized allergen mixture also correlated with eczema pattern, skin prick and specific IgE ($p < 0.01$). There was

Table 4. Sensitivity and specificity of different diagnostic methods in two studies with patients with AE. Better results are obtained with a seasonal allergen (data from [12] and [16])

Test	Sensitivity*	Specificity*
Single center study *n*=79, allergen: grass pollen		
Skin prick	100%	33%
RAST	92%	33%
APT	75%	84%
APT multicenter study *n*=253, 3 allergens		
Skin prick	69–82%	44–53%
RAST	65–94%	42–64%
APT	42–56%	69–92%

* Referring to predictive history of eczema exacerbations in pollen season or in direct contact with allergen, excluding questionable cases, depending on allergen.

also a significant concordance of standardized and unprocessed grass pollen APT. The fact that unprocessed pollen elicited eczematous skin reactions on not pretreated skin of atopic eczema patients with significant correlation to history suggests that pollen are involved in eczema flares in some patients. In healthy and rhinoconjunctivitis controls, no positive reactions were observed.

In a subgroup of our patients of the multicenter trial, specific activation of T cells in peripheral blood was compared with the patient's APT result. Also, specific lymphocyte proliferation was investigated in these patients [66]. Positive APT reactions were significantly more frequent in patients with elevated $CD54^+$ or $CD30^+$ T cells after in-vitro stimulation with the corresponding allergen. In addition, positive APT were associated with an allergen-specific lymphocyte proliferation ($p<0.001$). Positive APT reactions were not associated with disease severity in the SCORAD system [17, 66].

From APT biopsies, allergen specific T-cells have been cloned. In serial biopsies, T-cells showed a characteristic TH2 secretion pattern at 24 h, whereas after 48 h a TH1 pattern like in chronic AE lesions was predominant [39, 49, 61]. A similar cytokine pattern is found in natural lesions of atopic eczema characterized also by a predominance of CD-4 positive T cells [28]. Taken together, these findings argue against the interpretation of APT results as irritative or nonspecific.

The Future of the APT

As in bronchial asthma and rhinoconjunctivitis, the results of our studies support B. Wüthrich's concept of extrinsic/allergic versus intrinsic/idiopathic atopic eczema [68]. At least in a subgroup of patients with AE, IgE-dependent allergic reactions which are elicited by the transdermal route play a pathophysiological role. Appropriate allergy diagnosis in these patients is difficult due to the lack of specificity of the classical methods. The described APT methodology was evaluated in a large group of patients with AE. For patients with aeroallergen-triggered disease, the APT may provide an important diagnostic tool, a provocation test of the skin in analogy to the specific provocation methods in respiratory atopy.

Positive APT results in AE patients with negative skin prick tests and RAST were obtained. According to the above mentioned concept, these patients were classified as „intrinsic", however a role for allergens in their disease cannot be excluded. Controlled studies using specific provocation and elimination procedures in patients with positive and negative APT results are still necessary. Standardization of major allergen content is an important goal for the future. However, appropriate allergen specific avoidance strategies [11, 19, 27, 44, 57] are recommended in patients showing positive APT reactions. The diagnostic validity of APT in routine diagnosis of aeroallergen-triggered atopic eczema is investigated in ongoing further studies. We are currently coordinating a European multicenter study with biologically standardized APT extracts of the European Task Force on Atopic Dermatitis (ETFAD). Meetings of most European groups performing APT for clinical use on April 11, 1997, and June 30, 1998 in Munich resulted in a refined consensus APT reading key for describing the intensity of APT reactions, which will be further evaluated. The European multicenter trial also deals with the investigation of food allergen patch testing. Further aeroallergens of regional significance are to be standardized. A test for the clinical relevance of an aeroallergen sensitization that can be applied in the allergist's practice may evolve soon. The identified subgroup of patients may profit extraordinarily from allergen avoidance. More controversially, the APT may also prove valuable in selecting patients for specific immunotherapy.

References

1. Adinoff A, Tellez P, Clark R. Atopic dermatitis and aeroallergen contact sensitivity. J Allergy Clin Immunol 1988; 81: 736–742
2. Andersen KE, Benezra C, Burrows D, Dooms-Goossens A et al. The European environmental and contact dermatitis research group: contact dermatitis a review. Contact Dermatitis 1987;16:55–78
3. Barnetson RSTC, MacFarlane HAF, Benton EC. House dust mite allergy and atopic eczema: a case report. Br J Dermatol 1987;116:857–860
4. Bieber T, de la Salle C, Wollenberg A, Hakimi J, Chizzonite R, Ring J. Constitutive expression of the high affinity receptor for IgE (FCeR1) on human Langerhans-cells. J Exp Med 1992;175:1285–1290
5. Bieber T, Rieger A, Neuchrist C, Prinz JC, Rieber EP, Boltz-Nitulescu G, Scheiner O, Kraft D, Ring J, Stingl G. Induction of FCeR2/CD23 on human epidermal Langerhans-Cells by human recombinant IL4 and IFN. J Exp Med 1989; 170: 309–314
6. Bieber T. FCeRI on human Langerhans cells: a receptor in seach of new functions. Immunol Today 1994; 15: 52–53
7. Bruijnzeel-Koomen C, van Wichen D, Spry C, Venge P, Bruijnzeel P. Active participation of eosinophils in patch test reactions to inhalant allergens in patients with atopic dermatitis. Br J Dermatol 1988;118:229–238
8. Bruijnzeel-Koomen C, van Wichen DF, Toonstra J, Berrens L, Bruijnzeel PLB. The presence of IgE molecules on epidermal Langerhans-cells in patients with atopic dermatitis. Arch Dermatol Res 1986;278:199–205
9. Clark R, Adinoff A. Aeroallergen contact can exacerbate atopic dermatitis: patch test as a diagnostic tool. J Am Acad Dermatol 1989; 21: 863–869
10. Darsow U. Etablierte Diagnostikverfahren. In: Ring J. Neurodermitis. Ecomed, Landsberg, 1998, pp. 61–73
11. Darsow U, Abeck D, Ring J. Allergie und atopisches Ekzem: Zur Bedeutung des „Atopie-Patch-Tests". Hautarzt 1997; 48: 528–535
12. Darsow U, Behrendt H, Ring J. Gramineae pollen as trigger factors of atopic eczema: evaluation of diagnostic measures using the atopy patch test. Br J Dermatol 1997; 137:201–207
13. Darsow U, Vieluf D, Berg B, Berger J, Busse A, Czech W, Heese A, Heidelbach U, Peters KP, Przybilla B, Richter G, Rueff F, Werfel T, Wistokat-Wülfing A, Ring J. Dose response study of atopy patch test in children with atopic eczema. Pediatr Asthma Allergy Immunol 1999; 13: 115–122
14. Darsow U, Vieluf D, Ring J. Atopy patch test with different vehicles and allergen concentrations – an approach to standardization. J Allergy Clin Immunol 1995; 95: 677–684
15. Darsow U, Vieluf D, Ring J. The atopy patch test: an increased rate of reactivity in patients who have an air-exposed pattern of atopic eczema. Br J Dermatol 1996; 135: 182–186
16. Darsow U, Vieluf D, Ring J for the APT study group. Evaluating the relevance of aeroallergen sensitization in atopic eczema using the tool „atopy patch test": a randomized, double-blind multicenter study. J Am Acad Dermatol 1999; 40: 187–193
17. European Task Force on Atopic Dermatitis. Severity scoring of atopic dermatitis: the SCORAD index. Dermatology 1993; 186:23–31
18. Fisher AA. Contact Dermatitis. 3rd Edition. Lea & Febiger, Philadelphia, 1986: pp. 686–691
19. Fukuda H, Imayama S, Okada T. Mite-free room (MFR) for the management of atopic dermatitis. Jpn J Allergol 1991;40:626–632

20. Gondo A, Saeki N, Tokuda Y. Challenge reactions in atopic dermatitis after percutaneous entry of mite antigen. Br J Dermatol 1986; 115: 485–493
21. Grewe M, Gyufko K, Schöpf E, Krutmann J. Lesional expression of interferon-gamma in atopic eczema. Lancet 1994;I:25–26
22. Hanifin JM, Rajka G. Diagnostic features of atopic dermatitis. Acta Derm Venereol (Stockh) 1980;114:146–148
23. Hanifin JM. Clinical and basic aspects of atopic dermatitis. Semin Dermatol 1983;2:5
24. Imayama S, Hashizuma T, Miyahara H, Tanahashi T, Takeishi M, Kubota Y, Koga T, Hori Y, Fukuda H. Combination of patch test and IgE for dust mite antigens differentiates 130 patients with atopic dermatitis into four groups. J Am Acad Dermatol 1992;27:531–538
25. Jones HE, Inouye JC, McGerity JL, Lewis CW. Atopic disease and serum immunoglobulin-E. Br J Dermatol 1975;92:17–25
26. Langeland T, Braathen L, Borch M. Studies of atopic patch tests. Acta Derm Venereol (Stockh) 1989; Suppl 144: 105–109
27. Lau S, Ehnert B, Cremer B, Nasert S, Büttner P, Czarnetzki BM, Wahn U. Häusliche Milbenallergenreduktion bei spezifisch sensibilisierten Patienten mit atopischem Ekzem. Allergo J 1995;4:432–435
28. Leung DYM, Ghan AK, Schneeberger EE, Geha RS. Characterization of the mononuclear cell infiltrate in atopic dermatitis using mononuclear antibodies. J Allergy Clin Immunol 1983;71:47–56
29. Leung DYM, Rhodes AR, Geha RS, Schneider LC, Ring J. Atopic dermatitis (atopic eczema). In: Fitzpatrick TB, Eisen AZ, Wolff K, Freedberg IM, Austen KF (eds) Dermatology in general medicine, 4th edn., McGraw Hill, New York, 1993, pp. 1543–1563
30. Maeda K, Yamamoto K, Tanaka Y, Anan S, Yoshida H. House dust mite (HDM) antigen in naturally occurring lesions of atopic dermatitis (AD): The relationship between HDM antigen in the skin and HDM antigen-specific IgE antibody. J Derm Science 1992; 3: 73–77
31. Maurer D, Ebner C, Reininger B, Fiebiger E, Kraft D, Kinet Jp, Stingl G. The high affinity IgE receptor mediates IgE-dependent allergen presentation. J Immunol 1995; 154:6285–90
32. Mitchell E, Chapman M, Pope F, Crow J, Jouhal S, Platts-Mills T. Basophils in allergen-induced patch test sites in atopic dermatitis. Lancet 1982; I: 127–130
33. Morren MA, Przybilla B, Bamelis M, Heykants B, Reynaers A, Degreef H. Atopic dermatitis: triggering factors. J Am Acad Dermatol 1994; 31: 467–73
34. Norris P, Schofield O, Camp R. A study of the role of house dust mite in atopic dermatitis. Br J Dermatol 1988; 118: 435–440
35. Ohmen JD, Hanifin JM, Nickoloff BJ, Rea TH, Wyzykowski R, Kim J, Jullien D, McHugh T, Nassif AS, Chan SC. Overexpression of IL-10 in atopic dermatitis. Contrasting cytokine patterns with delayed-type hypersensitivity reactions. J Immunol 1995;154:1956–1963
36. Platts-Mills T, Mitchell E, Rowntree S, Chapman M, Wilkins S. The role of dust mite allergens in atopic dermatitis. Clin Exp Dermatol 1983; 8: 233–247
37. Przybilla B, Ring J. Food allergy and atopic eczema. Semin. Dermatol 1990; 9: 220–225
38. Rajka G. Essential aspects of atopic dermatitis. Berlin: Springer, 1989
39. Ramb-Lindhauer CH, Feldmann A, Rotte M, Neumann CH. Characterization of grass pollen reactive T-cell lines derived from lesional atopic skin. Arch Dermatol Res 1991; 283:71–76
40. Reitamo S, Visa K, Kaehoenen K, Käykhö A, Lauerna I, Stubb S, Salo OP. Patch test reactions to inhalant allergens in atopic dermatitis. Acta Derm Venereol (Stockh) 1989; 144:119–121
41. Reitamo S, Visa K, Kähönen K, Stubb S, Salo OP. Eczematous reactions in atopic patients caused by epicutaneous testing with inhalant allergens. Br J Dermatol 1986; 114: 303–309
42. Renz H, Jujo K, Bradley K, Domenico L, Gelfand EW, Leung DY. Enhanced IL-4 production and IL-4 receptor expression in atopic dermatitis and their modulation by interferon-gamma. J Invest Dermatol 1992; 99: 403–408
43. Ring J, Bieber T, Vieluf D, Kunz B, Przybilla B. Atopic eczema, Langerhans cells and allergy. Int Arch Allergy Appl Immunol 1991; 94: 194–201
44. Ring J, Brockow K, Abeck D. The therapeutic concept of „patient management" in atopic eczema. Allergy 1996;51: 206–215
45. Ring J, Kunz B, Bieber T, Vieluf D, Przybilla B. The „atopy patch test" with aeroallergens in atopic eczema (abstr). J Allergy Clin Immunol 1989; 82: 195

46. Ring J. Angewandte Allergologie, 2. Aufl. MMV Medizin Verlag, München, 1995
47. Ring J. Atopy: condition, disease, or syndrome? In: Ruzicka T, Ring J, Przybilla B (eds) Handbook of atopic eczema. Springer, Berlin, Heidelberg, New York, 1991: pp. 3–8
48. Rostenberg A, Sulzberger MD. Some results of patch tests. Arch Dermatol 1937; 35: 433–54
49. Sager N, Feldmann A, Schilling G, Kreitsch P, Neumann C. House dust mite-specific T cells in the skin of subjects with atopic dermatitis: Frequency and lymphokine profile in the allergen patch test. J Allergy Clin Immunol 1992; 89: 801–810
50. Sanda T, Yasue T. Oohashi M, Yasue A. Effectiveness of house dust-mite allergen avoidance with atopic dermatitis. J Allergy Clin Immunol 1992; 89: 653–657
51. Schäfer L, Kragballe K. Abnormalities in epidermal lipid metabolism in patients with atopic dermatitis. J Invest Dermatol 1991;96:10–15
52. Seidenari S, Manzini BM, Danese P, Giannetti A. Positive patch tests to whole mite culture and purified mite extracts in patients with atopic dermatitis, asthma and rhinitis. Ann Allergy 1992; 69: 201–206
53. Seidenari B, Manzini M, Danese P. Patch testing with pollens of Gramineae in patients with atopic dermatitis and mucosal atopy. Contact Dermatitis 1992; 27: 125–6
54. Seifert H, Wollemann G, Seifert B, Borelli S. Neurodermitis: Eine Protein-Kontaktdermatitis? Dtsch Derm 1987; 35: 1204–1214
55. Skov L, Baadsgaard O. Ultraviolet B-exposed major histocompatibility complex class II positive keratinocytes and antigen-presenting cells demonstrate a differential capacity to activate T cells in the presence of staphylococcal superantigens. Br J Dermatol 1996; 134: 824–830
56. Sowden J, Powell R, Allen B. Selective activation of circulating CD4+ lymphocytes in severe adult atopic dermatitis. Br J Dermatol 1992; 127: 228–232
57. Tan B, Weald D, Strickland I, Friedman P. Double-blind controlled trial of effect of housedust-mite allergen avoidance on atopic dermatitis. Lancet 1996; 347: 15–18
58. Tanaka Y, Anan S, Yoshida H. Immunohistochemical studies in mite antigen-induced patch test sites in atopic dermatitis. J Derm Science 1990; 1: 361–368
59. Tupker R, DeMonchy J, Coenraads P, Homan A, van der Meer J. Induction of atopic dermatitis by inhalation of house dust mite. J Allergy Clin Immunol 1996; 97: 1064–1070
60. Van Bever HP, Docx M, Stevens WJ. Food and food additives in severe atopic dermatitis. Allergy 1989; 44: 588–594
61. van Reijsen FC, Bruijnzeel-Koomen CAFM, Kalthoff FS, Maggi E, Romagnani S, Westland JKT, Mudde GC. Skin-derived aeroallergen-specific T-cell clones of TH2 phenotype in patiens with atopic dermatitis. J Allergy Clin Immunol 1992;90:184–192
62. van Voorst Vader PC, Lier JG, Woest TE, Coenraads PJ, Nater JP. Patch tests with house dust mite antigens in atopic dermatitis patients: methodological problems. Acta Derm Venereol (Stockh) 1991; 71(4): 301–305
63. Vercelli D, Jabara H, Lauener R, Geha R. IL-4 inhibits the synthesis of INF-gamma and induces the synthesis of IgE in human mixed lymphocyte cultures. J Immunol 1990; 144: 570–573
64. Vieluf D, Kunz B, Bieber T, Przybilla B, Ring J. „Atopy Patch Test" with aeroallergens in patients with atopic eczema. Allergo J 1993; 2: 9–12
65. Vocks E, Seifert H, Seifert B, Drosner M. Patch test with immediate type allergens in patients with atopic dermatitis. In: Ring J, Przybilla B, eds. New Trends in Allergy III. Berlin: Springer, 1991: 230–233
66. Wistokat-Wülfing A, Schmidt P, Darsow U, Ring J, Kapp A, Werfel T. Atopy patch test reactions are associated with T lymphocyte-mediated allergen-specific immune responses in atopic dermatitis. Clin Exp Allergy 1999; 29: 513–521
67. Wüthrich B. Minimal forms of atopic eczema. In: Ruzicka T, Ring J, Przybilla B, eds. Handbook of atopic eczema. Springer, Berlin, 1991, pp. 46–53
68. Wüthrich B. Neurodermitis atopica sive constitutionalis. Ein pathogenetisches Modell aus der Sicht des Allergologen. Akt. Dermatol 1983; 9:1–7

19 The Intrinsic Type of Atopic Dermatitis Is Characterised by a Low Expression of the High-Affinity IgE Receptor FcεRI on Epidermal Dendritic Cells

A. Wollenberg, T. Oppel, K. Reiser, M. Moderer, J. Haberstok, S. Günther, T. Bieber, E. Schuller

Abstract

Atopic dermatitis (AD) is a chronic inflammatory skin disease of unknown origin, characterised by a chronically relapsing course, a distinctive clinical appearance and severe pruritus. The diagnosis is made on clinical grounds. IgE-mediated presentation of environmental allergens by dendritic cells to antigen specific T cells is assumed to be the central immunopathogenetic event. An 'intrinsic' type (IAD) has been delineated from the more common 'extrinsic' disease form (EAD) by normal serum IgE levels, negative RAST tests and negative immediate type skin reactions towards environmental allergens. In these patients, a substitution of environmental allergens by the recently characterised autoantigen Hom s 1 has been attributed a paradigmatic role for the pathogenesis. On the other hand, more complex differences in the epidermodermal inflammatory environment may as well represent the pathogenetic background of intrinsic AD.

Here, we present our clinical and laboratory data of 7 IAD and 62 EAD patients. EAD patients tended to have an earlier onset of disease but similar disease duration and family history of atopic diseases. Epidermal dendritic cell (DC) phenotyping, a recently validated technique based on the three-colour flow cytometric analysis of Langerhans cells and the so-called inflammatory dendritic epidermal cells (IDEC) from epidermal single cell suspensions, was performed on samples from 69 AD and 94 control patients. Quantitative analysis of CD36 expression on DC as a marker of inflammation, as well as the percentage of IDEC in the CD1a+ epidermal DC pool, indicated a comparable disease activity in IAD and EAD. EAD was characterised by a significantly higher FcεRI expression on the CD1a+ epidermal DC than IAD. Using the FcεRI/FcγRII expression ratio as a disease marker for AD, values for IAD fell below the diagnostic cut-off level of 1.5 for this ratio.

In conclusion, immunodermatological differences between EAD and IAD could be demonstrated, indicating that these disease forms may have an at least in part different underlying pathophysiology. It remains elusive whether EAD and IAD represent extreme clinical manifestations of a continuous spectrum of AD, or if there are different disease mechanisms active in IAD and EAD. Thus, while IAD is clinically similar to EAD, the inflammatory microenvironment in this condition is different from classical EAD and can be distinguished by phenotyping of epidermal DC.

New Trends in Allergy V
J. Ring, H. Behrendt (Eds.)
© Springer-Verlag Berlin, Heidelberg 2002

Introduction

Atopic dermatitis (AD) is a common inflammatory skin disease with increasing incidence. It is characterised by a chronically relapsing course, a distinctive clinical appearance and severe pruritus. In addition, many AD patients are highly susceptible for viral infections and tend to develop allergic rhinoconjunctivitis or bronchial asthma. Laboratory markers include an elevated serum IgE and multiple positive prick test reactions to a variety of (mostly aero-) allergens [8, 13]. IgE-mediated uptake and antigen focusing of environmental allergens by IgE-bearing dendritic cells (DC) to antigen specific T cells is assumed to be a central immunopathogenetic event [3]. Recently, an increased expression of the high affinity receptor for IgE (FcεRI) on epidermal DC from nonlesional and lesional skin of AD patients was demonstrated [16]. Furthermore, the expression of FcεRI on epidermal DC was shown to be correlated to the serum IgE level [16].

Up to 20% of the patients with the clinical phenotype of AD belong to a subtype which is characterised by low serum IgE levels, and an absence of environmental-allergen-specific RAST tests and immediate type skin reactions. This subtype of disease has been described as the 'intrinsic' type of atopic dermatitis (IAD) by Wüthrich in 1983 [17, 18], as a counterpart to the classical 'extrinsic' type of disease (EAD). Diagnostic criteria have not formally been proposed, but in our opinion and that of Wüthrich (personal communication), these could be as follows:

- a clinical phenotype of AD, fulfilling the diagnostic criteria of Hanifin and Rajka [4],
- low or moderate total serum-IgE levels (<200 kU/l) in combination with negative in-vitro IgE-screening for aeroallergens (Sx1-RAST/CAP) and food allergens (Fx5-RAST) as well as negative skin prick test results for standard aero- and food-allergens and
- absence of other atopic diseases such as allergic rhinoconjunctivitis or allergic bronchial asthma.

Hence, patients may initially be suspected to have an IAD, but during the allergological work-up they need to be reclassified as EAD. As the immunopathogenesis of AD as such is still elusive [7, 13], there is even less known about the mechanisms leading to IAD [12].

Recently, the human protein Hom S 1 was characterised in AD skin and the authors hypothesised, that this structure may play the role of an autoantigen in the pathogenesis of IAD [9]. If this would be the case, no differences in the cytokine secretion pattern of lesional lymphocytes as well as in other markers of the inflammatory micromilieu of the lesions in IAD and EAD should be expected.

Epidermal DC phenotyping (EDCP) is a recently validated technique based on the cell surface receptor analysis of the CD1a$^+$ DC isolated from the epidermal compartment [16]. Diagnostic EDCP criteria for AD have been proposed as early as 1995 [15], and are based on the high expression of FcεRI and a corresponding low expression CD32/FcγRII. These criteria allow for a sensitive and specific identification of AD out of other chronic inflammatory skin diseases [16]. To investigate for potential differences in the inflammatory micromilieu of the

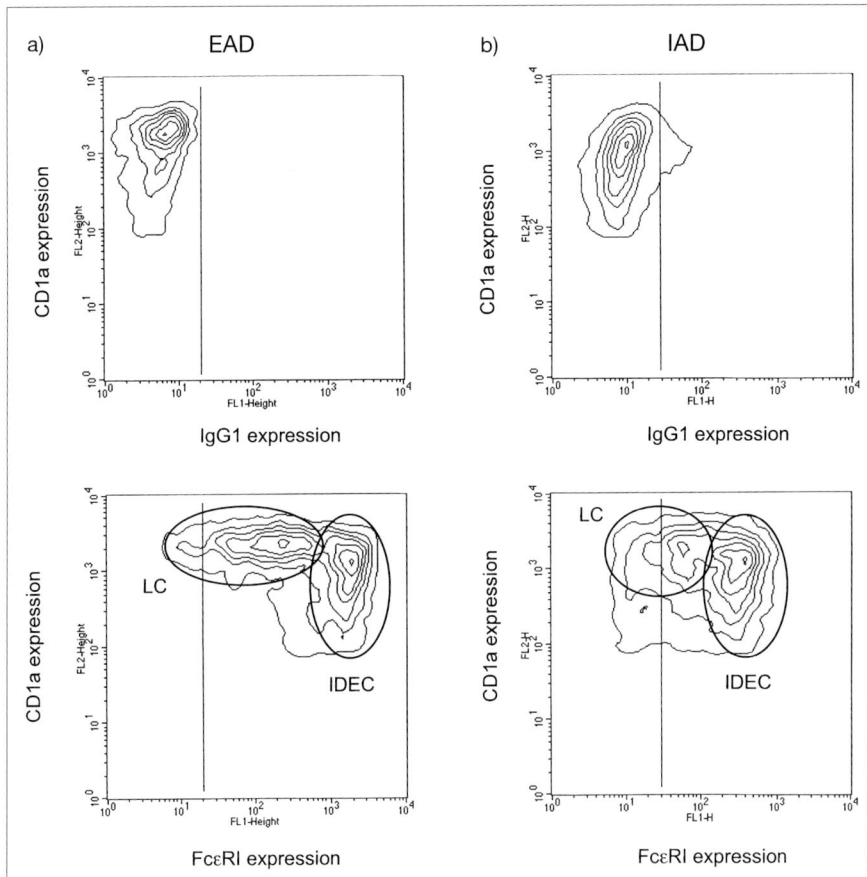

Fig. 1a, b. Contour plot analysis of epidermal dendritic cells from atopic dermatitis skin. Contour plot analysis of the CD1a+ epidermal DC. Cell suspensions were prepared from a sample of (**a**) EAD and (**b**) IAD skin. The Langerhans cell (*LC*) and inflammatory dendritic epidermal cell (*IDEC*) populations, as well as the respective gate settings, are indicated. The two epidermal dendritic cell populations in EAD are characterised by a higher FcεRI expression as compared IAD (Fl1 ~ FcεRI, Fl2 ~ CD1a)

epidermal compartment in IAD and EAD lesions, we correlated the clinical data of 69 AD patients with the immunophenotyping results from our EDCP data bank. The controls consisted of 14 biopsies of allergic contact dermatitis lesions (CD), 42 psoriasis vulgaris lesions (PV) and 38 normal human skin specimen (NS).

Clinical Characteristics of IAD Patients

AD was diagnosed according to the criteria of Hanifin and Rajka [4]. IAD was diagnosed, if the above mentioned criteria for IAD were met by a patient. All other

AD patients were classified as EAD. Out of the total number of 69 AD patients, 7 patients met the diagnostic criteria of IAD, which is a total of 11% of our 69 AD patients. This percentage is slightly lower than the 18% prevalence of IAD reported in a group of 93 AD patients from Davos, Switzerland [19].

The IAD patients tended to be younger of age (26.4±3.4 vs. 33.5±1.7), but had a similar duration of disease as compared to EAD (17.8±3.2 vs. 19.5±2.0). Interestingly, all 7 IAD patients were female, whereas the EAD group consisted of 26 female and 36 male patients. Most of our IAD patients (5/7) had acquired their disease in early childhood, whereas only 2 of them had a history of later onset between their 20th to 25th year of life. The onset of disease in our EAD patients varied between 1 and 81 years, but was higher in EAD (15.3±2.6 vs. 9.0±4.2) as compared to IAD. At the age of 1 year 31% and at the age of 25 years more than 80% of our patients suffered from EAD. In addition, 73% of our EAD patients suffered from allergic rhinitis, 47% from allergic asthma.

Per definition, none of the patients with IAD had a history of allergic rhinitis or allergic asthma. Furthermore, prick tests for aeroallergens (pollens, house dust mite, cat and dog epithelia) and food allergens revealed no immediate type skin reactions. In contrast, all of our EAD patients had positive prick test reactions for aeroallergens and/or food allergens.

In IAD, the total serum-IgE levels ranged from 5 to 187 kU/l (mean of 77±28 kU/l), whereas the serum-IgE levels of the EAD patients ranged from 55 to 47120 kU/l (mean of 8564±185 kU/l). Environmental-allergen-specific IgE (see above) was not detected in any of our IAD patients, whereas allergen-specific IgE was found in all our EAD patients.

About half of our patients with IAD stated a history of AD (4/7) or allergic rhinitis (3/7) in their families (parents, siblings or first grade cousins). In EAD, a comparable number of our patients (58%) had a positive family history of atopic diseases.

IAD Is Characterised by a Low Expression of FcεRI on CD1a+ Epidermal Dendritic Cells

The increased expression of FcεRI on the CD1a+ epidermal DC is an immuno-biological hallmark of AD [14,16]. Using EDCP, a high expression ratio of FcεRI/FcγRII, exceeding the threshold value of 1.5, has been demonstrated a novel diagnostic criterium for AD [16], but no data had been available concerning IAD and EAD.

We were able to detect high levels of FcεRI on epidermal DC in EAD, whereas a significantly ($p < 0.01$) lower FcεRI-expression was seen in IAD (Fig. 2c). Furthermore, the diagnostic ratio of FcεRI/FcγRII expression was highly elevated in EAD, leading to a correct identification of 80% of the EAD patients (Fig. 2d). In contrast, epidermal DC phenotyping did not label any of the IAD patients as AD (0/7), since the diagnostic FcεRI/FcγRII expression ratio in IAD remained low (Fig. 2d). The FcεRI-expression of allergic contact dermatitis and psoriasis was similar to IAD, and the FcεRI/FcγRII expression ratio was almost identical in IAD, CD and PV.

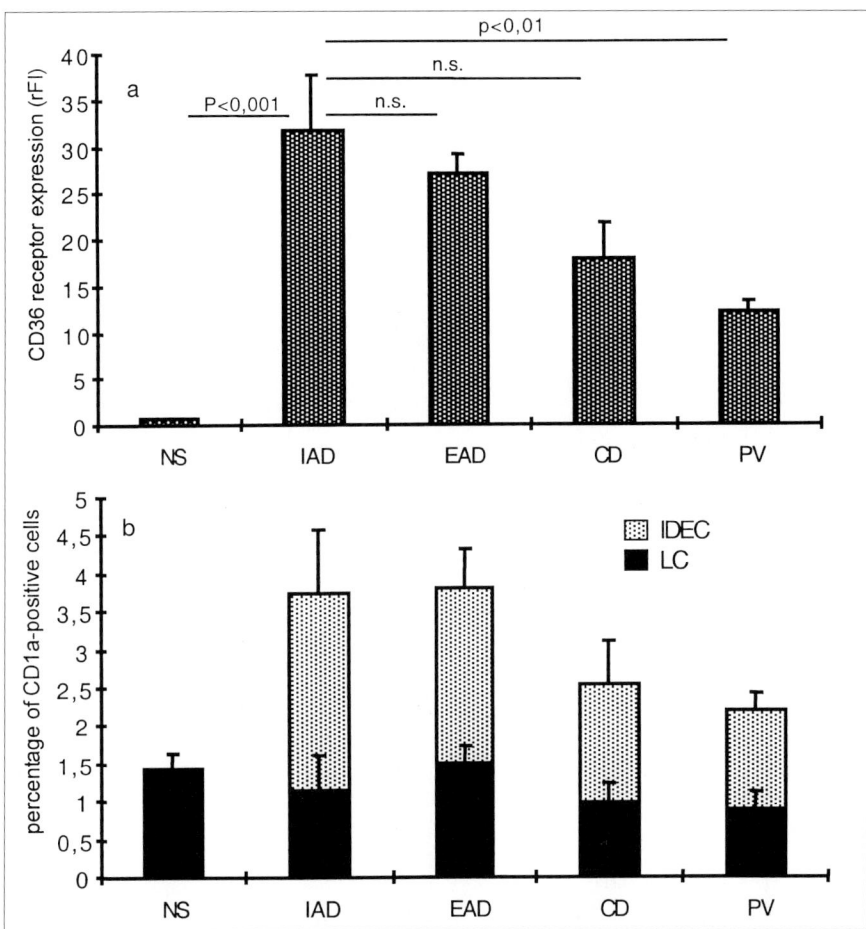

Fig. 2a, b. Statistical analysis of epidermal dendritic cell phenotyping. The results of epidermal DC phenotyping are shown for the different underlying diseases. *NS*, normal skin; *IAD*, intrinsic atopic dermatitis; *EAD*, extrinsic atopic dermatitis; *CD*, allergic contact dermatitis; *PV*, psoriasis vulgaris. All results are given as arithmetic mean±SEM, significances have been calculated with the Mann-Whitney *U* test. **a** A similar disease activity in both subgroups is indicated by a comparably high expression of the thrombospondin receptor CD36 on CD1a+ epidermal dendritic cells in EAD and IAD. **b** The percentage of both CD1a+ epidermal dendritic cell populations does not show significant differences between IAD and EAD.

It is known that LC contain significant amounts of preformed FcεRI-α chain in their cytoplasm, and that the surface expression is linked to the co-expression of the FcεRI-γ chain [6]. However, nothing is known about the molecular mechanisms of FcεRI regulation in IDEC, which represent the relevant FcεRI expressing epidermal cell population in inflammatory skin [14, 16]. Hence, the different inflammatory micromilieu in IAD and EAD lesions is reflected by the immunophenotype of the epidermal DC [16].

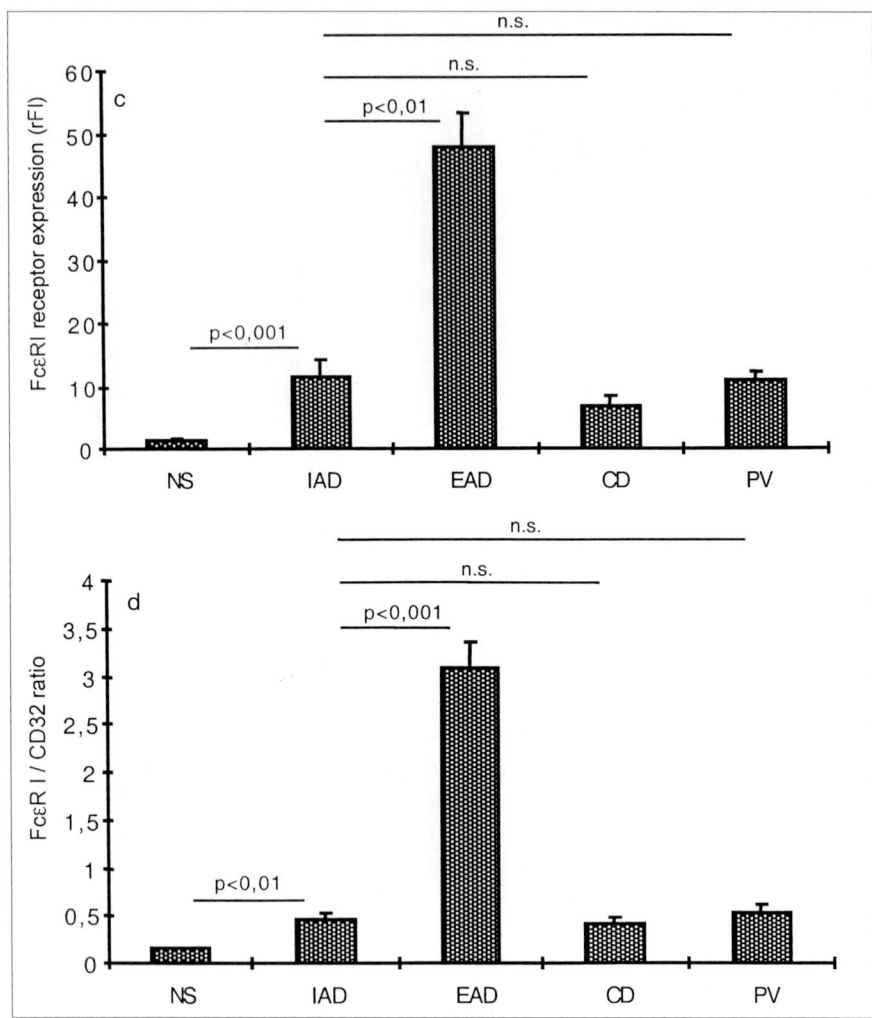

Fig. 2c, d. c Epidermal DC of EAD show a significant upregulation of the high-affinity IgE Receptor FcεRI, as compared to IAD and other inflammatory skin diseases. **d** The diagnostic expression ratio of FcεRI/FcγRII on epidermal DC is significantly elevated in the EAD samples, but not in the IAD samples

Valenta et al. have shown that AD patients frequently display IgE antibody reactivity against human proteins [9] and have suspected that a sensitisation against Hom s 1 might be the basis of intrinsic atopic dermatitis. However, the data published by others [1, 5, 10] and our own data presented here indicate further immunodermatological differences between EAD and IAD. These cannot be explained by a simple substitution of environmental allergens with the autoantigen Hom S 1. It may however be suspected, that autoantigens such as Hom S 1 may play a role in the chronicity of EAD in the absence of exogenous allergens.

IAD and EAD Show a Similar Inflammatory Activity Inside the Epidermal Compartment

Since our EDCP results might have been biased by differences in the inflammatory activity of the epidermal compartment, we analysed the expression of CD36 on CD1a$^+$ epidermal DC in all patient groups. The expression of CD36 on epidermal DC has been proposed as a marker for the inflammatory activity inside the epidermal compartment [16]. The quantitative analysis of CD36 (Fig. 2a) revealed a high expression in both EAD and IAD, thus indicating a comparable inflammatory activity. As compared to both forms of AD, all control groups had a, mostly significantly, lower expression of CD36 on their EDC.

In previous studies, we and others have demonstrated that beside Langerhans cells, a second CD1a$^+$ cell population lacking Birbeck granules is present inside the inflammatory epidermis [2, 14]. This second cell type, the inflammatory dendritic epidermal cells (IDEC), have been shown to be the relevant IgE-binding epidermal cell [16]. In both disease forms of AD, a similarly high percentage of IDEC was found in the CD1a$^+$ epidermal DC pool. However, the number of IDEC was raised in all of the inflammatory skin diseases (IAD, EAD, CD and PV) as compared to normal skin (Fig. 2b). The similar expression of CD36 as well as the similar percentage of IDEC in IAD and EAD indicate a comparable inflammatory disease activity in both subtypes of disease, thereby excluding a potential bias caused by the analysis of patients with a different severity grade of their lesions.

T Cell Analysis in IAD and EAD Patients

Previous studies have identified differences in the immunoregulatory mechanisms between EAD and IAD. Kägi et al. described a different cytokine pattern in peripheral blood lymphocytes of patients with the intrinsic and the extrinsic forms of AD [5]. Elevated levels for IL-4 and IL-5 were observed in the EAD patients, whereas IAD patients displayed a high IL-5 but low IL-4 secretion of their blood lymphocytes.

More recently, Akdis et al. demonstrated that skin derived T cells from EAD give effective B-cell help for IgE production, whereas T cells from IAD do not [1]. This was attributed to an increased IL-13 production of skin derived T cells from EAD, since the increased IgE production could be reduced by the addition of anti-IL-13 antibody to the cell cultures. Different immune mechanisms of EAD and IAD are also suggested by their finding of a high IL-13 content in skin derived T cells from EAD patients, whereas T cells from IAD patients showed a much lower IL-13 content [1].

Peripheral blood T cell activation and peripheral blood eosinophilia were described in both EAD and IAD [10], whereas elevated serum IgE levels and CD23$^+$ B cells were found only in the extrinsic type of AD [10]. This is suggestive of a different inflammatory micromilieu and cytokine profile in EAD and IAD. Beside IL-13, skin derived T cells from EAD and IAD patients produce significant amounts of IL-5 [1]. These elevated IL-5 levels in EAD and IAD might explain blood eosinophilia and increased eosinophil survival by delayed eosinophil programmed cell death [11].

In conclusion, our recent data indicate immunodermatological differences between EAD and IAD, suggesting that these two disease forms may have an at least in part different underlying pathophysiology. It remains elusive whether EAD and IAD represent extreme clinical manifestations of a continuous spectrum of AD, or if there are different disease mechanisms active in IAD and EAD.

References

1. Akdis CA, Akdis M, Simon D, Dibbert B, Weber M, Kratzl S, Kreyden O, Disch R, Wüthrich B, Blaser K, Simun HU (1999): T cells and T cell-derived cytokines as pathogenic factors in the nonallergic form of atopic dermatitis. J Invest Dermatol 113: 628–634
2. Baadsgaard O, Gupta AK, Taylor RS, Ellis CN, Voorhees JJ, Cooper KD (1989): Psoriatic epidermal cells demonstrate increased numbers and function of non-Langerhans antigen presenting cells. J Invest Dermatol 92: 190–195
3. Bieber T (1997): FceRI-expressing antigen-presenting cells: new players in the atopic game. Immunol Today 18: 311–313
4. Hanifin JM, Rajka G (1980): Diagnostic features of atopic dermatitis. Acta Derm Venereol (Stockh) Suppl 92: 44–47
5. Kägi MK, Wuthrich B, Montano E, Barandun J, Blaser K, Walker C (1994): Differential cytokine profiles in peripheral blood lymphocyte supernatants and skin biopsies from patients with different forms of atopic dermatitis, psoriasis and normal individuals. Int Arch Allergy Immunol 103: 332–340
6. Kraft S, Weßendorf JHM, Hanau D, Bieber T (1998): Regulation of the high affinity receptor for IgE on human epidermal Langerhans cells. J Immunol 161: 1000–1006
7. Leung DY (1999): Pathogenesis of atopic dermatitis. J Allergy Clin Immunol 104: S99–108
8. Rajka G (1989): Essential aspects of atopic dermatitis. Springer, Berlin
9. Valenta R, Natter S, Seiberler S, Wichlas S, Maurer D, Hess M, Pavelka M, Grote M, Ferreira F, Szepfalusi Z, Valent P, Stingl G (1998): Molecular characterization of an autoallergen, Hom s 1, identified by serum IgE from atopic dermatitis patients. J Invest Dermatol 111: 1178–1183
10. Walker C, Kagi MK, Ingold P, Braun P, Blaser K, Bruijnzeel Koomen CA, Wuthrich B (1993): Atopic dermatitis: correlation of peripheral blood T cell activation, eosinophilia and serum factors with clinical severity. Clin Exp Allergy 23: 145–153
11. Wedi B, Raap U, Lewrick H, Kapp A (1997): Delayed eosinophil programmed cell death in vitro: a common feature of inhalant allergy and extrinsic and intrinsic atopic dermatitis. J Allergy Clin Immunol 100: 536–543
12. Werfel T, Kapp A (1999): What do we know about the etiopathology of the intrinsic type of atopic dermatitis? Curr Probl Dermatol 28: 29–36
13. Wollenberg A, Bieber T (2000): Atopic dermatitis: from the genes to skin lesions. Allergy 55: 205–213
14. Wollenberg A, Kraft S, Hanau D, Bieber T (1996): Immunomorphological and ultrastructural characterization of Langerhans cells and a novel, inflammatory dendritic epidermal cell (IDEC) population in lesional skin of atopic eczema. J Invest Dermatol 106: 446–453
15. Wollenberg A, Wen S, Bieber T (1995): Langerhans cell phenotyping: A new tool for differential diagnosis of inflammatory skin diseases. Lancet 346: 1626–1627
16. Wollenberg A, Wen S, Bieber T (1999): Phenotyping of epidermal dendritic cells – clinical applications of a flow cytometric micromethod. Cytometry 37: 147–155
17. Wüthrich B (1983): Neurodermitis atopica sive constitutionalis. Ein pathogenetisches Modell aus der Sicht des Allergologen. Akt Dermatol 9: 1–7
18. Wüthrich B (1989): Atopic dermatitis flare provoked by inhalant allergens. Dermatologica 178: 51–53
19. Wüthrich B (1999): Clinical aspects, epidemiology, and prognosis of atopic dermatitis. Ann Allergy Asthma Immunol 83: 464–470

20 Staphylococcal Exotoxins as Trigger Factors of Atopic Dermatitis

K. Breuer, T. Werfel, A. Kapp

Summary

S. aureus has been identified as a trigger factor of atopic dermatitis. 30–60% of *S. aureus* strains are capable to produce exotoxins with superantigenic properties in patients with atopic dermatitis. In order to investigate if these exotoxins exacerbate atopic dermatitis (AD) primarily as superantigens or as „conventional" allergens, we generated exotoxin-reactive T cell lines (TCL) from skin and blood of three patients with atopic dermatitis, who were colonized with toxigenic *S. aureus* strains. Furthermore we determined the relationship between the severity of skin lesions and the sensitization to staphylococcal enterotoxins A and B in a group of 71 adult patients with atopic dermatitis.

Both superantigen-reactive and exotoxin-specific TCL were generated from skin and blood of the three patients colonized with toxigenic *S. aureus* strains, which points to the importance of the exotoxins not only as superantigens but also as allergens.

This finding and the recently published fact that patients sensitized to staphylococcal enterotoxin B have a higher disease activity than non-sensitized patients confirm the importance of allergen-specific responses to staphylococcal exotoxins.

Introduction

Atopic dermatitis is a chronic inflammatory skin disease which often begins in infancy and runs a course of remissions and exacerbations. Acute eczematous lesions are characterized by erythema, oozing and crusting, whereas chronic lesions show thickened skin and papules. Furthermore, intense pruritus and consequently sleeplessness are hallmarks of atopic dermatitis [1]. Environmental allergens and food allergens have been identified as major provocation factors of atopic dermatitis [2]. Allergen-specific T-cells play a prominent role at the cellular level: Allergen-specific T-cell-clones could be generated from biopsies of „atopy patch test" lesions and food-specific T-cell-clones were obtained from blood and skin lesions after oral food challenges [3–6]. Specific IgE-antibodies are thought to play a role in antigen presentation via Fc receptors for IgE (FcεR-I) on epidermal Langerhans cells [7]. Degranulation of dermal mast-cells by allergen-induced crosslinking of IgE-antibodies bound to FcεR on the cell surface may also contribute to the allergic inflammation in AD.

By the use of limiting dilution cultures, inhalant allergen-specific T-cells have been shown to represent only a minority (1 to 5%) of infiltrating T-cells in lesional

New Trends in Allergy V
J. Ring, H. Behrendt (Eds.)
© Springer-Verlag Berlin, Heidelberg 2002

skin [4, 8]. Therefore other factors, which lead to the activation of T-cells at the site of inflammation are probably involved in the pathogenesis of atopic dermatitis. There is increasing evidence, that cutaneous and nasal colonization with *S. aureus* contributes to the pathogenesis of atopic dermatitis. *S. aureus* can be isolated from the skin of 80–100% of AD patients [9–13], whereas only 5–10% of normal persons are colonized with this bacterium. Several studies could show, that 30–60% of *S. aureus* strains isolated from individuals with atopic dermatitis secrete exotoxins with superantigenic properties (SEA, SEB, SEC, SED, TSST-1) [12, 14–17]. Bacterial superantigens have been identified as potential mitogens for T-lymphocytes, since they are able to activate up to 20% of the T-cell pool in a MHC-unrestricted fashion, by binding to certain TCR-Vβ-chains on T-cells and outside the antigen-binding groove of the MHC-molecule on antigen-presenting cells [18]. In a previous study the application of SEB on the skin of normal individuals and patients with AD resulted in an inflammatory reaction at the application site [19] and skin biopsies from patch test sites showed a selective accumulation of SEB-reactive TCR-Vβ elements [20]. Leung et al. first proposed that superantigens may not only exacerbate atopic dermatitis in their function as superantigens, but also by acting as a new group of allergens, since specific IgE to SEA, SEB and TSST-1 could be detected in the sera from 57% of atopic dermatitis patients, most of whom were carriers of toxigenic staphylococcus aureus strains. Basophils of these patients were found to release histamine upon incubation with the respective toxin [12]. Thus, colonization with exotoxin-producing strains could lead to a permanent release of proinflammatory mediators from cutaneous mast cells, in this way acting as a trigger factor in atopic dermatitis. Bunikowski et al. could show, that the presence of IgE antibodies to SEA and SEB is correlated with the severity of skin lesions in childhood atopic dermatitis [17].

In order to investigate if the exotoxins exacerbate atopic dermatitis primarily as T-cell superantigens or as conventional allergens we investigated the role of exotoxin-specific IgE and the T-cell-response to staphylococcal exotoxins in adult patients with atopic dermatitis.

Methods

Patients

In total, 71 patients with mild to severe atopic dermatitis were investigated (median age 32 years, range 18 to 65 years). Diagnosis was performed following the criteria of Hanifin and Rajka. Clinical severity of AD was determined according to the SCORAD (range 14 to 103 points).

The T-cell response to staphylococcal exotoxins was investigated independently in three patients [patient 1 (T.S.) age 21 years, patient 2 (K.B.) age 26 years, patient 3 (T.A.) age 18 years] with severe atopic dermatitis (SCORAD 73.5, 41.5, and 44.5, respectively).

Total and Superantigen-Specific IgE

Levels of total IgE were determined in the sera from AD patients using the CAP RAST (Pharmacia and Upjohn, Freiburg, Germany). Specific IgE to SEA, SEB, SEC, SED and TSST-1 were determined with the CAP RAST according to the manufacturer's instructions (Pharmacia and Upjohn, Freiburg, Germany).

Eosinophil Mediators

Urine EPX

Urine samples were frozen immediately and stored at −20°C. EPX was measured with a competitive RIA according to the manufacturer's instructions (Pharmacia and Upjohn, Freiburg, Germany). Considering the patient's renal function, the EPX concentrations were referred to the urine creatinine concentration and expressed as μg/mmol creatinine.

Serum ECP

Blood samples were coagulated for 60 min at room temperature, followed by a 30-min incubation at 4°C. Samples were centrifuged for 10 min (4°C, 850×g). Sera were frozen immediately and stored at −20°C. ECP was determined by use of the CAP system ECP FEIA (Pharmacia and Upjohn, Freiburg, Germany) after the completion of the study.

Identification of Staphylococcal Toxins

In three patients with severe atopic dermatitis swabs were taken from the skin and the anterior nares for the identification of *S. aureus* and staphylococcal toxins. Bacterial cultures were performed. *S. aureus* was identified by testing typical colonies for coagulase activity. One colony each was selected and a subculture was grown for 24 h on blood agar. Ten colonies of the subculture were grow in RPMI-1640 protein-free cell culture medium for 18 h at 37°C. The bacteria were harvested by centrifugation and the filter-sterilized supernatants were tested for the presence of exotoxins with the TSST-1-RPLA and SET-RPLA latex agglutination test (Unipath, Hampshire, UK) according to the manufacturer's instructions. The detection limit was 7 ng/ml for TSST and 0.5 ng/ml for SEA-D.

Isolation of Lymphocytes from Blood and Skin Biopsies

PBMC were isolated from heparinized blood samples of three patients by density centrifugation on Ficoll Hypaque (Nycomed Pharma AS, Oslo, Norway).

Punch biopsies (5 mm diameter) were taken from lesional skin. The tissue was incubated in Hank's solution, containing 1% HEPES, 0.5% Gentamycin, 0.1% Collagenase, 0,1% Hyaluronidase, 0,01% DNAase, 1.2 U/ml dispase and 10% FCS for 5 h at 37°C. Cell suspensions were filtered through a nylon gauze and washed.

The percentage of T-cells was assessed by flow cytometry with an antibody to CD3 (Becton Dickenson, Heidelberg, Germany). T-cells represented about 10% of all cells in cutaneous cell suspensions. The ethical committee of the Hannover Medical University had approved taking skin biopsies from lesional skin.

Generation of T-Cell Lines

Responder cells from the patients skin and blood were added to limiting-dilution wells (96-well round bottom trays, Nunc GmbH, Roskilde, Denmark) in dilutions ranging from 500 cells/well to 25 cells/well together with 2×10^4 autologous, antigen-presenting cells (PBMC, irradiated with 55 Gy, ^{37}Cs). The cultures were kept in Iscove's medium (Biochrome KG), supplemented with 4% heat-inactivated AB serum (human serum), 2 mmol/l glutamine, 50 µg/ml gentamycin, 100 µg/ml penicillin, 100 µg/ml streptomycin, non-essential amino acids and 10 U/ml rIL-2 in the presence or absence of the respective superantigen, produced by staphylococci isolated from the patients skin, at a concentration of 1 µg/ml (highly purified SEC2, SED, Toxin Technology Inc., Sarasota, USA).

After 12 to 14 days, wells that demonstrated growth of >50 lymphoblasts were scored as positive and defined as a T cell line. Frequencies of reactive CD3+ T-cells were determined by the minimum chi square method according to Taswell [21].

After 14 days and 8–10 days thereafter, expansion of growing lines were performed in 24-well flat bottom plates with allogeneic, irradiated PBMC as feeder cells (1×10^6 cells per well), phytohaemagglutinin (10 µg/ml) and IL-2 (10 U/ml) in Iscove's medium.

Restimulation Assay

For assessment of the exotoxin-reactivity of T cell lines an 8 day interval between the last expansion step was allowed before cells were used in the restimulation assay. After repeated washings, 6.5×10^3 T-cells were incubated in the presence of 7.5×10^4 irradiated PBMC and were stimulated with 1 µ/ml exotoxin and without antigen as negative control. Each line was incubated with autologous and allogeneic PBMC.

After 5 days of culture the cells were pulsed with tritiated thymidine (^{3}H-thymidine) (0.5 µCi/well) for 4 h. The β-decay was counted in a liquid scintillation counter and results of triplicate cultures were expressed as mean cpm. Stimulation index (SI) was defined by a ratio of mean counts per minute of stimulated to unstimulated cultures. TCL were only selected, if the stimulation index in the presence of the exotoxins plus autologous APC was higher than 4 or if the SI was between 3 and 4 and more than double of the SI in the presence of allogeneic APC.

Phenotyping of T-Cell Lines

Expression of the T-cell surface antigens were investigated with FITC or PE-labelled antibodies recognizing CD3 and superantigen-reactive TCR-Vβ chains in a two-colour staining. After the staining procedure 1×10^4 cells per sample were analysed on a FACScan flow cytometer (Becton Dickenson, Heidelberg, Germany) using a gate for lymphocytes. Viable cells were identified by staining with propidium iodide.

First the cells were stained with a mixture of antibodies reactive to the different exotoxins. Positive cells were stained with each of the antibodies separately.

The distribution of the TCR-Vβ-elements was calculated and expressed as a percentage of $CD3^+$ cells.

Statistical Analysis

The comparison of the medians of non-parametral distributed results of different patient groups was performed with the Mann-Whitney rank sum test.

Results

Fifty-Six Percent of Adult Patients with Atopic Dermatitis Are Sensitized to SEA and/or SEB

The sera of 71 patients were analysed for the presence of specific IgE to SEA and SEB. Of these 71 patients, 40 (56%) were found to be sensitized to staphylococcal exotoxins (specific IgE concentrations of more than 0.35 kU/l). 19 of these patients (47.5%) were sensitized to both SEA and SEB, in 12 patients (30%) only IgE-antibodies to SEA and in 9 patients (22.5%) only IgE-antibodies to SEB were detected.

Patients sensitized to SEB had median serum-SEB-IgE levels of 2.06 kU/l (range 0.47 to 30.54 kU/l), whereas SEA-sensitized patients had median serum-SEA-IgE levels of 1.80 kU/l (range 0.37 to 80.46 kU/l).

We found higher levels of total IgE in patients sensitized to staphylococcus-derived exotoxins compared to non-sensitized patients. On the other hand IgE-antibodies with specificity to SEA or SEB were not detectable in patients with high amounts of total IgE and low SCORAD score, a fact which demonstrates the specificity of the assay.

A Sensitization to SEB, but Not to SEA, Is Associated with a High SCORAD Score

The statistical analysis revealed a statistically significant difference in clinical severity as determined by means of the SCORAD when SEB-IgE positive patients were compared with SEB-IgE negative patients (median values 50.4 and 33.3 points, respectively, $p < 0.0001$) (Fig. 1). There was no significant difference when

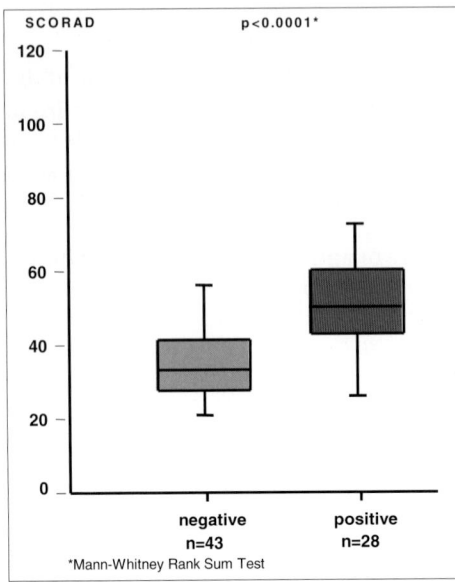

SCORAD   p<0.0001*

Fig. 1. Clinical severity of atopic dermatitis assessed by SCORAD score in patients sensitized to SEB compared with patients not sensitized to SEB. *Horizontal lines* indicate median values of SCORAD points, *boxes* show the 25th and 75th percentile. *Mann-Whitney rank sum test, $p<0.0001$

patients who were sensitized to SEA and patients who were not sensitized to SEA were compared (p=0.156).

A Sensitization to Staphylococcal Exotoxins
Is Associated with Elevated Eosinophil Protein Concentrations

ECP concentration was analysed in the sera of all patients (n=71, median value 13.8 µg/l, range 2.09 to 114.0 µg/l). Serum ECP levels were significantly higher in patients sensitized to SEB compared to non-sensitized patients (median values 22.7 and 12.9 µg/l, p=0.018) (Fig. 2a). There was also a significant difference when SEA-sensitized and non-sensitized patients were compared (median values 22.7 and 12.0 µg/l, p=0.0038).

Urine samples were obtained for analysis of EPX concentration from 35 of 71 patients (median value 103.1 µg/mmol creatinine, range 26.3 to 390 µg/mmol creatinine). Urine EPX levels were significantly higher in patients sensitized to SEB than in non-sensitized patients (median values 176.3 and 73.3 µg/mmol creatinine, p=0.0096) (Fig. 2b). A significant difference could not be shown when SEA-IgE positive/negative patients were compared (p=0.2338).

S. aureus-Reactive T-Cell Lines
Are Superantigen-Reactive and Exotoxin-Specific

T-cell lines were derived from lesional skin and peripheral blood of 3 patients with severe atopic dermatitis, who were colonized with toxigenic *S. aureus* strains (pa-

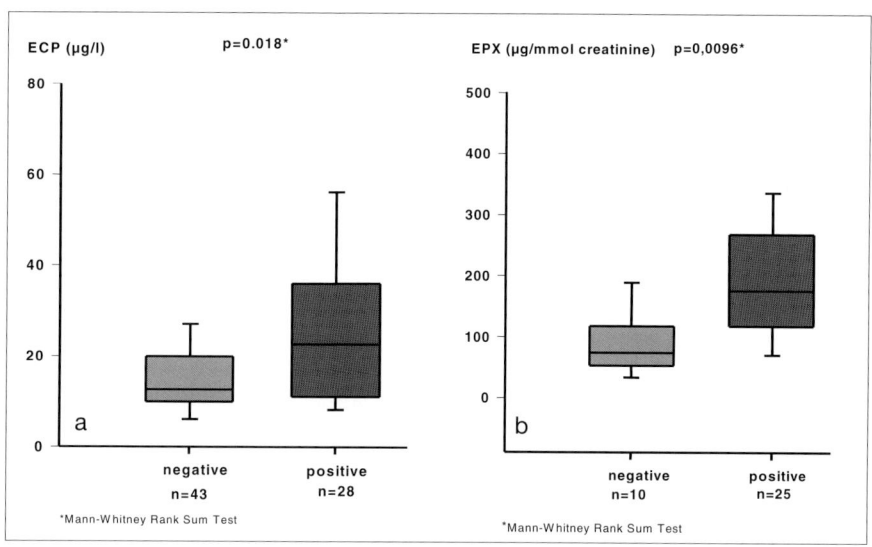

Fig. 2a,b. Serum ECP levels of patients sensitized to SEB in comparison with patients not sensitized to SEB. *Horizontal lines* represent median ECP levels, *boxes contain* the 25th and 75th percentile. *Mann-Whitney rank sum test, p=0.018. **b** Urine EPX levels of patients sensitized to SEB compared with patients who are not sensitized to SEB. *Horizontal lines* indicate median EPX concentrations, *boxes* represent the 25th and 75th percentile. *Mann-Whitney rank sum test, p=0.0096

tient 1: SEC, patient 2: SED, patient 3: SEC) Patient 1 and 2 were also sensitized to the respective toxin, patient 3 was not sensitized to the toxin detected on his skin. The partners of patient 1 and 2 were investigated for the colonization with toxigenic *S. aureus* strains. Interestingly, *S. aureus* could be isolated from the anterior nares and these strains produced the same toxins as the strains isolated from the patients.

T-cell lines growing in the presence of staphylococcal exotoxins were picked out of the lower cell concentrations and were restimulated with the respective exotoxin (patient 1, 3: SEC2, patient 2: SED) in the presence of autologous and allogeneic antigen presenting cells in separate cultures.

Taken together, 36 exotoxin-reactive TCL were obtained from the skin of patient 1, 2 and 3. Of these 36 lines, 12 (33,3%) could be stimulated only in the presence of autologous antigen-presenting cells (SI≥3) and were thus regarded as al-

Table 1. Exotoxin-reactive TCL derived from skin and blood of three patients with severe atopic dermatitis

Patient no.	Exotoxins produced by colonizing *S. aureus*	Skin Allergen-specific TCL	Superantigen-reactive TCL	Blood Allergen-specific TCL	Superantigen-reactive TCL
1	SEC	4/16 (25%)	12/16 (75%)	7/9 (77.8%)	2/9 (22.2%)
2	SED	4/13 (30.8%)	9/13 (69.2%)	0/7 (0%)	7/7 (100%)
3	SEC	4/7 (57.1%)	3/7 (42.9%)	5/12 (41.7%)	7/12 (58.3%)
All	SEC/SED	12/36 (33.3%)	24/36 (66.7%)	12/28 (42.9%)	16/28 (57.1%)

Table 2. Stimulation indices of cutaneous allergen-specific and superantigen-reactive TCL

	Autologous APC (S.I.) (mean±SD)	Allogeneic APC (S.I.) (mean±SD)
Patient 1		
Allergen-specific TCL	4.4±1.2 (*p=0.018*)*	1.6±0.4
Superantigen-reactive TCL	45.8±62.5 (*p=0.018*)*	18.4±52.0
Patient 2		
Allergen-specific TCL	4.9±1.8 (*p=0.037*)*	1.8±0.95
Superantigen-reactive TCL	17.9±11.8 (*p=0.037*)*	12.8±8.1
Patient 3		
Allergen-specific TCL	6.6±2.6 (*p=0.025*)*	2.5±0.96
Superantigen-reactive TCL	35.1±18.4 (*p=0.025*)*	52.9±81.2

*Mann-Whitney rank sum test.

lergen-specific. 24 (66.7%) could be stimulated with autologous and allogeneic antigen-presenting cells and were thus regarded as superantigen-reactive (Table 1). 28 TCL were generated from the peripheral blood. 12 (48.9%) of these TCL proved to be allergen specific, 16 (57.1%) were superantigen-reactive. The data for each of the three patients are presented in detail in Table 1.

The stimulation indices of the superantigen-reactive cells were significantly higher than the indices of allergen-specific lines when restimulated in the presence of autologous APC in cutaneous and blood derived TCL. Table 2 shows the stimulation indices of the cutaneous TCL derived from patient 1.

Expression of TCR-Vβ Elements on Skin- or Blood-Derived TCL

TCL derived from lesional skin and blood of patient 1 were randomly selected for phenotyping of TCR-Vβ elements. The superantigen-reactive TCL were found to express the SEC-reactive TCR-Vβ elements on their surface, the allergen-specific TCL did not express any SEC-reactive TCR-Vβ element (Table 3).

Table 3. T-cell lines derived from skin and blood of patient 1 and their expression of TCR-Vβ elements

	Autologous APC S.I.	Allogeneic APC S.I.	TCR-Vβ
Blood			
B 10	4.6	2.6	*
B 1	5.5	6.1	13
Skin			
H 9	4.3	1.6	*
H 23	10.5	19.0	13.17

*No superantigen-reactive TCR-Vb elements could be detected.

Discussion

Our results demonstrate that staphylococcal exotoxins exacerbate atopic dermatitis not only as superantigens but to a great extent also as „conventional" allergens.

Numerous studies have investigated the pathophysiological mechanisms leading from the colonization with toxigenic *S. aureus* strains to cutaneous inflammation. T-lymphocytes have been proven to play a central role in this process. There is strong evidence that at least two different mechanisms are involved in the activation of T-cells by staphylococcal exotoxins, which have been shown to penetrate into the dermis when applied on the skin of healthy and atopic subjects [19, 20]: firstly, the exotoxins may act as superantigens, secondly, they may induce the generation of exotoxin-specific T-cells able to promote the generation of exotoxin-specific IgE antibodies in their function as conventional allergens. Different studies suggest, that both pathways are involved in the pathogenesis of atopic dermatitis. However, it is not clear to date, if one of these mechanisms predominates and if subgroups of patients differ concerning the mechanism by which exotoxins exacerbate their atopic dermatitis.

To investigate to which extent staphylococcal exotoxins activate T-cells as superantigens or as allergens we generated exotoxin-reactive TCL from lesional skin and blood of three adult patients suffering from a longstanding severe atopic dermatitis who were colonized with exotoxin-reactive *S. aureus* strains.

Both allergen (exotoxin)-specific and superantigen-reactive TCL could be generated from skin and blood of these patients, which confirms the involvement of both mechanisms in the process of T-cell activation.

Due to the strong mitogenic potential of superantigens, one would expect a large proportion of the cutaneous TCL to be superantigen-reactive, i.e. to proliferate upon incubation with exotoxins in the presence of autologous and allogeneic APC in restimulation experiments. In two of our patients about 70% (75%/69.2%) and in one patient 42.9% of all cutaneous exotoxin-reactive TCL were superantigen-reactive. The stimulation indices of the superantigen-reactive TCL were significantly higher compared to the stimulation indices of the allergen-specific TCL when stimulated in the presence of autologous APC, which points to a higher degree of activation. Strickland et al could demonstrate that the colonization with toxigenic *S. aureus* strains is associated with an expansion of T-cells expressing the appropriate TCR-Vβ chains among the CLA positive T-cell subset in the peripheral blood [22]. Recently, a shift in the intradermal TCR-Vβ repertoire corresponding to the respective superantigen was found in lesional skin of children with atopic dermatitis by immunohistochemical staining [15] and skin biopsy specimens obtained from SEB-treated areas demonstrated a selective accumulation of T cells expressing SEB-reactive TCR-Vβ elements [20]. Our results confirm this mechanism. Furthermore we investigated superantigen-reactive and allergen-specific TCL isolated from skin and peripheral blood of patient 1, who was colonized with SEC producing strains for the expression of TCR-Vβ elements. Superantigen-reactive TCL were found to express the SEC-reactive TCR-Vβ-chains 13 and 17 on their surface, which confirms the immunohistological features found in lesional skin by Bunikowski and Skov et al. In contrast, allergen-specific TCL did not express any SEC-reactive TCR-Vβ elements.

Surprisingly, a relatively high proportion (33.3%) of cutaneous TCL were allergen-specific and could be stimulated with exotoxins only in the presence of autologous APC. These data demonstrate, that there is also a significant exotoxin (allergen)-specific cutaneous T-cell response in these patients, who had toxin-specific IgE in the peripheral blood in two cases. One can speculate, that staphylococcal exotoxins may exacerbate skin lesions in atopic dermatitis through the same mechanism which is now widely accepted for inhalant allergens. We determined toxin-specific IgE in a group of 71 adult patients with mild to severe atopic dermatitis and could show that sensitizations to staphylococcal enterotoxin B (SEB) is associated with severe atopic dermatitis in adults. The severity of skin lesions was quantified with the SCORAD index. In addition to the SCORAD, serum ECP and urine EPX levels were elevated in patients sensitized to SEB. The serum concentration of ECP has been shown to be a sensitive measure of disease activity in allergic asthma and atopic dermatitis [23–25]. A clear relationship could also be demonstrated between urine EPX concentration and disease activity in asthma [26] and in atopic dermatitis [27]. For anti-SEA specific IgE, we could demonstrate an association only with serum ECP concentrations and not with EPX concentrations as with SCORAD. In keeping with our results, Nomura et al. were able to show that the severity of atopic dermatitis is related to the level of SEB-specific IgE, and not to the level of SEA- and TSST-1-specific IgE in children and adolescents with AD [28].

These findings suggest a higher immunogenicity of SEB than SEA in patients with atopic dermatitis. Staphylococcal enterotoxins can be differentiated into two groups due to their amino-acid sequence. SEA and SED are similar, as are SEB and SEC [18]. Therefore SEB and SEC might be more immunogenic due to their molecular structure. However, Bunikowski et al found a relationship between a sensitization to the staphylococcal exotoxins A and B and the severity of atopic dermatitis in children [17]. The presence of exotoxins on the skin could lead to a release of proinflammatory mediators from cutaneous mast cells and a subsequent pruritus and scratching. Furthermore the toxins may bind to specific IgE on the surface of Langerhans cells thus leading to the activation of specific T cells.

Interestingly, a relatively high proportion of allergen-specific TCL could be isolated from the skin of patient 3, who had no specific IgE to the respective toxin, as compared to patients 1 and 2 who were also sensitized to the cutaneous exotoxins. Therefore T-cell-dependent mechanisms which do not involve the production of specific IgE antibodies are likely to contribute to the cutaneous inflammation. Recently, Akdis et al could show that SEB induced a significant proliferation of T-lymphocytes derived from lesional skin of patients with both the extrinsic and the intrinsic form of atopic dermatitis in a dose dependent manner [29]. In contrast to T-lymphocytes derived from the skin of patients with the extrinsic form of AD, cells from patients with intrinsic atopic dermatitis failed to produce significant amounts of IL-13 upon incubation with SEB, which could therefore be unable to offer help to B cells to produce specific IgE in these patients.

In summary our results confirm the importance of *S. aureus* and staphylococcal exotoxins as important trigger factors of adult atopic dermatitis. We could demonstrate that both superantigen-reactive T-cells and exotoxin (allergen)-specific T-cells play a crucial role in the pathogenesis of atopic dermatitis. Furthermore we found a relationship between the severity and a sensitization to staphylococcal enterotoxin B. We conclude that the staphylococcal exotoxins exacerbate atopic dermatitis not only as superantigens but to a great extent also as „conventional" allergens leading to the generation of exotoxin-specific IgE. Furthermore, our data suggest, that exotoxin (allergen)-specific T-lymphocytes perpetuate the chronic inflammation via pathways which do not involve the induction of specific IgE antibodies.

Further studies have to characterize the T-cell response to staphylococcal exotoxins specifically in the IgE-independent (intrinsic) form of atopic dermatitis.

References

1. Kapp A. Atopic dermatitis – the skin manifestation of atopy. Clin Exp Allergy 1995;25:210–9.
2. Werfel T, Kapp A. Environmental and other major provocation factors in atopic dermatitis. Allergy 1998;53:731–9.
3. Reekers R, Schmidt P, Kapp A., Werfel T. Evidence of a lymphocyte response to birch pollen related food antigens in atopic dermatitis. J Allergy Clin Immunol 1999;104:466–72.
4. Sager N, Feldmann A, Schilling G, Kreitsch P, Neumann C. House dust mite-specific T cells in the skin of subjects with atopic dermatitis: Frequency and lymphokine profile in the allergen patch test. J Allergy Clin Immunol 1992;89:801–10.
5. van Reijsen FC, Bruijnzeel-Koomen CA, Kalthoff FS, Maggi E, Romagnani S, Westland JK et al. Skin derived aeroallergen-specific T-cell clones of Th2 phenotype in patients with atopic dermatitis. J Allergy Clin Immunol 1992;90:184–93.
6. Werfel T, Ahlers G, Schmidt P, Boeker M, Kapp A, Neumann C. Milk-responsive atopic dermatitis is associated with a casein-specific lymphocyte response in adolescent and adult patients. J Allergy Clin Immunol 1997;99:124–33.
7. Mudde GC, von Reijsen FC, Boland GJ, Gast GC, Bruijnzeel PL, Bruijnzeel-Koomen CA. Allergen presentation by epidermal Langerhans cells from patients with atopic dermatitis is mediated by IgE. Immunology 1990;69:335–41.
8. Werfel T, Morita A, Grewe M, Renz H, Wahn U, Krutmann J et al. Allergen-specificity of skin-infiltrating T-cells is not restricted to a type 2 cytokine pattern in chronic skin lesions of atopic dermatitis. J Invest Dermatol 1996;107:871–6.
9. Aly R. Bacteriology of atopic dermatitis. Acta Dermatol Venereol Stockh 1980;Suppl.92:16–8.
10. Hauser C, Wuethrich B, Matter L, Wilhelm JA, Sonnabend W, Schopfer K. Staphylococcus aureus skin colonization in atopic dermatitis. Dermatologica 1985;170:35–9.
11. Leyden JE, Marples RR, Kligmann AM. Staphylococcus aureus in the lesions of atopic dermatitis. Br J Dermatol 1974;90:525–30.
12. Leung DYM, Harbeck R, Bina P, Reiser R, Yang E, Norris DA et al. Presence of IgE antibodies to staphylococcal exotoxins on the skin of patients with atopic dermatitis. J Clin Invest 1993;92:1374–80.
13. Williams REA, Gibson AG, Aitchison TC, Lever R, Mackie RM. Assessment of contact plate sampling technique and subsequent quantitative bacterial studies in atopic dermatitis. Br J Dermatol 1990;123:493–501.
14. Akiyama H, Toi Y, Kanzaki H, Tada J, Arata J. Prevalence of producers of enterotoxins and the toxic shock syndrome toxin-1 among Staphylococcus aureus strains isolated from atopic dermatitis lesions. Arch Dermatol Res 1996;288:418–20.
15. Bunikowski R, Mielke M, Skarabis H, Worm M, Anagnostopoulos I, Kolde G et al. Evidence for a disease-promoting effect of Staphylococcus aureus-derived exotoxins in atopic dermatitis. J Allergy Clin Immunol 2000;105:814–9.

16. McFadden JP, Noble WC, Camp RDR. Superantigenic exotoxin-secreting potential of staphylococci isolated from atopic ekzematous skin. Br J Dermatol 2000;128:631-2.
17. Bunikowski R, Mielke M, Skarabis H, Herz U, Bergmann RL, Wahn U et al. Prevalence and role of serum IgE antibodies to S. aureus-derived superantigens SEA and SEB in children with atopic dermatitis. J Allergy Clin Immunol 1999;103:119-24.
18. Marrack P, Kappler J. The staphylococcal exotoxins and their relatives. Science 1990;248:705-11.
19. Strange P, Lone S, Lisby S, Nielsen PL, Baadsgaard O. Staphylococcal enterotoxin B applied on intact normal and intact atopic skin induces dermatitis. Arch Dermatol 1996;132:27-33.
20. Skov L, Olsen JV, Giorno R, Schlievert PM, Baadsgaard O, Leung DYM. Application of staphylococcal enterotoxin B on normal and atopic skin induces up-regulation of T cells by a superantigen-mediated mechanism. J Allergy Clin Immunol 2000;105:820-6.
21. Taswell C. Limiting dilution assays for the determination of immunocompetent cell frequencies. J Immunol 1981;126:1614.
22. Strickland I, Hauk PJ, Trumble A, Picker LJ, Leung DY. Evidence for superantigen involvement in skin homing of T cells in atopic dermatitis. J Invest Dermatol 1999;112:249-53.
23. Kapp A, Czech W, Krutmann J, Schöpf E. Eosinophil cationic protein in sera of patients with atopic dermatitis. J Am Acad Dermatol 1991;24:555-8.
24. Koller DY, Herouy Y, Götz M, Hagel E, Urbanek R, Eichler I. Clinical value of monitoring eosinophil activity in asthma. Arch Dis Child 1995;73:413-7.
25. Kapp A. The role of eosinophils in the pathogenesis of atopic dermatitis – eosinophil granule proteins as markers of disease activity. Allergy 1993;48:1-5.
26. Kristjansson S, Strannegard IL, Strannegard O, Peterson C, Enander I, Wennegren G. Urinary eosinophil protein X in children with atopic asthma: a useful marker of antiinflammatory treatment. J Allergy Clin Immunol 1996;97(1179):1187.
27. Pucci N, Lombardi E., Novembre E, Farina S, Bernardini R, Rossi E et al. Urinary eosinophil protein X and serum eosinophil cationic protein in infants and children with atopic dermatitis: correlation with disease activity. J Allergy Clin Immunol 2000;105:353-7.
28. Nomura I, Tanaka K, Tomita H, Katsunama T, Ohya Y, Ikeda N et al. Evaluation of staphylococcal exotoxin and its specific IgE in childhood atopic dermatitis. J Allergy Clin Immunol 1999;104(441):446.
29. Akdis CA, Akdis M, Simon D, Dibbert B, Weber M, Gratzl S et al. T cells and T cell-derived cytokines as pathogenic factors in the non-allergic form of atopic dermatitis. J Invest Dermatol 1999;113:628-34.

Food Allergy and Anaphylaxis

21 Peanut Allergy: Are Clinical Symptoms Associated with IgE-Reactivity to Certain (Recombinant) Peanut Allergens?

W.M. Becker, T. Kleber-Janke, U. Lepp

Abstract

Data on the prevalence of food allergy are limited but estimated at 1.4–1.8% of the general population and at nearly 7% of the child population. The IgE mediated food allergy is caused by aeroallergen associated food allergens and by „real" food allergens, without such association.

It is the current opinion, that most food allergies caused by the first group elicit mild clinical symptoms, whereas the group of food allergens without aeroallergen association are factors in causing severe to fatal clinical reactions. This opinion should be revised. Progress in the identification of allergens in allergenic source material shows that typical birch pollen associated foods such as apple or peach contain amongst others Lipid Transfer Proteins (LTP) which may cause strong clinical symptoms whereas peanuts, one of the strongest allergenic sources, contain profilin which may be the reason why patients eating peanut react only with mild symptoms. Moreover, peanuts elicit a number of different allergic symptoms with differing degrees of severity. These clinical symptoms are amongst others the oral allergy syndrome, atopic dermatitis, asthma, diarrhoea, and/or anaphylactic reactions. Since peanuts contain several allergenic components, the question arises whether these components are associated with distinct clinical symptoms or the severity of the clinical reaction. This would improve diagnostics, it would allow monitoring of the development of the disease and it would improve prevention. The non plus ultra would be the identification of anaphylaxis inducing allergens.

A prerequisite of answering these questions is the identification and characterisation of the whole set of peanut allergens on a molecular level. With the aid of the phage display system we were able to clone six different allergens. Two of them were the well known major allergens of peanut Ara h 1 and Ara h 2. Ara h 4, Ara h 5 (profilin), Ara h 6 and Ara h 7 are first described in their structure deduced from the DNA-sequence.

Correlation of clinical data of peanut allergic patients with the IgE reactivity to certain peanut allergens are not revealed without further analysis. Whether the measurement of intensity of IgE reactivity to certain peanut allergens by binding assays provides clearer associations between clinical symptoms and these allergens is now under investigation. If the outcome of this study is not sufficient, then we will try to improve the peanut allergy diagnostis on the basis of allergen substructures, e.g. linear versus conformational epitopes.

New Trends in Allergy V
J. Ring, H. Behrendt (Eds.)
© Springer-Verlag Berlin, Heidelberg 2002

Introduction

The most urgent problems in food allergy are diagnostics and therapy. According to the well known questionnaire of Young and co-workers [1] nearly 20% of respondents feel ill from food allergy, whereas only 1.8% of the population of the study suffer from food allergy as verified by allergists. These findings are in accordance with our own study, which could only confirm food allergy in 10% of patients referred with such a diagnosis [2]. However, a clear diagnosis is important from the point of view of allergen avoidance in order not to restrict the prohibited food stuff beyond the absolutely necessary level. In this context the study of Bernhisel-Broadbent and Sampson [3] is enlightening. They evaluated the clinical relevance of patients' cross-reactivity to various legumes by using the double blind placebo controlled food challenge (DBPCFC). They found that out of 43 patients tested only two reacted with a second legume regardless of extensive immunologic cross-reactivity among legume antigens on immunoblot.

There are three desirable results from in vitro diagnostis of type-1-allergy, giving optimally:
1. Identification of the offending allergen with 100% sensitivity and specificity
2. Prediction of the severity of the disease and
3. Duration of the allergy, i.e. transient or persistent

Until now the most important part of the diagnostics of allergies has been to evaluate the case history of patients, followed by in vitro and in vivo tests whereby the double blind placebo controlled challenge test has for some allergists the ranking of a golden standard. However this procedure is inconvenient for patients, time consuming and only practicable for special medical facilities. Therefore improvement of in vitro diagnostics is urgent needed. Ultimately success in creating tests with 100% sensitivity and specificity is likely to be found in single allergenic components or allergen substructures up to linear epitopes. An absolute precondition of achieving this result are sera of patients diagnosed to a very high clinical standard and controls in statistically sufficient numbers. This will be the crucial point in setting up assays for predicting the severity of the disease and the duration of the allergy, i.e. transient or persistent.

The Quality of In Vitro Tests

According to Ortolani [4] and others [5, 6] the in vitro tests for diagnosing food allergy have a poor predictive value since in vitro tests with a 100% sensitivity and specificity are hardly available [7] (Tables 1, 2).

This is owing to the poor quality of food extracts [7], cross reactivity between extracts or substances like carbohydrates with unknown clinical relevance [8].

One way of improving the in vitro diagnostic is to enhance the quality of the extracts or to use single allergenic components purified from natural extracts or recombinant allergens and their substructures. There is a growing body of evidence that clinical symptoms may be associated with allergenic structures.

Table 1. Clinical validation of in vitro assays: definitions [7]

Diagnostic sensitivity (SE):
   Diseased
   Number of true positive test results
   Number of true positive and number of false negative test results
Diagnostic specificity (SP):
   Not diseased
   Number of true negative test results
   Number of true negative and number of false positive test results
Positive predictive value (PPV):
   Number of true positive test results (diseased)
   Number of true positive (diseased) and of false positive (not diseased) test results

Table 2. Sensitivity and specificity of Cap tests of some food allergens (references)

Cap test	% Sensitivity	% Specificity
Cod	100	87 (6)
Egg white	100	100 (4)
	100	79 (5)
Egg yolk	89	83 (5)
Peanut	100	38 (4)
Soya	100	62 (4)
Wheat	100	41 (4)

Are Clinical Symptoms of Type-1 Allergy Associated with Certain Allergens?

We know that Bet v 1 analogous structures in apple or peach are associated with the Oral Allergy Syndrome (OAS) whereas rare but severe reactions to peach are caused by Lipid Transfer Proteins [9]. Thus the oversimplified view that aero-allergen associated foods elicit mild allergic reactions like the Oral Allergy Syndrome has to be corrected. Conversely real food allergens like peanut, which has the potency to cause severe allergic reactions contain allergenic components such as profilin which has the reputation for eliciting only mild symptoms.

Hence we can hypothesise that in future in vitro diagnostic based on single allergenic components will be an improvement if clinical symptoms are predictable and followed by therapeutic implications. The therapeutic implications are provision for the patients with an emergency kit for self medication, an immunotherapy against certain hazardous allergens if available or a clear avoidance strategy.

That this hypothesis is not a complete fiction was shown by findings of Cooke and Sampson who could associate transient egg allergy to conformational epitopes of ovomucoid (Gal d 1) whereas persistent egg allergy showed significant quantities of IgE to linear epitopes of Gal d 1 [10]. For α_{s1}-casein Chatchatee et al. could show similar findings on epitope level, where persistent milk allergy was correlated with IgE reactivity to linear epitopes [11].

The State of In Vitro Diagnostics of Peanut Allergy

Peanut allergy is an ideal paradigm for the verification of this hypothesis since peanut elicits a wide spectrum of clinical symptoms such as urticaria, eczema, sneezing, cough, asthma, OAS, vomiting, diarrhoea or anaphylaxis which become manifest on different organs. It focuses on the question, whether certain symptoms are associated with certain allergens or their substructures and whether the severity of the symptoms are correlated with the amount of specific IgE. A prerequisite of answering these questions is the identification and characterisation of these components on molecular level.

An ideal method of cloning the allergenic entities completely is the phage display system where patients' IgE is the selection and enrichment agent. In this system the presented allergen and its gene containing phages are selected by patients' IgE using the panning method. The selected phages are multiplied in *E. coli* and in the next cycle selected and enriched and so on. After five cycles we were able to clone six different allergens [12].

Two of them were the well known major allergens of peanut Ara h 1 and Ara h 2. Ara h 4, Ara h 5 (profilin), Ara h 6 and Ara h 7 are first described in their structure deduced from the DNA-sequence. Ara h 4, Ara h 6 and Ara h 7 show significant sequence similarities to seed storage proteins whereby Ara h 6 and 7 belongs to the conglutin family. They are not isoforms of Ara h 2 but independent gene products. Ara h 3 is an isoform of Ara h 4 with 91% identity whereby Ara h 4 has the priority over Ara h 3 with regard to the time of registration in the data base and announcement to nomenclature subcommittee of the IUIS [13]. Testing the IgE reactivity of peanut allergic patients by Western blotting we found that Ara h 1, Ara h 2 and Ara h 4 was recognised by more than 50% of 49 tested patients. Thus, in accordance with literature [14] Ara h 1, Ara h 2 and Ara h 4 (Ara h 3) belong to the major allergens of peanut. Ara h 5, Ara h 6 and Ara h 7 are identified by more than 10% of the patients and are of intermediate frequency.

As source of recombinant allergens performing Western blots we used cell lysates of the expression system. However, for quantifying assays purified recombinant allergen is needed. Apart from the peanut profilin (Ara h 5) we have difficulties in expressing the other recombinant peanut allergens with a satisfactory yield. As cause we identified a different codon usages between *E. coli* and peanut with regard to arginine.

We overcame the codon usage problem by using BL21 (DE3) Codon Plus RIL cells (Stratagene) providing the needed rare tRNAs for the proper expression. In these cells we were able to express Ara h 2 and Ara h 1 and Ara h 6 in excellent yields [15]. That opens the way to investigate the question whether certain peanut allergens are associated with clinical symptoms and the severity of the clinical reactions.

On the basis of eight clinically characterised peanut allergic patient we found at the first glance no difference in the IgE reaction pattern of shock patients and patients with OAS to peanut extract. The fact that recombinant Ara h 6 is detected by patients with shock symptoms and urticaria but not by patients with an isolated Oral Allergy Syndrome (OAS) may be a hint that Ara h 6 is a candidate to be associated with severe clinical reactions. This is underlined by the findings of Sellers, a co-worker of Teubers group [16], who could show that Ara h 6 is resistant to pepsin degradation. It is obvious that it is not possible to establish a sensitive and specific diagnostic for at least ten distinct clinical symptoms on the basis of six allergens. Thus we have to ask which factors influence the clinical reaction? First of all the allergen and its place of contact with the organism: That may be the skin, the mucosa of the upper gastrointestinal tract, of the lower gastrointestinal tract or the respiratory tract by generation of aerosols: eating with open mouth and breathing or for example the exposure to peanuts when served in aeroplanes.

On molecular level this tackles the fate of degradation of the allergen, its pathway of degradation in the organism and the interaction with the immune system. How is the allergen presented to the immune system, as intact molecule or in fragments?

Is There a Possibility of Differentiating Clinical Symptoms by Substructures of Peanut Allergens?

We know from Burks and co-workers that the peanut allergens Ara h 1, 2 and 3 contain at least 23, 10 or 4 linear epitopes respectively [17–19] in contrast to tree pollen allergens such as Bet v 1 or Profilin which present preferably conformational epitopes. Thus these substructures may have a predictive value.

Why should peanut allergens not contain conformational and linear epitopes on the same molecule? Why should the different reactions of patients to peanut allergen not have a molecular basis?

For instance, patients with mild mouth itching might react with a conformational epitope of a certain allergen; even under denaturing conditions like cooking or baking or degradation of the allergen patients' IgE may react to parts of the conformational epitope but with lower affinity of the IgE. Thus the maturing immune system has a chance to develop other immunoglobulin-isotypes with higher affinity competing with the IgE resulting in the well known phenomenon of growing out of the allergy.

Conclusion

The improvement of diagnostics and therapy especially of food allergy is urgently needed. On the paradigm of peanut allergy it was shown that this problem is not solvable on the basis of extracts but hopefully on single allergenic components or their substructures.

Future Prospects

We have now the instruments to solve the problems of diagnostics and therapy of food allergy. The time of immunoblots without validity and unreadable sequences is over. Now the quality of diagnostics is part of the clinicians. The patients need the cooperation between bench workers and clinicians because the progress in diagnostics and therapy definitively depends on the quality of the clinical diagnostic and convincing arguments to persuade patients to cooperate with research.

References

1. Young E, Stoneham MD, Petruckevitch A, Barton J, Rona R (1994). A population study of food intolerance. Lancet 343:1127–1130
2. Lepp U, Birke R, Schlaak M (1997). Selbstdiagnose „Nahrungsmittelallergie": Grund zu differenzierter Diagnostik. Allergo J 6:412–416
3. Bernhisel-Broadbent J, Taylor S, Sampson HA (1989). Cross-allergenicity in the legume botanical family in children with food hypersensitivity. II. Laboratory correlates. J Allergy Clin Immunol 84:701–709
4. Ispano M, Colafrancesco M, Ansaloni R, Vighi G, Ortolani C (1996). Comparison of the Results of Skin Prick Tests, CAP System and ENEA System in the Diagnosis of Food Allergy. In Highlights in Food Allergy, Wüthrich B, Ortolani C (eds): . Monogr Allergy. Basel, Karger, vol 32, pp 181–186
5. Norgaard A (1992).Type I allergy to egg and milk in adults (PhD thesis). National University Hospital, University of Copenhagen, Copenhagen
6. Hansen TK Bindslev-Jensen C, Skov PS, Poulsen LK (1996).Codfish allergy in adults. Specific tests for IgE and histamine release versuss double blind placebo controlled challenges. Clin Exp Allergy 26:1276–12856
7. Bindslev-Jensen C, Poulsen LK (1997). In vitro diagnostic methods in the evaluation of food hypersensitivity. In Food Allergy. Adverse reactions to foods and food additives. Metcalfe DD, Sampson HA Simon RA (eds)Blackwell Science, Oxford, UK, pp 137–150
8. Aalberse RC, van Ree R (1996). Cross-reactive carbohydrate determinants.In Highlights in Food Allergy, Wüthrich B, Ortolani C (eds): . Monogr Allergy. Basel, Karger, vol 32, pp 78–83
9. Pastorello EA, Farioli L, Pravettoni V, Ortolani C, Ispano M, Monza M, Baroglio C, Scibola E, Ansaloni R, Incorvaia C, Conti A: The major allergen of peach (Prunus persica) is a lipid transfer protein. J Allergy Clin Immunol 1999; 103:520–526
10. Cooke SK, Sampson HA (1997). Allergenic properties of ovomucoid in man. J Immunol159: 2026–2032
11. Chatchatee P, Kirsit -Marjut J, Bardina L, Beyer K, Sampson HA (2001). identification of IgE and IgG-binding epitopes on casein: Differences in patients with persistent and transient cow's milk allergy. J Allergy Clin Immunol 107: 379–383
12. Kleber-Janke T, Crameri R, Appenzeller U, Schlaak M, Becker WM: Selective cloning of peanut allergens, including profilin and 2S albumins, by phage display technology. Int. Arch. Allergy Immunol. 1999;119:265–274
13 Becker WM Becker, Kleber-Janke T, Lepp U (2001). Four novel recombinant peanut allergens: more information – more problems. Int Arch Allergy Immunol 124:100–102
14. Bannon GA, Besler M, Hefle SI, Hourihane JO'B SichererSH (2000). Allergen Data collection: Peanut (Arachis hypogaea). Internet Symposium on Food Allergens 2:87–123. http://www.food-allergens.de
15. Kleber-Janke T and Becker W-M (2000). Use of modified BL21(DE3) E. coli cells for high level Expression of recombinant peanut allergens affected by poor codon usage. Protein Express Purif 19 :419–24
16. Sellers CL, Teuber SS, Buchanan BB, Chen L (2000). Peanut protein digestibility: a gastric and intestinal model. J Allergy Clin Immunol 105:140
17. Burks AW, Shin D, Cockrell G, Stanley JS, Helm RM, Bannon GA (1997). Mapping and mutational analysis of the IgE-binding epitopes on Ara h 1, a legume vicilin protein and a major allergen in peanut hypersensitivity. Eur J Biochem 245:334–339

18. Stanley JS, King N, Burks AW, Huang SK, Sampson H, Cockrell G, Helm RM, West CM, Bannon GA (1997). Identification and mutational analysis of the immunodominant IgE binding epitopes of the major peanut allergen Ara h 2. Arch Biochem Biophys 342:244–253
19. Rabjohn P, Helm EM, Stanley JS, West CM, Sampson HA, Burks AW, Bannon GA (1999). Molecular cloning and epitope analysis of the peanut allergen Ara h 3. Clin Invest 103:535–42

22 Challenge Tests with Food Additives and Aspirin in the Diagnostics of Chronic Urticaria. A Case of Immediate Cutaneous Hypersensitivity to Sodium Bisulphite (E-222) Confirmed by Patch Testing

M. Kurek, E. Grubska-Suchanek

Abstract

Various symptoms and diseases are attributed to intolerance or allergy to food additives. Both are phenomena of individual hypersensitivity although allergies only are triggered by specific immunological mechanisms. Some food additives and some drugs, especially aspirin, have been accused of exacerbating chronic urticaria and angioedema, asthma, or provoking anaphylactoid reactions. We investigated 37 patients with chronic, active urticaria and histories suggestive of food or/and aspirin related exacerbations. Double blind, placebo controlled challenges with tartrazine, methyl-paraben, p-hydroxy-benzoate, sodium benzoate, indigotine, quinolone yellow, sodium glutamate, sodium bisulphite, and acetyl salicylic acid were performed in 18 patients who became symptom-free during the elimination diet. Skin tests with food additives were performed in all patients following the prick and patch test technique. Positive reactions to single, or multiple oral challenges were found in 8 patients. In one case, positive reaction to oral challenge with sodium bisulphite was associated with a local wheal and flare skin reaction by patch testing corresponding to IgE-mediated sulphite hypersensitivity. The discrepancy between the responsiveness to additive-free diet and the positive rate of oral challenges with individual additives was remarkable. This strongly suggests that food additives, which are not labelled, or natural food compounds might exacerbate chronic urticaria.

Introduction

The food additives used first were sulphating agents. The Romans burned sulphur to produce sulphur dioxide, which was then bubbled through wine to prevent further fermentation and microbial contamination. An increase in additive intake occurred in the 19th and 20th century. This was related to tinned food, with a very rapid increase since the 1950s arising from the fast-food restaurants. Today, there are preservatives, stabilisers, conditioners, colourings, flavourings, sweeteners, antioxidants, and other natural or artificial additives used in mass-produced, pre-packed foods. Estimates are that 2,000 to 20,000 agents are used in the food industry [1]. The most frequently recognised as able to elicit pseudo-allergic reactions are additives labelled with the E-numbers. For other agents, such

New Trends in Allergy V
J. Ring, H. Behrendt (Eds.)
© Springer-Verlag Berlin, Heidelberg 2002

documentation is poor, and for some, it is rare or uncertain. These are mostly intolerance reactions although it has been reported that IgE-mediated allergies to some ingested dyes and sulphites appear sporadically [2, 3]. There are many difficulties in identifying adverse reactions to food additives, not least because of the difference between popular concepts of food allergy and the results of objective tests. The prevalence of adverse reactions to food additives, which are labelled, has been calculated to be between 0.01–0.23% of the whole population, and approximately 2.0% in atopic children [4, 5]. The prevalence has been found to be higher, in studies performed with selected dyes and preservatives, in patients with chronic urticaria or asthma including aspirin intolerance [1, 4, 5]. Despite many studies that have attempted to establish the prevalence of food additive related exacerbations of chronic urticaria and angioedema, the true incidence of those reactions remains poorly evaluated. Unfortunately, properly controlled studies have been few. There are problems with criteria of patient selection, evaluation of urticaria-activity at the time of study, discontinuation of medications with antihistamines, and the design of oral challenges schedule [3]. We selected 37 patients with chronic, active urticaria and/or angioedema following the criterion of the history of food and/or aspirin related symptoms. Medication with antihistamines and corticosteroids was stopped, and additive-free diet was applied. For quantification of symptoms, scoring was used before the introduction of additive-free diet, and after double blind placebo controlled challenges (DBPCFC) with individual additives and aspirin [6].

Patients and Methods

These are 37 adult patients aged from 17 to 73 years (30 female and 7 male) with chronic, active urticaria and/or angioedema, in whom a standardised diagnostic and therapeutic regimen was performed. All patients reported exacerbations related to the intake of particular foods ($n=16$), particular foods and aspirin ($n=6$), unspecified foods ($n=10$), unspecified foods and aspirin ($n=2$), aspirin only ($n=1$), aspirin and other drugs ($n=2$). The patients experienced a history of urticaria/angioedema between 3 months and 27 years (54% urticaria only, 30% urticaria and angioedema, 16% angioedema only). Antihistamines and corticosteroids were stopped 7 days and 4 weeks before hospitalisation, respectively.

Evaluation of Urticaria and Angioedema Symptoms

A record of visible symptoms was performed before the introduction of additive-free diet, and after oral challenges with food additives and aspirin. For quantification of symptoms, scoring proposed by Zuberbier et al [7] was used: 0=no symptoms, 1=mild (<10 wheals or an angioedema, diameter <2 cm), 2=moderate (disseminated, non-confluent wheals of limited extension; up to 3 lesions of angioedema, each <10 cm diameter), 3=intense (large areas of confluent wheals; diameter of angioedema >10 cm). The evaluation of the challenge results was scored and performed when increasing doses of tested substances were given.

Laboratory Tests and Tests for Cold, Factitious, and Cholinergic Urticaria

On admission, blood, urine and stool tests were performed in all patients: total blood count and differential, ESR, electrolytes, glucose, liver enzymes, creatinine, urea, serum protein electrophoresis, thyroid antibodies, antinuclear antibodies (ANA), cryoglobulins, HBS-antigen, urine analysis, and culture. Three consecutive stool specimens were tested for eggs and parasites. In cases suspected of associated cold urticaria, factitious urticaria, and cholinergic urticaria, the ice cube test, test with weighted rods, or exercise to the point of sweating were performed, respectively. In patients with history suggesting chronic gastritis or gastric and/or duodenal ulcerous disease, gastroscopy followed by Helicobacter pylori urease test was performed. Specific IgE screening with common inhalative and food allergens (Phadiatop, F5x, Pharmacia CAP System) was performed in patients responding to additive-free diet only.

Additive-Free Diet

Standardised diet was given to all patients for 7 days. These were only freshly cooked, unsulphited potatoes, polished rice, water, and salt [15].

Skin Testing

Skin testing was performed in patients responding to additive-free diet. Prick (SPT) and patch tests (PT) were performed for screening of type I and type IV sensitisations in all patients. For SPT, common allergens (mites, pollens, cat and dog epithels, cow's milk, egg and fish) of commercial origin (Alergopharma, Rainbeck, Germany) were used, as well as food additives (0.01 M tartrazine, 0.01 M brilliant black, 0.01 quinollone yellow, 0.2 M sodium benzoate, 0.01 M sodium bisulphite and, 0.1% methyl-paraben) obtained from Sigma, Deisenhofen, Germany. The SPT were performed on the volar forearm. Reactions were read at 15 min, and the SPT were assessed as positive if the wheal was > 3 mm without any reaction of the negative control. As a positive control, 10 mg/ml histamine dihydrochloride was used. For patch testing, food additives 1% tartrazine, 1% brillant black, 0.1% quinolone yellow, 3% methyl-parabene, 2% sodium benzoate and 1.0% sodium bisulphite in petrolatum, and 2.0%, 10.0% in saline were used respectively. The occlusion time was 48 h. The results were read 20 min and 24 h. after the removal of the tested substances. To interpret the PT, a classification of + for erythema and slight infiltration, ++ for erythema and papules, and +++ for erythema and vesicles was used [8].

Oral Challenge Tests

The tested substances were applied orally in non-transparent gelatine capsules (Apipol-Farma, Myslenice, Poland) under double-blind, placebo-controlled con-

Table 1. Challenge schedule. Tested agents and sequential doses [6]

Day	Tested agents (mg)	8.00 h	10:00 h	12:00 h
1	Tartrazine	10	Placebo	50
2	Methylparabene	200	Placebo	400
3	Sodium benzoate	50	200	500
4	Non-azo dyes Indigotine 10 mg Quinolone yellow 10 mg	5+5	Placebo	10+10
5	Sodium glutamate	Placebo	100	500
6	Sodium bisulphite	10	50	100
7	Acetyl salicylic acid	50	250	500

ditions (DBPCFC). Potato starch in identical capsules was used as placebo. Placebo was given in relation 1:4 to verum in a randomised manner. Table 1. All objective and subjective symptoms were recorded for 24 h after the beginning of the challenges. The reaction was considered positive only when the original burst of urticaria/angioedema appeared (score > 1). When a doubtful reaction appeared, the dose was increased if previously provided. Other questionable reactions (flare, itching, or subjective symptoms only) were re-tested under the same conditions. After a clearly positive reaction, no challenges were performed with other substances for the subsequent 48 h. in order to avoid testing in a period of tachyphylaxis.

Table 2. Challenge schedule and effective doses in patient responding to methyl-paraben, glutamate, sodium benzoate and sodium bisulphite. Results of patch-testing with sodium bisulphite [6]

DBPCFC-tested agents and doses (mg)				Skin patch tests with sodium bisulphite		
Day/agent/time	8 h	10 h	12 h	Effective doses	Patch test	Patch open
1. Tartrazine	10	Placebo	50			0.2% Aqua-negative
2. Methyl-PHB	200	Placebo	400	200→400 mg	After 48 h	0.5% Aqua-negative
3. Sodium benzoate	50	200	500	200→500 mg	Wheal, flare	1.0% Aqua-negative
4. Non-azo dyes	5+5	Placebo				2% Aqua-wheal, flare
	10+10			→500 mg	After 72 h	5% Aqua-wheal, flare
5. Glutamate	Placebo	100	500	50→100 mg	Flare only	1% Petrolatum-wheal, flare
6. Sodium bisulphite	10	50	100			
7. Aspirin	50	250	500			

Results

Of the 37 patients tested, the symptoms disappeared totally in 18 (48%) within 7 days under the additive-free diet. Except for low positive ANA in one case (without clinical relevance, with a titre 1:320), other laboratory findings such as: oxyuriasis, positive tests for associated cold, factitious and cholinergic urticaria and Helicobacter infection refer to the patients not responding to the additive-free diet. In 22% ($n=4$) patients who had responded to the diet, SPT and/or sIgE screening was informative. Patch testing with food additives was informative in

Table 3. Anamnestical data and results of skin testing and sIgE screening in patients responding to additive-free diet. Individual substances eliciting positive reactions by oral testing are marked [6]

No.	Histories of food and/or aspirin related urticaria/oedema	Prick tests or/and sIgE when positive. Atopic disease when performed	Mean score before diet introduction [1–3]	DBPCFC findings when informative
1	Unspecified legumes	D. pteronyssinus Pollen weeds Allergic rhinitis	2	
2	Unspecified foods		2	
3	Aspirin		2	
4	Aspirin Unspecified fruits		2	Aspirin Sodium glutamate
5	Wine, soft drinks, tinned foods	D. pteronyssinus D. farinae, cat	1	Aspirin Sodium glutamate
6	Aspirin, egg	Egg, pollen weeds, cat Food allergy	2	Aspirin
7	Unspecified food	Pollens trees, pollens grasses, pollens weeds	2	
8	Tinned foods		1	Sodium benzoate
9	Tinned foods		2	
	Tinned foods		2	Methyl-parabene
10	Spiced foods Unspecific foods			Natrium benzoate Sodium benzoate Sodium bisulphite
11	Soft drinks, milk, aspirin		2	Aspirin Natrium glutamate
12	Soft drinks, smoked fish, grapes		2	Methyl-paraben Sodium benzoate Sodium bisulphite Tartrazine
13	Smoked meats Sausage		2	Aspirin
14	Soft drinks		2	
15	McDonald's food, blue cheese		1	
16	Instant coffee, dried fruit and nuts		2	
17	Unspecific		2	
18	Unspecific		2	

Table 4. Evaluation of urticaria/angioedema severity by score, doses of individual substances eliciting positive reactions and cumulated by oral challenge tests [6]

No	Mean score before diet introduction [1–3]	Substances delivering positive reactions	Doses eliciting first symptoms or positive reaction (mg)	Cumulated doses of tested substances (mg)	Mean score after challenges [1–3]	Associated subjective or objective symptoms
4	2	Aspirin	500→60 min	800	1	
		Sodium glutamate	500→60 min	600	1*	Numbness of the tongue[a]
5	1	Aspirin	500→120 min	800	1	
		Sodium glutamate	500→240 min	600	1	
6	2	Aspirin	500→15 min	800	2	
8	1	Sodium benzoate	500→240 min	750	1*	Metallic taste[a]
10	2	Methyl-paraben	200→120 min	600	2	
		Sodium glutamate	500→60 min	600	2	
		Sodium benzoate	200→60 min	750	2	
		Sodium bisulphite	50→60 min	160	2	
11	2	Aspirin	250→5 min	300	3*	Laryngeal oedema[a]
		Sodium glutamate	500→60 min	600	1	
12	2	Tartrazine	50→360 min	60	2	
		Methyl-paraben	400→240 min	600	2	
		Sodium benzoate	500→60 min	750	2	
		Sodium bisulphite	100→120 min	160	2	
13	2	Aspirin	250→60 min	300	2	

[a] Subjective symptoms associated to ingestion of tested substance.

one case only. This was a wheal and flare reaction to 1% sodium bisulphite (in petrolatum) noted after 48 h by usual patch test. This was confirmed 1 week later with the open patch test (Table 2). Anamnestical data, results of skin testing and sIgE screening in patients responding to additive-free diet and individual substances eliciting positive reactions by oral testing are given in Table 3. In 44% patients (*n*=8) who had improved on additive-free diet, individual additives and/or aspirin caused objective urticaria and/or angioedema symptoms on oral challenge tests. For the most part, reactions occurred between 5 and 120 min, and in 5 cases combinations of two to four individual substances were noted. All reactions resolved spontaneously within 24 h, and these were generally mild or moderate urticaria bursts. Only one patient (no. 11) developed severe angioedema with stridor, and emergency treatment with adrenaline and steroids was required (Table 4).

Conclusions

Exacerbation of chronic urticaria and angioedema may be due to intolerance of some food additives, or associated with aspirin intolerance. About 5–10% aspirin-sensitive patients react to additives as well [1]. On the other hand, toxic food reactions, congenital or induced enzyme deficiencies including abnormalities in histamine pharmacodynamics and others might be involved [9] (Table 5). Considering that the proposed mechanisms for reactions to tartrazine, sodium benzoate, sulphites, glutamate and aspirin are so different, the association of reactions to multiple additives and aspirin remains unclear [10]. We found a case of positive skin reaction to sodium bisulphite which correlated to the positive result of the oral challenge test. Although this strongly suggests IgE-mediated sul-

Table 5. Some mechanisms proposed for pseudo-allergic (PAR) symptoms occurring in patients with toxic reactions and intolerances of some foods and food additives [10]

Intolerance	Food constituents	Trigger mechanism	Symptoms
Pharmacological intolerance	Monosodium glutamate	Affected transmitter release in peripherical and central nervous sysytem	PAR
	Sulphites		
Enzyme deficiency:	Lactose	Lactase deficiency	
Congenital	Sulphites	Oxidase deficiency?	
	Cholinergic reflex?		
Induced	Histamine and drugs, alcohol, nitrites	IgE-mediated allergy?	
		DAO inhibition	PAR
	Tyramine and drugs	MAO inhibition	
Release of mediators	Natural foods and products of digestion	Non-immunologically mediated activation of effector system for allergy and inflammation	
	Aspirin and NSAID		
	Azo and non-azo dyes benzoates		
Toxic reactions	Histamine		
	Tyramine	Typical pharmacological effects	PAR
	Others		
Psychogenic reactions	Natural foods and food additives	Release of mediators due to conditioned Pavlovian reflex?	PAR

DAO, diamine oxidase; MAO, monoamine oxidase; NSAID, non-steroidal anti-inflammatory drugs.

phite hypersensitivity, this phenomenon seems to be extremely rare [3]. Histories of food additive related exacerbations of chronic urticaria or angioedema are usually poorly informative. The concordance of positive challenges and histories suggesting a causal role of additive-containing foods and/or aspirin was found in 5 of 18 our patients responding to diet only. In patients with chronic urticaria, oral aspirin challenges are usually safer than in asthmatic patients. The association between reactions to aspirin and food additives seems to be of considerable practical interest for allergists and dermatologists. History of aspirin related exacerbations of chronic urticaria may be an indication for both, oral challenges with aspirin and food additives. Although a strict additive-free diet without common allergens and pharmacologically active compounds was used, a remarkable discrepancy between responsiveness to diet and challenge results was found. This discrepancy might be related to dose dependency, or combined effects of additives, or their interactions with other natural or synthetic food compounds. However, the existence of hitherto unknown pseudoallergens can not be excluded [11, 12]. Following this concept, Zuberbier et al. found pseudo-allergic properties of aromatic compounds of tomato in patients with chronic urticaria [13]. In addition, oral challenges with individual food additives are of limited value in chronic urticaria not least because of their limited repeatability. This might be due to the fact that starting with small doses might induce a phenomenon of rush hyposensitization [14]. This is why additive-free, stringently controlled diet seems to provide a reasonable means of diagnosis and therapy in some patients with food dependent chronic urticaria [15].

References

1. Frey PC (1989) Changing habits in food and drug additives (Europe). In: Pichler WL et al. (eds) Progress in Allergy and Clinical Immunology. Hogrefe&Huber, Toronto pp 474–477
2. Moneret-Vautrin DA, Kanny G (1993) Intolérance et immunotoxicité des additifs alimentaires. Méd et Hyg 51: 881–890
3. Simon RA, Stevenson DD (1993) Adverse reactions to food and drug additives. In: Middleton E, Reed CE, Ellis EF, Adkinson NF, Youngiger JW, Busse WN, (eds) Allergy principles and practice. 4th Edition, St Louis Mosby, pp 1687–1704
4. Young E, Patel S, Stoneham MD, Rona R, Wilkonson JD (1987) The prevalence of reactions to food additives in a survey population. J Royal Coll Physicians (London) 21: 241–247
5. Dutau G, Rancé F, Fejji A, Juchet F, Brémont P, Nouilhan P (1996) Intolérance aux additifs alimentaires chez l'enfant: mythe ou réalité? Rev Fr Allergol lImmunol Clin 36: 129–142
6. Kurek M, Grubska-Suchanek E (2001) Challenge tests with food additives and aspirin in the diagnostics of chronic urticaria. Rev Fr Allergol Immunol Clin 41: 463–469
7. Zuberbier T, Chantraine-Hess S, Hartmann K, Czarnetzki B (1997) Pseudoallergen-free diet in the treatment of chronic urticaria. Acta Derm Venerol (Stockh) 75: 484–487
8. Bandmann HJ, Dohn W (1967) Die Epikutantestung. München, Bergmann
9. Kanny G, Moneret-Vautrin DA, Schohn H, Feldman L, Mallie JP, Gueant JL (1993) Abnormalities in histamine pharmacodynamics in chronic urticaria. Clin Exp Allergy 23: 1015–1020
10. Kurek M (1996) Pseudoallergic reactions. Intolerance to natural and synthetic food constituents masquerading as food allergy. Ped Pol 9: 743–752
11. Moneret-Vautrin DA, Kanny G (1993) Intolérance et immunotoxicité des additifs alimentaires. Méd et Hyg 51: 881–890
12. Kurek M, Janowska E (2001): Allergische und pseudoallergische Reaktionen auf Aromastoffe in der Nahrung. Z Hautkr 76: 699–703

13. Zuberbier T, Ehlers I, Pfrommer C, Bastl R, Vieths S, Henz BM (1998) Aromastoffe – bisher unbekannte Auslöser von Nahrungsmittelpseudoallergien bei chronischer Urticaria. In: Garbe C, Rassner G (eds) Dermatologie: Leitninien und Qualitätssicherung für Diagnostik und Therapie. Berlin, Springer pp 124–126
14. Lessof MH (1987) Adverse reactions to food additives. J Royal Coll Physicians (London) 21: 237–242
15. Werfel T, Wedi B, Kleine-Tebbe J, Niggemann B, Saloga J, Sennekamp J, Vieluf I, Vieths S, Zuberbier T, Jaeger L (1998) Vorgehen bei Verdacht auf eine pseudo-allergische Reaktion durch Nahrungsmittelinhaltsstoffe. Positionspapier von DGAI und ÄDA. Allergo J 8 : 135–141

23 Serum Sickness as a Clinical Model for Food Intolerance

V.A. Marinkovich

Many people, as much as 40% of the population, have symptoms which they attribute to eating specific foods [1]. Testing for specific IgE to foods in a majority of these patients is negative and they are classed among the food intolerant. The clinical model most often cited for food intolerance is the patient with a lactase deficiency who develops abdominal distress including bloating, flatulence and crampy diarrhea after consuming milk. But most patients with food intolerance do not have primarily gastrointestinal problems after consuming their problem food. Rather they complain of joint stiffness and soreness, migraine headaches, exacerbation of asthma, fatigue, malaise, nasal and sinus congestion, rashes and cardiac arrhythmias. They complain of symptoms, which are more likely, the result of circulating immune complexes.

Immune complex formation is the necessary prelude to immune clearance of foreign antigens that enter the circulation. Circulating immune complexes are able to reach all organs of the body and when deposited can activate complement and trigger inflammation. They are rapidly removed from the circulation by the reticuloendothelial system of the spleen, liver, bone marrow, lymph nodes and by tissue macrophages thus limiting their inflammatory impact. This is a normal mechanism for clearing foreign molecules from the body to control their health-threatening potential. When complexes are formed in large numbers such as occurs during the immune response to an injection of horse serum, the clearing mechanisms are temporarily overwhelmed and symptoms of serum sickness follow. As clearance is completed, symptoms and inflammation end.

If serum injections are repeated, the burden on the clearing mechanisms may become chronically overwhelmed and chronic symptoms ensue. The circulating complexes become deposited in various organs beginning with arterial walls (vasculitis) and by extension affect normal function of the skin (e.g. eczema), kidneys (e.g. glomerulonephritis), cerebral vasculature (migraine headaches), lungs (pneumonitis-asthma), etc. In most cases the immune complex pathology seems to be a secondary phenomenon, the result of an altogether different basic dis-

Table 1. Clinical features of serum sickness (based on a survey of the medical literature)

Malaise/prostration	Neurological symptoms: headache, cerebral, neuritic
Fever	Lymphadenopathy
Rash	Myocardial ischemia
Arthritis	Transient renal disease
GI symptoms: nausea, vomiting, diarrhea, abdominal pain	

New Trends in Allergy V
J. Ring, H. Behrendt (Eds.)
© Springer-Verlag Berlin, Heidelberg 2002

ease process, but nonetheless of special importance in causing symptoms. Understanding the mechanisms of immune complex formation and their nature can help elucidate the basis for many chronic diseases. This is essential to effective therapeutic intervention (Table 1).

The pathogenesis of immune complex disease was first described by Von Pirquet in 1905, from his observations on patients receiving horse anti-sera for the successful treatment of diphtheria and streptococcal scarlet fever [2]. He correctly deduced that the symptoms the patients developed several days after surviving the potentially fatal crisis of their infections were the result of the host's immune system reacting with the circulating horse serum and forming immune complexes.

He called this immune complex illness. In the decades that followed, a great deal of research into serum sickness, as it came to be known, was conducted and reported in the medical literature. By 1965 there was no substantial change in the original conclusions of Von Pirquet. Then in 1966, IgE was discovered and the great previous interest in immune complexes virtually ended. The basic mechanisms of serum sickness are shown in the next slide taken from Cochrane's work [3] (Fig. 1). Of historical interest, Dr. Ishizaha who discovered IgE while working in Denver had previously spent several years with Professor Dan Campbell at Caltech studying the pathology of immune complex diseases.

The time has come to reawaken our attention to the role of immune complexes in producing human illness. I propose that the medical model for immunologically mediated, non-IgE food reactions is chronic serum sickness. Instead of reacting to injected horse serum as in Von Pirquet's work, patient's with food intolerance are reacting to large quantities of food antigens crossing the intestinal mucosa because of an underlying gastrointestinal malfunction. It must be un-

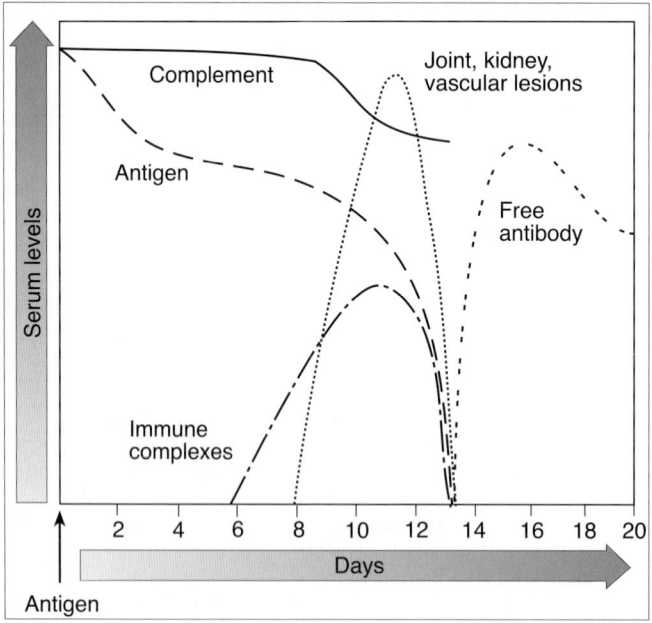

Fig. 1. Immunological responses in experimental acute serum sickness

Table 2. Model for non-IgE food reactions in chronic serum sickness

Increased intestinal permeability
General immune response
Immune complex formation
Macrophage overload
Circulating complexes
Tissue deposition
Symptoms

derstood that immune complex formation is a constant and ongoing part of immune surveillance and such complexes do not cause illness unless formed in large number, not cleared well, and finally deposited in various organs. Tissue deposition leads to inflammation which produces symptoms reflecting the organs involved and generally involving vasculitis. The necessary sequence of events leading to symptoms is shown in Table 2.

If food reactions are primarily due to the protective response of the immune system to high uptake of food antigens caused by a digestive tract disorder, it is likely that the single most helpful clinical guide to an elimination diet that would reduce complex formation and the burden on the macrophage clearing mechanisms is measurement of specific IgG antibody to foods [4]. In order to test this hypothesis, a study was undertaken using a test system in which food antigens are covalently bonded to cellulose filaments and otherwise run as a typical ELISA without the variability caused by the insecure adhesion of food allergens to microtiter plates (Hitachi Chemical Diagnostics, Inc., Mountain View, California; CLA food and mold specific IgG panel). The panel, which has been cleared by the FDA years ago for measuring specific IgE antibodies to Foods, was converted to a specific IgG test following a developmental process involving 139 selected normal blood donors at the Stanford Blood Services Facility. Each of the donors was selected following a personal interview in which all possible manifestations of immune complex illness were ruled out. The antibody levels to foods measured in these selected healthy donors were considered normal among the local population. In studying these blood samples it was determined that a 300-fold dilution of serum would reduce a majority of the normal food specific IgG levels found in healthy controls below the detection level (Table 3).

A blinded study was conducted using 63 consecutive patients seen in clinic who had food-associated symptoms, negative IgE tests and elevated specific IgG

Table 3. Specific IgG for foods (from [4])

	Normal controls (139)	Patients (63)
Positive at class 4	0.2%	0.3%
Positive at class 3	0.5%	1.7%
Positive at class 2	2.2%	7.2%
Positive at class 1	6.2%	16.7%
Total positive	9.1%	25.9%

Table 4. Study results (31 patients followed the prescribed diet, 24 chose not to diet)

	Dieters	Non-dieters
Patients	31	24
>25% Drop in IgG titer	27 ($p<0.0001$)	0
>25% Drop in blank readings	21 ($p<0.01$)	6
Clinical improvement	28 ($p<0.01$)	7

antibody titers to foods in the newly adapted CLA specific IgG test. The patients were all told what foods were likely to be involved in causing their symptoms and how to avoid these foods in the diet. Most of the foods selected for exclusion were foods most often eaten by the patients and were preferred foods. Accepting the elimination diets was difficult for the patients. 33 patients chose to diet, 30 did not diet but participated in other non-dietary, palliative, symptom-directed treatments. After one year, the patients were reevaluated for clinical improvement and re-tested for specific IgG to the same foods previously tested. 8 patients were lost to follow-up. The patients who stayed on the elimination diet showed significant differences from non-dieters in symptom relief and antibody levels to the problem foods (Table 4).

Each of the CLA IgG panels contains a blank filament to which human serum albumin is covalently bound. Patients often showed substantial elevations in the blank reading over controls. This was later shown to be a semi-quantitative measure of circulating immune complexes. This measure also showed a significantly greater drop among dieters than among non-dieters, as would be expected. This study clearly showed that diet played some role in the patient's symptoms and that specific IgG antibody titers to commonly eaten foods could serve as a basis for effective dietary manipulation.

The characteristics of IgE based food allergy symptoms and those caused by immune complex (non-IgE) based symptoms are quite distinct (Table 5). In IgE allergy the symptoms are quick to appear after ingestion of the allergenic food (minutes) and are triggered by small amounts (mgs) of food. They are relatively short-lived (hours), they usually involve only one food, are usually life-long, and have some genetic basis. Immune complex based symptoms are delayed in appearance (hours), have a prolonged duration (days to weeks), and are the result

Table 5. Symptom characteristics IgE vs IgG (mixed immunological)

	IgE	IgG
Onset	Rapid (minutes)	Delayed (hours)
Duration	Brief (hours)	Prolonged (days)
Mechanism	Mast cell	Circulating complexes (macrophage overload)
Quantity of food	Tiny	Dose-dependent
Food	Any (rare)	Common foods
Patient awareness	Always	Never
Persistence of antibody	Lifelong	Months after elimination

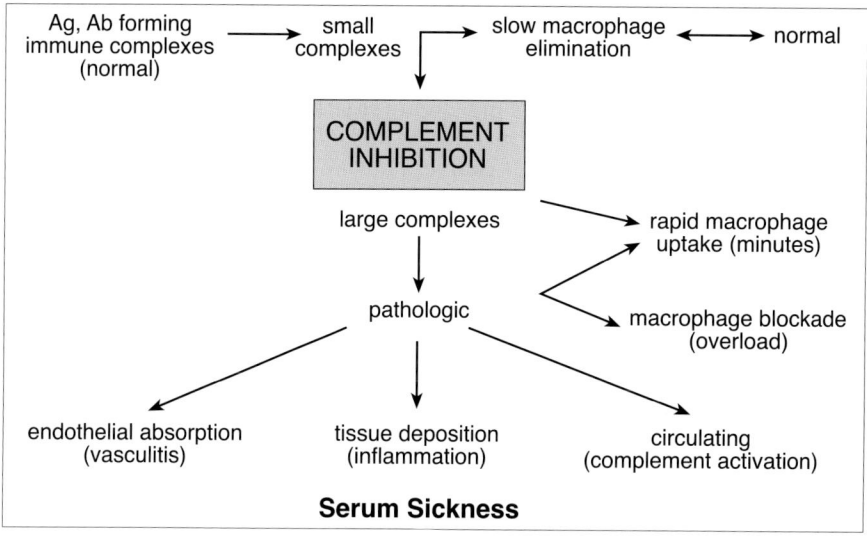

Fig. 2. Type III (Coombs and Gell) immunopathology

of a digestive or permeability problem in the gut. The illness, therefore, involves multiple foods, involves foods that are most often eaten by the patients, is dose dependent usually requiring large quantities to be triggered, is not life long and is not basically a problem of the immune system. It represents a normal immune response to increased antigenic uptake across the intestinal wall. Once the macrophages responsible for immune clearance are overwhelmed by the sheer magnitude of immune complex formation, symptoms ensue. The causes for increased antigenic uptake in the intestines can range from immaturity to alcoholism, to pancreatic insufficiency to others. One interesting cause is an undiagnosed or ignored IgE-based allergy to a specific food which increases membrane permeability through the local release of histamine. This can also occur in allergic individuals during their pollen season when all membrane permeability increases due to high circulating histamine levels. One way of viewing the mechanisms of non-IgE immunopathology is presented in Figure 2. As long as the complement system is operative and preventing the growth of immune complexes, complexes remain small and are removed from the circulation by macrophages with minimal symptoms. This function of complement is strictly temperature dependent and fades as the temperature falls below 37°C. This may explain Raynauld's phenomena in which the extremities become cooled, favoring the growth and deposition of immune complexes in the skin of the extremities where the risk of impairment of vital body functions is less. The malar flush seen in lupus erythematosus may be an example of this phenomenon, exposing complexes to the ultraviolet rays of sunlight striking the malar regions of the face. Proteins absorb energy in the ultraviolet spectrum (e.g. 280 mu) and can be more easily denatured.

Another interesting phenomena observed in this illness resembling chronic serum sickness is that symptoms often abate with the elimination of a single food from the diet to which there is a large IgG antibody titer even when other foods with measurable IgG antibody titers remain in the diet. Although the antigen antibody interaction is highly specific, the complex-macrophage interaction is not. Therefore the elimination of any highly reactive food from the diet unburdens the clearing mechanism to that degree and allows faster processing and inactivation of other complexes. Of course, a more comprehensive elimination of highly reactive foods produces better clinical results but considerations of proper nutrition and patient compliance need to be allowed. In conclusion, I propose chronic serum sickness as the correct medical model for food hypersensitivity reactions („leaky gut syndrome") and that specific IgG determinations are the best single markers of the foods most involved in the production of symptoms. Effective treatment in the short run is diet exclusion of the foods involved. Long-term successful therapy requires attention to the basis for the increased antigen uptake in the gut.

References

1. Sampson, HA, Food Allergy, Part 1: Immunopathogenesis and Clinical Disorders. Journal of Allergy and Clinical Immunology 1999; 103: 717–28: Part 2 Diagnosis and Management, 981–89.
2. Von Pirquet, CP, Schick, B 1908 Serum Sickness, Leipzig und Wien, Franz Deuticke.
3. Cochrane CG. Immune complex-mediated tissue injury. In Cohen, S., Ward, PA and McCluskey, RT (editors) Mechanisms of Immunopathology, Werbel and Peck, New York, 1979, pp 29–48.
4. Marinkovich, V, Specific IgG Antibodies as markers of adverse reactions to foods. In: Wuthrick, B, Ortolani, C, editors, Highlights in Food Allergy. Monographs of Allergy, Basel: Karger: 1996: 32: 221–5.

24 Role of Tryptase in Anaphylaxis

B. Przybilla, D. Ludolph-Hauser

Introduction

A central pathogenetic event in anaphylaxis is the rapid release of mediators from mast cells and basophils upon exposure to a stimulus. The reaction can be initiated by an immunological mechanism (mostly IgE-mediated) or non-immunologically („pseudo-allergy"). The clinical picture is characterized by the sudden onset of symptoms ranging from mere skin involvement (flush, urticaria), minor to moderate cardiovascular, respiratory or gastrointestinal symptoms to full shock, which may have a fatal outcome in some cases.

Mast cells can release a large array of mediators (Table 1), among which histamine is thought to be pathophysiologically most important in acute anaphylaxis. In recent years the protease tryptase, which constitutes a significant amount of the mast cell protein content, has gained increasing interest.

Characteristics of Tryptase

The serine endoprotease tryptase (EC 3.4.21.59) is highly specific to mast cells, its concentration in basophils is only less than one hundredth [1]. Tryptase has a molecular weight of 134,000, it is a tetramer with one active site per subunit (molecular weight 33,000 to 37,000). There are several isoenzymes, one α- and three β-tryptases have a sequence identity of more than 95% [2–4]. The structure of β-tryptase has been characterized [5]. Evidently, α-tryptase is secreted continuously, whereas β-tryptase is localized to the mast cell granules complexed with heparin and other proteoglycans in an enzymatically active form [6,7]. Recently, also the existence of γ-tryptases was reported [8]. Besides β-tryptase the mast cell granules contain the serum proteases chymase [9], cathepsin G (or a very similar protease) [10], and carboxypeptidase A [11]. Depending on the presence

Table 1. Mediators from human mast cells

Biogenic amine	Histamine
Proteases	Tryptase, chymase, carboxypeptidase A, cathepsin G-like protease
Proteoglycans	Heparin, chondroitin sulfate, heparan sulfate
Lipid mediators	LTC_4, LTB_4, PGD_2, PAF
Cytokines	TNF-α, IL-4/-5/-6/-8/-13/-16
Chemotactic factors	ECF, NCF

New Trends in Allergy V
J. Ring, H. Behrendt (Eds.)
© Springer-Verlag Berlin, Heidelberg 2002

of these proteases, three phenotypes of mast cells can be discerned: Some contain only tryptase [9, 12], some tryptase, chymase, cathepsin G and carboxpeptidase A [11, 13], rarely there is only chymase [13].

Active tryptase was demonstrated in the extracellular space as well as in the circulation. Enzymatic activity depends on the integrity of the tetrameric structure, which is stabilized by heparin. Inactivation probably is due to the decomposition of this complex. Up to now, no natural human inhibitor of tryptase has been identified.

Functions of Tryptase

The biological functions of mast cell tryptases in humans are largely unknown. The properties of tryptases even from various mammals differ, results from animal studies cannot be applied directly to human tryptase. As a specific tryptase inhibitor is not yet available for clinical studies, biological functions cannot be assessed in vivo. Available data suggest that tryptase may play a role in inflammatory processes, including immediate type allergic reactions, as well as in tissue remodeling; a short survey is given in Table 2. As recently reported, some of the actions of tryptase may be initiated via the proteinase–activated receptor 2 [29].

With regard to anaphylaxis, the ability of tryptase to form C3a by cleavage of C3 and to release badykinin from kininogens may be relevant [14, 15]. Also, tryptase was found to stimulate vascular leakage and to induce mast cell activation [16], which both could be related to the forementioned actions. The lack of fibrin deposition at sites of immediate type reactions might be related to the anticoagulant properties of tryptase [17, 18]. Also, tryptase could be involved in the development of late phase reactions by stimulating the synthesis of ICAM-1 and

Table 2. Potential biological functions of tryptase

Inflammation	
L.B. Schwartz et al. [14]	Cleavage of C3, C3a formation
T. Imamura et al. [15]	Release of bradykinin from kininogens
S. He et al. [16]	Increase of capillary permeability
M.S. Stack et al. [17]	Activation of plasminogen activator (urokinase)
S. Ren et al. [18]	Degradation of fibrinogen
J.A. Cairns et al. [19]	Stimulation of synthesis of IL-8 and ICAM-1
S. He et al. [20]	Induction of neutrophil-/eosinophil-rich Infiltrate
G.H. Caughey et al. [21]	Degradation of VIP
A.F. Walls et al. [22]	Attenuation of vasodilator activity of CGRP
Tissue remodeling	
S.J. Ruoss et al. [23]	Mitogen for fibroblasts
J.K. Brown et al. [24]	Mitogen for smooth muscle cells
J.A. Cairns et al. [19]	Mitogen for epithelial cells
J.A. Cairns et al. [25]	Stimulation of type I collagen synthesis
R.J. Blair et al. [26]	Stimulation of angiogenesis/vascular tube formation
B.L. Gruber et al. [27]	Activation of pro-matrix-metalloproteinase (MMP)-3
M. Lees et al. [28]	Activation of MMP-1 via activation of pro-MMP-3

IL-8 [19] and by induction of a cellular infiltrate [20]. In addition, tryptase could modulate neurogenic inflammation by degradation of VIP and CGRP [21, 22].

Measurement of Tryptase

Various immunoassays, using enzymatic or radioactive labeling, were employed to measure tryptase by polyclonal or monoclonal antibodies in body fluids [30, 31]. Recently a commercial fluoroenyzme immunoassay has become available which has a detection limit <1 µg/l (Unicap Tryptase, Pharmacia & Upjohn). The assay detects both α- and β-tryptase. According to the data given by the manufacturer, the 95th upper percentile in controls is 13.5 µg/l.

Tryptase in Anaphylaxis

Although the pathophysiologic role of tryptase in anaphylaxis is not clear, its applicability as a marker of mast cell activation, as it occurs in anaphylaxis, is well established. Whereas in many mastocytosis patients permanently elevated levels of α-tryptase are found in the circulation, in anaphylaxis β-tryptase, which is virtually absent from the blood of healthy individuals, is released in large quantities and can be temporarily detected in plasma or serum [7, 32]. Tryptase levels in patients with anaphylactic or anaphylactoid symptoms peak between less than 30 minutes [33–35] and more than five hours [35] after onset of the reaction; peaking of tryptase levels only after one to two hours was frequent [36]. The cause of these differences is still unclear. They may arise from methodological variations, specific effects of certain exposure conditions leading to anaphylaxis, or from different reactivity of individual patients. There is also some correlation of

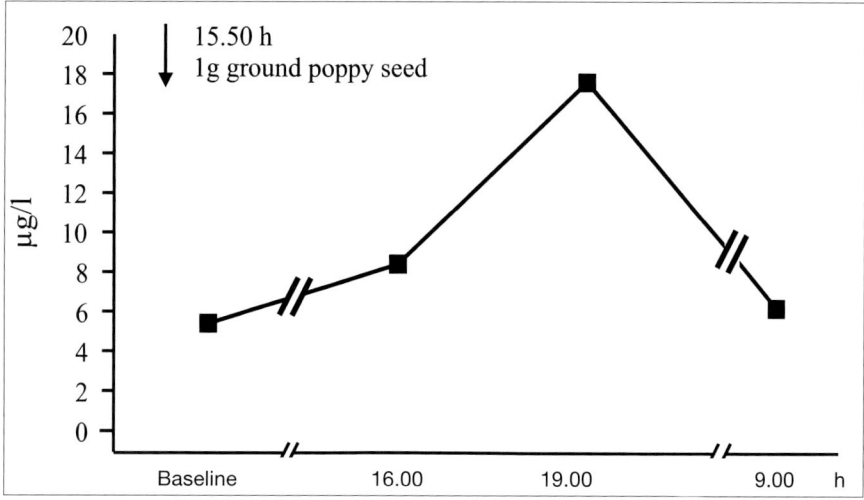

Fig. 1. Serum tryptase levels in a patient with anaphylaxis upon oral challenge with poppy seed

tryptase levels with the severity of symptoms, although an increase of tryptase was not seen in all reactions [33–35, 37].

Increases of tryptase levels in the circulation have been observed in immediate type reactions to insect stings [33, 34], antibiotics [35], nonsteroidal antiinflammatory drugs [35, 38], drugs used during anesthesia or operation [37, 39–43], natural rubber latex [44, 45], food [46], amniotic fluid [47] or chlorhexidine [48]. The time course of serum tryptase concentrations in a poppy seed-allergic patient with anaphylaxis to a challenge test is shown in Figure 1.

Measurement of tryptase may aid also in the post-mortem diagnosis of anaphylaxis. Elevated serum tryptase concentrations were found after fatal anaphylaxis [49, 50], in about 13% of victims of sudden unexpected death [51] and in sudden infant death [52, 53]. However, increased tryptase levels were also found in about 12% in deaths of other causes [54].

Severe Anaphylaxis in Patients with Elevated Baseline Serum Tryptase Levels

Schwartz and co-workers reported that in untreated Hymenoptera venom allergic patients, who developed hypotensive reactions to a sting challenge, baseline serum tryptase levels before the sting were significantly higher than in those with less severe or without systemic symptoms [31]. The cause of these constitutively elevated tryptase levels was not reported by these authors.

We have performed a study to assess a possible relationship between the severity of anaphylactic reactions to field stings and the baseline serum tryptase levels [55]. Each forty consecutive patients with systemic anaphylactic reactions to wasp or honeybee stings were allocated to three groups according to their most severe symptoms [after 56]: Only generalized skin reactions such as flush or urticaria (mild reactions); loss of consciousness (severe reactions); or intermediate symptoms as cardiovascular, respiratory and/or gastrointestinal symptoms without loss of consciousness (moderate reactions). The diagnosis of Hymenoptera venom allergy was based on history, skin tests with bee and wasp venom, and measurement of bee and wasp venom specific IgE in the serum. Patients in the three severity groups did not differ significantly with regard to age, gender, diagnosis of bee or wasp venom allergy, or use of beta-blockers or ACE inhibitors at the time of their most severe sting reaction. Also, there were no significant differences concerning prick test reactivity or levels of specific serum IgE antibodies to the eliciting venom.

Baseline tryptase levels were measured by a fluoroenzyme immunoassay (Unicap Tryptase) in sera that had been kept frozen at −20°C after preparation from blood samples taken at least two weeks after the last sting reaction. Tryptase concentrations >13.5 µg/l were considered as to be elevated. Some patients had to be excluded because of incomplete data, leaving a total of 114 patients. Twelve patients exhibited elevated serum tryptase levels ranging from 14.9 to 149 µg/l. Nine of these 12 patients (75.0%), but only 28 of 102 (27.5%) with lower tryptase levels had experienced severe sting reactions ($p=0.004$). In addition, two of the severely reacting patients had cutaneous mastocytosis without elevated tryptase levels.

As constitutively elevated tryptase levels in the circulation are a characteristic feature of mastocytosis, all of the Hymenoptera venom allergic patients with serum tryptase levels >13.5 µg/l were re-examined. In this context it is important to know that on occasion of their first admission to the hospital the whole skin surface of all patients had been routinely examined. Re-examination of the 12 patients yielded unexpected findings: two patients had urticaria pigmentosa which was easy to recognize and was already known; however, in nine of the 12 patients there were lesions of cutaneous mastocytosis which were very inconspicuous and had been evidently missed at the first examination without knowledge of the elevated tryptase levels („mastocytosis occulta"). The clinical presentation of these patients resembled a very faint form of teleangiectasia macularis eruptiva perstans, which was already reported in a single patient with very severe allergic reactions to wasp stings [57]. Skin biopsies could be taken from seven of the 11 patients with constitutively elevated tryptase levels and skin involvement, mastocytosis was proven histologically in all of them. Only in one patient with a baseline serum tryptase level of 22 µg/l no signs of cutaneous mastocytosis were present. This suggests mastocytosis of other organs than the skin or, alternatively, facilitated mast cell mediator release due to yet unknown factors. Also a diffuse increase of skin mast cells not causing macules or papules could underlie this elevated tryptase level.

As 75% of the patients with constitutively elevated tryptase levels had experienced very severe reactions, this finding indicates an increased risk to develop life-threatening anaphylaxis. The cause is probably the increased number of mediator-releasing cells in mastocytosis, alternatively enhanced liberation of mast cell mediators due to as yet unidentified reasons could play a role. Up to now, only few patients with mastocytosis and Hymenoptera venom allergy have been reported [57–60]. In the publication of a larger series of such patients, the simultaneous occurrence of both conditions was considered to be co-incidental [60]. Our findings point towards a causal relationship between mast cell disease associated with elevated baseline tryptase levels and severe reactions to Hymenoptera stings. Whether also mastocytosis without elevated tryptase levels constitutes a risk of particularly severe anaphylaxis has to be assessed by further studies.

Venom immunotherapy protects nearly all allergic patients from further systemic symptoms and can thus be life-saving. This treatment was tolerated by patients with mastocytosis as by other patients, side effects were not found to be increased [60]. Usually, venom immunotherapy can be discontinued after three to five years. We suggest that patients with mast cell disease should be treated lifelong, as fatal anaphylaxis was reported in patients with mastocytosis after stopping immunotherapy [59]. Also, one should consider increasing the usual maintenance dose of 100 µg/4 weeks, as a higher dose yields better protection [61, 62]. As immunotherapy with the routine 100-µg-dose seems less effective in bee than in wasp venom allergy, such a higher routine treatment dose of 200 µg/4 weeks is recommended at least for patients with bee venom allergy and mast cell disease.

Conclusions

Tryptase is a protease specific to mast cells. Its determination is a useful research tool to differentiate the contribution of mast cells or basophils to allergic reactions. The biological functions of tryptase in humans have not yet been definitely elucidated. The enzyme is likely to exert various actions in inflammatory reactions, including anaphylaxis, and in tissue remodeling. As specific inhibitors of human tryptase become available, they may not only help to better characterize the biological functions of this protease, but may also offer new therapeutic options.

The diagnosis of anaphylaxis is usually based on clinical features and/or simple parameters of organ function such as blood pressure or heart rate. However, not always the full characteristic spectrum of symptoms does develop (e.g. loss of consciousness without other apparent symptoms), and parameters of organ function are often not available when the patient presents for allergological diagnostics after the event. In addition, there are many differential diagnoses of anaphylaxis, e.g. cardiovascular events including vaso-vagal collapse, seizure disorders, or hyperventilation. For long, increased histamine levels in the circulation or elevated urinary histamine or N-methylhistamine excretion have been the only available objective parameters of mast cell and basophil activation characteristic of anaphylaxis. As levels of tryptase rise in anaphylaxis, their measurement can support diagnosing such reactions. Compared with histamine measurements, determination of tryptase levels is more reliable and easier to perform, as tryptase can be detected much longer in the circulation and plain serum samples can be used without the intricate procedures needed for histamine determination. Serial measurements of tryptase are recommended, as the course of tryptase concentrations may vary with peak levels between less than 30 min and more than 5 h after the onset of symptoms. A definite baseline tryptase level has to be obtained in order not to mistake a constitutively elevated tryptase level for an indicator of anaphylaxis. Measurement of tryptase may also support the post-mortem diagnosis of anaphylaxis. However, in no case a diagnosis of anaphylaxis can be made or excluded only by assessing serum tryptase levels alone. Clinical symptoms, circumstances of the reaction and other potential clues have to be considered carefully and constitute the basis of the diagnosis.

To detect mast cell disease, measurement of serum tryptase levels and a meticulous skin examination are necessary in all patients with Hymenoptera venom allergy. In the presence of mast cell disease standard treatment protocols have to be modified accordingly. Further investigations are needed to clarify if the relationship between mast cell disease and particularly severe anaphylactic symptoms applies only to Hymenoptera venom allergy or also to anaphylaxis due to other elicitors.

References

1. Castells MC, Irani AM, Schwartz LB (1987) Evaluation of human peripheral blood leukocytes for mast cell tryptase. J Immunol 138: 2184–2189

2. Miller JS, Moxley G, Schwartz LB (1989) Cloning and characterization of a complementary DNA for human tryptase. J Clin Invest 84: 1188–1195
3. Miller JS, Moxley G, Schwartz LB (1990) Cloning and characterization of a second complementary DNA for human tryptase. J Clin Invest 86: 864–870
4. Vanderslice P, Ballinger SM, Tam EK, Goldstein SM, Craik CS, Caughey GH (1990) Human mast cell tryptase multiple cDNAs and genes reveal a multigene serine protease family. Proc Natl Acad Sci USA 87: 3811 – 3815
5. Pereira PJ, Bergner A, Macedo-Ribeiro S, Huber R, Matschiner G, Fritz H, Sommerhoff CP, Bode W (1998) Human beta-tryptase is a ring-like tetramer with active sites facing a central pore. Nature 392: 306–311
6. Schwartz LB (1994) Tryptase: a mast cell serine protease. Meth Enzymol 244: 88–100
7. Schwartz LB, Sakai K, Bradford TR, Ren S, Zweimann B, Worobec AS (1995) The alpha form of human tryptase is the predominant type present in blood at baseline in normal subjects and is elevated in those with systemic mastocytosis. J Clin Invest 96: 2702–2710
8. Caughey GH, Raymond WW, Blount JL, Hau LW, Pallaoro M, Wolters PJ, Verghese GM (2000) Characterization of human gamma-tryptases, novel members of the chromosome 16p mast cell tryptase and prostasin gene families. J Immunol 164: 6566–6575
9. Irani AM, Schechter NM, Craig SS, DeBlois G, Schwarz LB (1986) Two types of human mast cells with distinct neutral protease compositions. Proc Natl Acad Sci USA 83: 4464–4468
10. Schechter NM, Irani AM, Sprows JL, Abernathy J, Wintroub B, Schwarz LB (1990) Identification of a cathepsin G-like proteinase in the MC_{TC} type of human mast cells. J Immunol 145: 2652–2661
11. Irani AM, Goldstein SM, Wintroub BU, Bradford T, Schwartz LB (1991) Human mast cell carboxypeptidase. Selective localization to MCTC cells. J Immunol 147: 247–253
12. Irani AM (1995) Tissue and developmental variation of protease expression in human mast cells. In: Caughey GH (ed) Mast cell proteases in immunology and biology. Marcel Decker, New York, 127–143
13. Weidner N, Austen KF (1993) Heterogeneity of mast cells at multiple body sites. Fluorescent determination of avidin binding and immunofluorescent determination of chymase, tryptase, and carboxypeptidase content. Pathol Res Pract 189: 156–162
14. Schwartz LB, Kawahara MS, Hugli TE, Vik D, Fearon DT, Austen KF (1983) Generation of C3a anaphylatoxin from human C3 by human mast cell tryptase. J Immunol 130: 1891–1895
15. Imamura T, Dubin A, Moore W, Tanaka R, Travis J (1996) Induction of vascular permeability enhancement by human tryptase: dependence on activation of prekallikrein and direct release of bradykinin from kininogens. Lab Invest 74: 861–870
16. He S, Walls AF (1997) Human mast cell tryptase: a stimulus of microvascular leakage and mast cell activation. Eur J Pharmacol 328: 89–97
17. Stack MS, Johnson DA (1994) Human mast cell tryptase activates single-chain urinary-type plasminogen activator (pro-urokinase). J Biol Chem 269: 9416–9419
18. Ren S, Lawson AE, Carr M, Baumgarten CM, Schwartz LB (1997) Human tryptase fibrinogenolysis is optimal at acidic pH and generates anticoagulant fragments in the presence of the anti-tryptase monoclonal antibody B12. J Immunol 159: 3540–3548
19. Cairns JA, Walls AF (1996) Mast cell tryptase is a mitogen for epithelial cells. Stimulation of Il-8 production and intercellular adhesion molecule-1 expression. J Immunol 156: 275–283
20. He S, Peng Q, Walls AF (1997) Potent induction of a neutrophil and eosinophil-rich infiltrate in vivo by human mast cell tryptase: selective enhancement of eosinophil recruitment by histamine. J Immunol 159: 6216 –6225
21. Caughey GH, Leidig F, Viro NF, Nadel G (1988) Substance P and vasoactive intestinal peptide degradation by mast cell tryptase and chymase. J Pharmacol Exp Ther 244: 133–137
22. Walls AF, Brain SD, Desai A, Jose PJ, Hawkings E, Church MK, Williams TJ (1992) Human mast cell tryptase attenuates the vasodilator activity of calcitonin gene-related peptide. Biochem Pharmacol 43: 1243 –1248
23. Ruoss SJ, Hartmann T, Caughey GC (1991) Mast cell tryptase is a mitogen for cultured fibroblasts. J Clin Invest 88: 493–499

24. Brown JK, Tyler CL, Jones CA, Ruoss SJ, Hartmann T, Caughey GH (1995) Tryptase, the dominant secretory granular protein in human mast cells is a potent mitogen for cultured dog tracheal smooth muscle cells. Am J Respir Cell Mol Biol 13: 227–236

25. Cairns JA, Walls AF (1997) Mast cell tryptase stimulates the synthesis of type I collagen in human lung fibroblasts. J Clin Invest 99: 1313–1321

26. Blair RJ, Meng H, Marchese MJ, Ren S, Schwartz LB, Tonnensen MG, Gruber BL (1997) Human mast cell tryptase stimulates vascular tube formation. Tryptase is a novel, potent angiogenic factor. J Clin Invest 99: 2691–2700

27. Gruber BL, Marchese MJ, Suzuki K, Schwartz LB, Okada Y, Nagase H, Ramamurthy NS (1989) Synovial procollagenase activation by human mast cell tryptase: dependence upon matrix metalloproteinase 3 activation. J Clin Invest 84: 1657–1662

28. Lees M, Taylor DJ, Woolley DE (1994) Mast cell proteinases activate precursor forms of collagenase and stromelysin, but not of gelatinases A and B. Eur J Biochem 223: 171–177

29. Steinhoff M, Vergnolle N, Young SH, Tognetto M, Amadesi S, Ennes HS, Trevisani M, Hollenberg MD, Wallace JL, Chaughey GH, Mitchell SE, Williams LM, Geppetti P, Mayer EA, Bunnett NW (2000) Agonists of proteinase-activated receptor 2 induce inflammation by a neurogenic mechanism. Nature Med 6:151–158

30. Enander I, Matsson P, Nystrand J, Andersson AS, Eklund E, Bradford TR, Schwartz LB (1991) A new radioimmunoassay for human mast cell tryptase using monoclonal antibodies. J Immunol Meth 138: 39–46

31. Schwartz LB, Bradford TR, Rouse C, Irani AM, Rasp G, van der Zwan JK, van der Linden PWG (1994) Development of a new, more sensitive immunoassay for human tryptase: use in systemic anaphylaxis. J Clin Immunol 14: 190–204

32. Schwartz LB, Metcalfe DD, Miller JS, Earl A, Sullivan T (1987) Tryptase levels as an indicator of mast-cellactivation in systemic anaphylaxis and mastocytosis. N Engl J Med 316: 1622–1626

33. van der Linden PWG, Hack CE, Poortman J, Vivié-Kipp YC, Struyvenberg A, van der Zwan JK (1992) Insect-sting challenge in 138 patients: relation between clinical severity of anaphylaxis and mast cell activation. J Allergy Clin Immunol 90: 110–118

34. Eberlein-König B, Ullmann S, Thomas P, Przybilla B (1995) Tryptase and histamine release due to a sting challenge in bee venom allergic patients treated successfully or unsuccessfully with hyposensitization. Clin Exper Allergy 25: 704–712

35. Ordoqui E, Zubeldia JM, Aranzábal A, Rubio M, Herrero T, Tornero P, Rodriguez VM, Prieto A, Baeza M (1997) Serum tryptase levels in adverse drug reactions. Allergy 52: 1102–1105

36. Schwartz LB, Yunginger JW, Miller J, Bockhari R, Dull D (1989) Time course of appearance and disappearance of human mast cell tryptase in the circulation after anaphylaxis. J Clin Invest 83: 1551–1555

37. Laroche D, Vergnaud MC, Sillard B, Soufarapis H, Bricard H (1991) Biochemical markers of anaphylactoid reactions to drugs. Comparison of plasma histamine and tryptase. Anesthesiology 75: 945–949

38. Butterfield JH, Kao PC, Klee GC, Yocum MW (1995) Aspirin idiosyncrasy in systemic mast cell disease: a new look at mediator release during desensitization. Mayo Clin Proc 70: 481–487

39. Matsson P, Enander I, Andersson AS, Nystrand J, Schwartz L, Watkins J (1991) Evaluation of mast cell activation (tryptase) in two patients suffering from drug-induced hypotensoid reactions. Agents Actions 33: 218–220

40. Laroche D, Lefrancois C, Gerard JL, Dubois F, Vergnaud MC, Gueant JL, Bricard H (1992) Early diagnosis of anaphylactic reactions to neuromuscular blocking drugs. Br J Anaesth 69: 611–614

41. Watkins J (1994) Adverse reaction to neuromuscular blockers: frequency, investigation, and epidemiology. Acta Anaesthesiol Scand (Suppl) 102: 6–10

42. Cottineau C, Drouet M, Costerousse F, Dussaussoy C, Sabbah A (1996) Importance of plasma (histamine and tryptase) and urinary (methylhistamine) in peri-anesthetic anaphylactic and/or anaphylactoid reactions. Allerg Immunol (Paris) 28: 273–276

43. Takenoshita M, Sugiyama M, Okuno Y, Inagaki Y, Yoshiya I, Shimazaki Y (1996) Anaphylactoid reaction to protamine confirmed by plasma tryptase in a diabetic patient during open heart surgery. Anesthesiology 84: 233–235

44. Ownby DR, Tomlanovich M, Sammons N, Mc Cullough J (1991) Anaphylaxis associated with latex allergy during barium enema examinations. Am J Roentgenol 156: 903–908
45. Volcheck GW, Li JT (1994) Elevated serum tryptase level in a case of intraoperative anaphylaxis caused by latex allergy. Arch Intern Med 154: 2243–2245
46. Ohtsuka T, Matsunaru S, Uchida K, Onobori M, Matsumoto T, Kuwahata K, Arita M (1993) Time course of plasma histamine and tryptase following food challenges in children with suspected food allergy. Ann Allergy 71: 139–146
47. Benson MD, Lindberg RE (1996) Amniotic fluid embolism, anaphylaxis and tryptase. Am J Obstet Gynecol 175: 737
48. Okuda T, Funasaka M, Arimitsu M, Umeda T, Wakita K, Koga Y (1994) Anaphylactic shock by ophthalmic wash solution containing chlorhexidine. Masui 43: 1352–1355
49. Yuninger JW, Nelson DR, Squillace DL, Jones RT, Holley KE, Hyma BA, Biedrzycki L, Sweeney KG, Sturner WQ, Schwartz LB (1991) Laboratory investigation of deaths due to anaphylaxis. J Forensic Sci 36: 857–865
50. Ansari MQ, Zamora JL, Lipscomb MF (1993) Postmortem diagnosis of acute anaphylaxis by serum tryptase analysis. A case report. Am J Clin Pathol 99: 101–103
51. Schwartz HJ, Yuninger JW, Schwartz LB (1995) Is unrecognized anaphylaxis a cause of sudden unexpected death? Clin Exp Allergy 25: 866–870
52. Holgate ST, Walters C, Walls AF, Lawrence S, Shell DJ, Variend S, Fleming P, Berry PJ, Gilbert RE, Robinson C (1994) The anaphylaxis hypothesis of sudden infant death syndrome (SIDS): mast cell degranulation in cot death revealed by elevated concentrations of tryptase in serum. Clin Exp Allergy 24: 1115–1122
53. Platt MS, Yuninger JW, Sekula-Perlman A, Irani AM, Smialek J, Mirchandani HG, Schwartz LB (1994) Involvement of mast cells in sudden infant death syndrome. J Allergy Clin Immunol 94: 250–256
54. Randall B, Butts J, Halsey JF (1995) Elevated postmortem tryptase in the absence of anaphylaxis. J Forensic Sci 40: 208–211
55. Ludolph-Hauser D, Ruëff F, Fries C, Schöpf P, Przybilla B (2001) Constitutively raised serum concentrations of mast-cell tryptase and severe anaphylactic reactions to hymenoptera stings. Lancet 357: 361–362
56. Ring J, Messmer K (1977) Incidence and severity of anaphylactoid reactions to colloid volume substitutes. Lancet i: 466–469
57. Biedermann T, Ruëff F, Sander CA, Przybilla B (1999) Mastocytosis associated with severe wasp sting anaphylaxis detected by elevated serum mast cell tryptase levels. Brit J Dermatol 141: 1110–1112
58. Kors JW, van Doormaal JJ, de Monchy JG (1993) Anaphylactoid shock following Hymenoptera sting as a presenting symptom of systemic mastocytosis. J Intern Med 233: 255–258
59. Oude Elberink JNG, de Monchy JRG, Kors JW, van Doormal JJ, Dubois AEJ (1997) Fatal anaphylaxis after a yellow jacket sting, despite venom immunotherapy, in two patients with mastocytosis J Allergy Clin Immunol 99: 153–154
60. Fricker M, Helbling A, Schwartz L, Müller U (1997) Hymenoptera sting anaphylaxis and urticaria pigmentosa: clinical findings and results of venom immunotherapy in ten patients. J Allergy Clin Immunol 100: 11–15
61. Bousquet J, Menardo JL, Velasquez G, Michel FB (1988) Systemic reactions during maintenance immunotherapy with honey bee venom. Ann Allergy 61: 63–68
62. Müller U, Helbling A, Bischof M (1989) Predictive value of venom-specific IgE, IgG and IgG subclass antibodies in patients on immunotherapy with honeybee venom. Allergy 44: 412–418

25 Practical Approach to Adverse Food Reactions

I. Vieluf, M. Besler, A. Paschke, H. Steinhart, D. Vieluf

Introduction

Parallel to the increasing prevalence of other atopic diseases as allergic rhinitis, asthma and atopic eczema, adverse reactions to foods have become a more frequent problem in daily practice, although limited epidemiological data are available. Adverse reactions to food may be life-threatening and food allergy is estimated to affect 1–2% of the adult population, and its prevalence is higher in infants and children. Therefore food allergy is one of the most problematic issues that food manufacturers must confront with. In the last few years an increasing interest in consumer protection and in improvement of food safety has been arisen.

Classification

There are many controversies about the terminology of adverse food reactions. Some patients are convinced that they are allergic to foods, although this cannot be verified by objective measures. Many unspecific complaints as fatigue, headache, abdominal pain, and disturbances of concentration and behavior are misdiagnosed as food-allergy. These reactions are often identified by the appropriate allergological examination as psychological reactions.

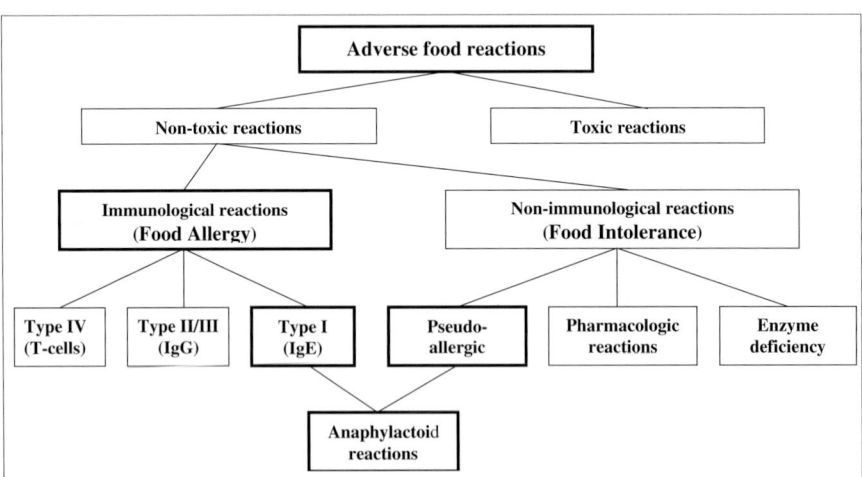

Fig. 1. Adverse food reactions (*AFR*): classification

New Trends in Allergy V
J. Ring, H. Behrendt (Eds.)
© Springer-Verlag Berlin, Heidelberg 2002

According to the position paper of the subcommittee on adverse food reactions of the European Academy of Allergy and Clinical Immunology adverse reactions to food can be divided into toxic and non-toxic reactions (see Fig. 1) [1]. Toxic reactions will occur in any exposed individual provided that the dose is high enough. The occurrence of non-toxic reactions depends on individual susceptibility to a certain food. They are either immune mediated or non-immune mediated. For immune-mediated reactions, the term „food allergy" is recommended, while non-immune-mediated reactions are referred to as „food intolerance". Food allergy can be further divided into IgE-mediated and non-IgE-mediated reactions. When the symptoms mimic those seen in allergic reactions, though no specific immunologic sensitization can be demonstrated, we call them „pseudo-allergic reactions".

Clinical Manifestations

In relation to the function of the gastrointestinal tract or pathologic disturbances many foods or food ingredients can cause allergic reactions in sensitive individuals. They can lead to allergic reactions on the skin (e.g. as urticaria or atopic eczema), the gastrointestinal tract (e.g. vomiting, abdominal pain and/or diarrhea),

Table 1. Clinical manifestations of adverse food reactions (AFR)

I. **Skin reactions:**
   Contact urticaria
   Urticaria/angioedema
   Flush, pruritus
   Oral allergy syndrome (local itching and tingling and/or edema of lips, tongue, palate and pharynx)
   Protein contact dermatitis
   Atopic eczema

II. **Reactions of the respiratory system:**
   Rhinoconjunctivitis
   Asthma bronchiale
   Laryngeal and/or pharyngeal edema
   Hoarseness

III. **Reactions of the gastrointestinal tract:**
   Abdominal pain (cramping)
   Abdominal distension
   Nausea, vomiting
   Gastritis
   Gastroenteritis with diarrhea
   Anorexia
   Flatulence
   Colitis

IV. **Reactions of the cardiovascular system:**
   Cardiac dysrhythmia
   Hypotension
   Vascular collapse
   Anaphylactic shock

the respiratory tract (e.g. bronchial asthma) or the cardiovascular system (hypotension, tachycardia, loss of consciousness, anaphylactic shock), and even to fatal reactions (see Table 1) [2]. In consequence of direct contact with the skin or mucosa foods can cause local urticaria, contact eczema or edema of mouth and throat. In rare cases vapors or steams from certain food e.g. fish, crustaceans and potatoes give rise to respiratory symptoms as asthma or rhinitis.

Epidemiology

The exact prevalence of food allergy is unknown because properly performed epidemiologic studies are rare. Nutritional habits which show regional differences are important for the frequency of individual foods as allergens. E.g. seafood and milk cause most episodes of food-related anaphylaxis in children in Italy, whereas, in the UK and the USA, the most common causes of food-related anaphylaxis in children and adults are peanut and tree nuts [3].

Furthermore the prevalence of allergy to foods varies with the dietary habits and the development of the immune system in different ages. In childhood cow's milk, hen's egg, soybean, wheat and peanut are the most important food allergens. The frequency of cow's milk allergy varies in different studies from 0.7–7% [4, 5], and up to 80% of the children „outgrow" their allergy before the 3rd year of life. In adults the estimated prevalence of food allergy or intolerance is about 2% [6–9]. The most frequent offending allergens in adulthood are fruits with cross sensitivity to birch pollen (e.g. apple, cherry), (raw) vegetables (celery, carrot etc.), spices, herbs, tree nuts, seeds, fish and seafood. With the increasing consumption of „health food" and the availability of foreign foods throughout the year, rare food allergens (e.g. kiwi, buckwheat, sesame seed) become more important as causes of food allergy.

In rare cases allergic contact dermatitis to foods is documented (e.g. protein contact dermatitis to fish or raw potatoes in food handlers or a generalized contact dermatitis due to intake of food containing nickel in sensitized individuals) [10, 11].

The exact prevalence of adverse reactions to food additives in the general population is unknown, but it is certainly overestimated. In relation to immune mediated food allergies pseudo-allergic reactions (e.g. urticaria, angioedema, bronchial asthma, anaphylactoid reactions) are rare (estimated prevalence in the general population about 0.1–0.23%, more frequent in adults between 20 to 40 years). The most common offending agents are food additives as preservatives (e.g. benzoates, sulphites), azo dyes (e.g. tartrazine), taste- and flavor-enhancers (monosodium glutamate), flavorings and sweeteners.

Diagnosis

Because of the possibly large variety of food ingredients, which are consumed in relation to an adverse food reaction, it is often difficult to determine the offending allergen(s). Therefore the clinician needs the patient's cooperation. The di-

Table 2. Diagnostic procedures of AFR

1. Case history:
Ingested foods and their ingredients
Description of symptoms
Timing of onset of symptoms
Quantity of food to produce symptoms
Frequency of reactions and reproducibility
Most recent occurrence
Accompanying factors (e.g. exercise, intake of other foods, drugs, coffee, alcohol, infections, stress etc.)
⇒ Diary reporting symptoms and food intake is necessary !

2. Skin tests:
(Skin application food test, SAFT)
Skin-prick test (SPT)
„Prick-prick" test
(Scarification test)
(Intradermal skin test)
(Atopy Patch Test)

3. In vitro assays:
Determination of total IgE
Determination of specific IgE antibodies to food allergens (e.g. RAST, CAP-RAST, EAST)
(Basophil histamine release)
(Western-blot)

4. Elimination/reintroduction diets:
Baseline registration of symptoms
Diet period

5. Provocation tests:
Open oral challenge with native foods/-additives
Single or double blinded oral challenge with selected foods/-additives (DBPCFC)
(Intragastral provocation under endoscopic control [IPEC])
(Colonoscopic allergen provocation test [COLAP])

Table 3. Threshold doses of food allergens in DBPCFC

Allergens	Amount	Estimated protein content[b]	Literature
Milk	0.5–8 g[a] up to 200 ml	125 mg–2 g up to 6.6 g	Bock et al. 1978
Milk	5–50 ml	165 mg–1.65 g	Host and Samuelsson 1988
Milk	5 g–250 g	165 mg–8.25 g	Norgaard and Bindslev-Jensen 1992
Egg	25 mg–8 g[a]	12 mg–4 g	Bock et al. 1978
Egg	50 mg–50 g	6 mg–6 g	Norgaard and Bindslev-Jensen 1992

Table 3. Continued

Allergens	Amount	Estimated protein content[b]	Literature
Egg white	<100 mg (30% of 40 patients)	<11 mg	Moneret-Vautrin et al. 1998
	100–1000 mg (30%)	11–110 mg	
	1–7 g (30%)	110 mg–780 mg	
	>10 g (10%)	>1.1 g	
Cod fish	6 mg–6.7 g	1 mg–1 g	Hansen and Bindslev-Jensen 1992
Shrimp	4 g–64 g[c]	700 mg–12 g	Daul et al. 1988
Beef	250 mg–60g	48 mg–11.5 g	Werfel et al. 1997
Peanut	100 mg–8 g[a]	26 mg–2 g	Bock et al. 1978
Peanut	ca. 4–100 mg (after ca. 200 µg subjective symptoms)	2–50 mg (after 100 µg subjective symptoms)	Hourihane et al. 1997b
Peanut	<100 mg (25% of 50 patients)		Moneret-Vautrin et al. 1998
	100–1000 mg (62.5%)		
	1–7.1 g (12.5%)		
Soy bean	1 g–8 g[a] up to 200 ml	0.3 g–2.7 g	Bock et al. 1978
Cashew nut	0.5 g – 8 g[a]	88 mg–1.4 g	Bock et al. 1978
Pecan nut	1 g[a]	93 mg	Bock et al. 1978
Pistachio	500 mg[a]	88 mg	Bock et al. 1978
Sesame seed	100 mg–10 g	18 mg–1.8 g	Kanny et al. 1996
Sesame seed	16 g (9–23 g)	2.8 g (1.6–4 g)	Majamaa et al. 1999
Fruits (apricot, cherry, peach, plum)	500 mg (subjective symptoms)	3–4.5 mg (subjective symptoms)	Pastorello et al. 1994
	4–8 g[d]	24–72 mg	
Apple	4–32 g[d]	12 mg–96 mg	Pastorello et al. 1999
Celery	700 mg (48% of 21 patients)	11 mg	Ballmer-Weber et al. 2000
	1.9–5.6 g (10%)	30–90 mg	
	13.3 g (5%)	213 mg	
	28.5 g (29%)	456 mg	
Hazelnut	Mean provocative dose:		
	1.4 g (patients in Copenhagen)	196 mg	Ortolani et al. 2000
	2.7 g (patients in Zurich)	378 mg	
	15.3 g (patients in Milan)	2.14 g	

[a] Applied to dry mass.
[b] Calculated according to food tables (Souci, Fachmann, Kraut).
[c] No lower doses tested.
[d] Open provocation.

agnostic procedure in adverse food reactions is based on a detailed case history, skin tests, in vitro assays and in selected cases provocation tests (see Table 2) [1, 9, 12].

It is evident, that in highly sensitized individuals small traces of allergenic proteins may be sufficient to cause severe allergic reactions. However, very few attempts have been made to define precisely the dose-response relationship for allergenic foods [13]. Some studies with double-blind, placebo-controlled food challenges indicated that the threshold dose for objective symptoms ranged from 1 to 50 mg (see Table 3) [14–18]. More data are needed to allow a more precise definition of the dose-response relationship for the commonly allergenic foods.

Therapy

The best treatment of food allergy is the complete avoidance of the offending allergen (see Table 4). This categorical recommendation for avoidance assumes a correct diagnosis and the identification of the responsible specific allergen. The avoidance is not a problem, if the patient is allergic to exotic foods as mango or lobster. But it is more difficult, if elementary foods like cows' milk or hens' egg are involved, especially in children. In such cases detailed dietary advice is necessary to avoid malnutrition in children [9].

But advising the severely allergic patient to avoid the offending food does not always guarantee safety. There are many reports of food induced anaphylactic shock and even deaths in subjects who had inadvertently eaten a food to which they were allergic. In most cases, the offending food was found to be a minor ingredient or contaminant in other foods. These so called „hidden" allergens (unsuspected but legitimate presence of a food material that is not declared on the label) can be found inadvertently in most composed and pre-packaged foods or

Table 4. Therapy of AFR

Specific elimination of offending foods:
  Correct identification of the foods and additives
  Knowledge of potential hidden sources of the food items
  Consideration of possible cross-reactivity between foods and other allergens
  ⇒ Supervision of elimination diets with regard to nutritional requirements, particularly in growing children!

Rescue medication (for patients with a history of severe anaphylactoid reactions):
  Oral antihistamines
  Oral or rectal corticosteroids
  Self-administerable epinephrine

Oral sodium cromoglycate (DNCG):
  If avoidance is difficult or impossible

Immunotherapy (IT):
  Studies about specific parenteral IT with pollen allergens in patients with pollen associated food allergy
  Studies about subcutaneous IT in patients with peanut allergy
  Oral IT (e.g. cow's milk)

are legally not declared or not sufficiently declared on the label. The main reasons for hidden allergens are:
- Contaminations during the processing of foods (improper clean up, cross contaminations by dust or by pieces of the allergen remaining in the processing facilities)
- Misclassification of raw material or misformulation
- Replacement of ingredients due to change of the recipe
- Insufficient or erroneous labelling.

Common food allergens as milk, egg, soybean and wheat are frequently hidden in pre-packaged foods, but are not declared sufficiently. This can be fatal for the allergic consumer. Therefore the name of the food ingredient shall indicate the true nature of the food and normally be specific and not generic. Terms as „caseine", „spices", „herbs", „lecithine" should be avoided and replaced and/or extended by the exact declaration of the ingredients source (e.g. milk, celery, soybean, peanut).

According to the 25% rule, a compound ingredient that is not considered an additive and for which a name has been established in a Codex standard or in national legislation need not be mentioned on the label if it makes up less than 25% of the total food [19]. Therefore it is possible, that an ingredient found in small quantities in a food must be declared, whereas the same substance found in large quantities as a compound ingredient need not to be declared. Legumes (e.g. soybean, peanut, pea), tree nuts, milk, egg, wheat, celery and seeds are the common inducers of inadvertent reactions to concealed food allergens [20, 21, 22].

Modifications of Allergenicity

With the increasing consumption of the so called „convenience food" the influence of various methods of food processing on the allergenicity of food allergens has to be considered (see Table 5).

The intrinsic properties of the food protein, the overall composition of the food, and the past processing history (especially thermal processing) all have an effect on the allergenic potential. The thermal modification of proteins is important because heat treatment may lead to substantial changes in their allergenic nature. A degree of resistance to digestion is a clear requirement for an allergenic dietary protein, because allergens must be absorbed intact (or as substantial fragments) through the gut mucosa, if they are able to stimulate an allergic response. Troublesome allergenic epitopes are mainly linear, because these are more likely to survive denaturation in the gut, as well as heating. Thus, heating can increase or decrease allergenicity, depending upon the protein involved and on the individual patient. Most food allergens have a molecular weight more than 10 kDa.

Various methods of food processing (e.g. mechanical processing, preservation, cooling, chemical hydrolysis) can alter the allergenicity of food allergens, but there are poor data about this topic [23]. Only some studies about the influence of thermal processing and enzymatic hydrolysis exist (see Tables 6, 7) [24,

Table 5. Methods of food processing, which may modify the allergenic potential of food allergens

Preparation:
  Washing, peeling, storing

Processes of crushing:
  Cutting, rough-grinding, grinding

Thermal processing:
  Drying, heating (baking, blanching, broiling, steaming, cooking, roasting, pasteurization, ultra-high heating, sterilization), cooling, freezing, freeze-drying

Biochemical processing:
  Fermentation (with lactic acid or acetic acid, clarification, tenderizing etc.)

Methods for isolation and cleaning:
  Melting, pressing, extraction, destillation, raffination, filtration, centrifugation, sifting, polishing

Chemical conservation:
  Alcohol, pickling, salt, sugar, preservatives

Additional processings/methods:
  Mixing, suspending, emulgation, homogenization, stabilization, extrudation, texturizing, bleaching etc.

Table 6. Stability of Food Allergens from animal origin

Allergens	Heat stability	Stability against enzymatic hydrolysis	Importance as hidden allergen
Milk and milk products	Mostly stable	Partially stable	High
Egg and egg products	Stable	Stable	High
Fish and fish products	Stable	Partially stable	Low
Crustaceans and products	Stable	No data	Low
Meat and meat products	Partially stable	Low	Low

Table 7. Stability of food allergens from plant origin

Allergens	Heat stability	Stability against enzymatic hydrolysis	Importance as hidden allergen
Peanut and peanut products	Stable	Partially stable	High
Soy and soy products	Partially stable	Partially stable	High
Nuts and nut products	Stable	Partially stable	High
Sesame seed and products	No data	No data	High
Cereals and cereal products	Partially stable	No data	High
Fruits of the Rosaceae family	Mostly unstable	unstable	Low
Latex associated fruits	No data (Avocado stable?)	No data (Avocado stable!)	Low
Celery and celery products	Partially stable	Mostly unstable	High
Carrot and carrot products	unstable	No data	Low

25]. Protein denaturation from heating can lead to a decrease or an increase of the allergenic potency: Fruits and certain vegetables are labile to heat. Cow's milk, rice, soybean, celery, cereals, spices, mustard, and almond show a partial decrease, peanut, hazelnut, fish, hens' egg and crustaceans no modification of the allergenicity after heating. Oxidative processes due to mechanical crushing can cause changes of the proteins. „Enzymatic browning" raises a decrease of allergenicity in fruits and vegetables.

Genetic engineering is a new method of food processing, which is controversially discussed. Among other food safety aspects, the genetically modified foods have to be proved according to their allergenicity [26–29]. The producers have to take care that allergenicity is not transferred into a genetically modified food or ingredient. Each genetically modified product has to be tested for suspected allergens by in vivo and in vitro methods. Stability of a protein or of protein fragments to digestion simulated by gastric fluid may be used to assess the potential allergenicity of a protein. Due to the possibility of new proteinaceaous allergens in genetically modified foods there may be an increased risk for the allergic consumer. Otherwise genetic engineering methods could be helpful in the prevention of food allergies, because this method can be used to prepare hypoallergenic foods. For example, Matsuda et al. [30] were able to produce transgenic rice containing less major allergen. Other methods for producing hypoallergenic foods are listed in Table 8.

Table 8. Production of hypoallergenic food

Food allergen	Treatment	Hypoallergenic product
Casein, whey proteins	Enzymatic hydrolysis, heating, ultra-filtration	Extensively hydrolysed milk-based formulas: Peptides <8 kDa (Halken & Host 1997)
Wheat flour	Extraction with saline solution	Decreased allergen content (Ikezawa et al. 1994)
Wheat flour	Enzymatic hydrolysis with bromelaine	Elimination of an IgE-binding epitope of Glutenin (Tanabe et al. 1996)
Rice	Enzymatic hydrolysis (actinase), extraction with tensid solution	Decreased content of 16- and 50-kDa allergens (Ikezawa et al. 1992)
Rice	Genetic engineering: Antisense strategy	Decreased content of 16-kDa major allergens (Matsuda et al. 1996)
Rice	Basic hydrolysis	Decreased content of 16-kDa major allergen (Ikezawa et al. 1999)
Rice	Over-pressure treatment	Reduction of the content of Globuline and Albumin (Juji et al. 1999)
Soy milk	Protein precipitation with sodium sulfate solution	Decreased content of the major allergen Gly m Bd30 K (Samoto et al. 1994)

Labelling

Patients and their relatives, physicians, dieticians, consumers, manufacturers and authorities need sufficient information regarding the nature of food allergens, their occurrence, the risk of exposure and the exact composition of each product. This information is important for the consumer in general and vital for the allergic one.

Food-allergic patients should be cautioned to read the ingredient label on all foods and they should repeat this procedure every time they shop, as ingredients of the same product may change without warning. Patients should also learn the scientific and technical names for foods that may appear on labels. Many ambiguous labelling practices persist that may camouflage the presence of an allergen. Some foods may appear to be so straightforward that the patient may not feel it necessary to scrutinize the label for hidden allergens. Alternatively, they may be so complex that the label is merely perused, or the food product is considered so unlikely to be allergenic that the label is never reviewed at all.

When food not personally prepared and served in one's home is consumed, the risk of encountering a hidden allergen increases. It is essential that food-allergic individuals develop a polite assertiveness while eating outwards. Particular care should be taken to make inquiries about ingredients as specific as possible.

A sufficient and correct labelling of food allergens is the most important measure in the prevention of allergic reactions to foods. Over 170 foods have been documented in the literature as causing allergic reactions. It is evident that it is impossible to deal with all of these. For practical purposes the food manufacturer should concentrate the attention on dealing effectively with „major allergens". Therefore a list of the most common allergenic foods to be labelled is necessary. This list has to be based on scientific data regarding prevalence and severity of adverse food reactions and must be useful for manufacturers and (allergic) consumers. The criteria are as follows:
- Prevalence of allergic reactions
- Frequency of consumption
- Frequency of application in foods
- Stability of allergens
- Severity of symptoms
- Documentation of defined allergic anaphylactic reactions or deaths due to the offending allergen (food challenge performed as DBPCFC)
- Severe reactions due to low allergen doses

Based on these criteria our recommendation for a list of the most common food allergens for mandatory labelling are (see Table 9):
- Cows' milk
- Hens' egg
- Tree nuts (e.g. hazelnut)
- Peanut
- Soybean
- Fish

Table 9. Summarized rating of the most important food allergens

Allergens	Frequency of reactions (F, frequently; R, rare)	Severity of reactions (D, death; A, anaphylaxis)	Stability/hidden allergen	Necessity of declaration
Milk	F	D, A	+/+	+
Egg	F	A	+/+	+
Fish	F	D, A	+/−	+
Crustacean	R	D, A	+/−	+
Meat	R	A	−/−	−
Peanut	F	D, A	+/+	+
Soybean	F	D, A	+/+	+
Nuts	F	D, A	+/+	+
Sesame seed	R	A	?/+	+
Other seeds	R	A	?/+	+
Wheat	R	A	+/+	+
Other cereals	R	−	?/?	+[a]
Fruits (Rosaceae)	F	A	−/−	−
Latex associated fruits	R	A	?/?	−
Celery	F	A	+/+	+
Spices	F	A	?/?	−

[a] Recommendation for gluten-containing cereals provoking gluten-sensitive enteropathy.

- Wheat
- Crustaceans/molluscs
- Celery
- Seeds (sesame, poppy, sunflower)

Physicians and dieticians need detailed information about the occurrence of certain food allergens, the changes of their allergenicity and possible cross-reactions to advise the allergic patients. Many measures are needed to improve the situation of the consumer suffering from adverse food reactions. Technical development, as well as the development of new products, increases the need for appropriate labelling, as many products and ingredients are unknown to the consumer, and their presence in a particular product might be unexpected. In the secondary prevention of adverse food reactions, better labelling of foods, that are capable of causing serious illness or even fatalities in some consumers or causing reduced quality of life in many others, should be given high priority.

References

1. Bruijnzeel-Koomen C, Ortolani C, Aas K, Bindslev-Jensen C, Björkstén LB, Wüthrich LB. Adverse reactions to food. Position paper of the European Academy of Allergology and Clinical Immunology. Allergy 1995; 50:623–635
2. Sampson HA. Food allergy. Part 1: Immunopathogenesis and clinical disorders. J Allergy Clin Immunol 1999a; 103:717–728

3. Hourihane JO'B. Prevalence and severity of food allergy–need for control. Allergy 1998; 53 (Suppl 46):84–88
4. Høst A, Halken S. A prospective study of cow milk allergy in Danish infants during the first 3 years of life. Allergy 1990; 45:587–596
5. Schrander JJP, van den Bogart JPH, Forget PP, Schrander-Stumpel CTRM, Juijten RH, Kester ADM. Cow's milk protein intolerance in infants under 1 year of age: a prospective epidemiological study. Eur J Pediatr 1993; 152:640–644
6. Niestijl Jansen JJ, Kardinaal AFM, Huijbers GH, Vlieg-Boerstra BJ, Martens BPM, Ockhuzen T. Prevalence of food allergy and intolerance in the adult Dutch population. J Allergy Clin Immunol 1994; 93:446–456
7. Young E, Stoneham MD, Petruckevitch A, Barton J, Rona R. A population study of food intolerance. Lancet 1994; 343 (8096):1127–1130
8. Metcalfe DD. Food allergy in adults. In: Metcalfe DD, Sampson HA, Simon RA (eds) Food Allergy: Adverse Reactions to Foods and Food Additives, 2nd edn. Blackwell Science, 1997; Oxford
9. Sampson HA. Food allergy. Part 2: Diagnosis and management. J Allergy Clin Immunol 1999b; 103:981–989
10. Hjorth N, Roed-Petersen J. Occupational protein contact dermatitis in food handlers. 1976; 2:28–42
11. Klaschka F. Hämatogenes Kontaktekzem durch Nahrungsmittel. Allergologie 1987; 10:93–96
12. Holgate ST, Church MK. Allergy. Gower Medical Publishing 1993; London, New York
13. Bousquet J, Björkstén B, Bruijnzeel-Koomen CAFM, Huggett A, Ortolani C, Warner JO, Smith JM. Scientific criteria and the selection of allergenic food for product labelling. Allergy 1998; 53:3–21
14. Bock SA, Lee WY, Remigio LK, May CD. Studies of hypersensitivity reactions to foods in infants and children. J Allergy Clin Immunol 1978; 62:327–334
15. Norgaard A, Bindslev-Jensen C. Egg and milk allergy in adults. Diagnosis and characterization. Allergy 1992; 47:503–509
16. Moneret-Vautrin DA, Rance F, Kanny G, Olsewski A, Gueant JL, Dutau G, Guerin L. Food allergy to peanuts in France–evaluation of 142 observations. Clin Exp Allergy 1998; 28:1113–1119
17. European Commission. Scientific co-operation on questions relating to food. Task 7.2. „Consideration of the epidemiological basis for appropriate measures for the protection of public health in respect of food allergy" Scoop/Nutr/Report/2; 2th May 1998
18. Malmheden Yman I. Hidden allergens in food detected and quantitated by specific antibodies. The 5th International Conference Agri-Food Antibodies '99, Norwich 14–17 September 1999
19. Codex Alimentarius Commission. Food labelling- complete texts. Joint FAO/WHO Food Standards Programme, FAO/WHO, Rome, 1999
20. Sampson HA, Mendelson LM, Rosen JP. Fatal and near-fatal anaphylactic reactions to food in children and adolescents. N Engl J Med 1992; 327:380–384
21. Malmheden Yman I, Eriksson A, Everitt G, Yman L, Karlsson T. Analysis of food proteins for verification of contamination or mislabelling. Food Agric Immunol 1994; 6:167–172
22. Malmheden Yman I. Serious reaction to food. Be aware of soy protein and peanuts. Var Föda 1997; 5:8–9z.
23. Besler M, Steinhart H, Paschke A. Stability of food allergens and allergenicity of processed foods. J Chromatogr 2001 (in press)
24. Fischer K, Vieths S, Dehne LI, Bögl KW. Verarbeitungsbedingte Einflüsse auf die Allergenität von Lebensmitteln. Eine Übersicht. 1993 Soz Ep-Heft 6
25. Davis PJ, Williams SC. Protein modification by thermal processing. Allergy 1998; 53 (Suppl 46):102–105
26. Metcalfe DD, Fuchs RL, Townsend R, Sampson HA, Taylor SL, Fordham JR. Allergenicity of foods produced by genetic modification. Crit Rev Food Sci Nutr (Suppl) 1996; 36:29–53
27. Metcalfe DD, Astwood JD, Townsend R et al. Assessment of the allergenic potential of foods derived from genetically modified food plants. Crit Rev Food Sci Nutr (Suppl) 1999; 36:165–186

28. Vieths S. Allergenic potential of genetically modified plant foods–how reliable is the proposed assessment strategy? In: Proceedings of the International Symposium on Novel Foods Regulation in the European Union- Integrity of the Process of Safety Evaluation. Berlin: Federal Institute of Consumer Health Protection and Veterinary Medicine, 1998: 295–310
29. Jany KD, Greiner R. Gentechnik und Lebensmittel. Berichte der Bundesforschungsanstalt für Ernährung. Bundesforschungsanstalt für Ernährung (ed) Karlsruhe,1998
30. Matsuda T, Nakase M, Adachi T, Nakamura R, Tada Y, Shimada H, Takahashi, Fujimura TJ. Allergenic proteins in rice: strategies for reduction and evaluation. In: Food Allergies and Intolerances. Symposium (Eisenbrand, G, Dayan AD, Ring J, Aulepp H, Elias PS, Grunow W, Schlatter J, eds) 1996; pp 161–9, VCH Weinheim

Occupational and Environmental Aspects

26 Multiple Chemical Sensitivity and Others: Allergological, Environmental and Psychological Investigations in Individuals with Indoor Air-Related Complaints

B. Eberlein-König, B. Przybilla, P. Kühnl, G. Golling, I. Gebefügi, J. Ring

Abstract

Background: Clinical observations point to an expanding group of individuals attributing hypersensitivity phenomena to indoor air pollution. *Objective*: It was the aim of this study to characterize such subjects by an approach of interdisciplinary investigations. *Methods*: 65 individuals, recruited by a public campaign, were investigated by a thorough allergological examination and a structured psychological interview. Measurements of common indoor pollutants in the air and in the dust were performed in rooms of several selected patients. *Results*: 42 patients (65%) revealed a sensitization to common allergens, out of these 32 (49%) to house dust mites. 38 (58%) patients showed a psychosomatic or psychotic disorder. Increased concentrations of at least one of the measured substances were found in 11 out of 13 patients. According to these results, four groups of patients could be identified: 17 patients (26%) had „classic" allergic diseases treated inadequately. In 19 patients (29%) allergic diseases were superimposed by strong psychosomatic interactions. An exclusive psychosomatic or psychotic cause of the complaints was found in 19 (29%). 10 subjects (16%) had „classic" allergic diseases (e.g. allergic rhinoconjunctivitis, urticaria), however, there were additional indications of hypersensitivity reactions to components other than classical allergens. *Conclusion*: Patients presenting with hypersensitivity phenomena attributed by themselves to indoor air pollution are a heterogeneous group and need a diligent work-up including intense allergological examination. The role of increased concentrations of indoor air pollutants has to be elucidated further.

Introduction

In recent years, air pollution as well as allergy have raised much interest in the general public, and there are increasing numbers of patients attributing hypersensitivity phenomena to indoor air exposures. There are a number of disorders that are associated with indoor pollutants. The sick building syndrome is characterized by symptoms of mucous membrane irritation, neurotoxic effects, asthma and asthma-like symptoms, skin dryness and irritation, gastrointestinal complaints and other ailments associated with certain modern buildings [1]. The multiple chemical sensitivity (MCS) syndrome is a complex, chronic disorder with multisystemic symptoms occurring in response to a wide variety of chemical

New Trends in Allergy V
J. Ring, H. Behrendt (Eds.)
© Springer-Verlag Berlin, Heidelberg 2002

odours or low-level exposures [2]. The term „clinical ecology syndrome" („eco-syn-drome") was suggested for a group of patients suffering from polysomatic complaints with a subjective feeling of allergy against environmental noxious agents [3].

It has been shown that asthma and rhinitis can be exacerbated by respiratory irritants [4, 5]. In a random general telephone survey the prevalence of sensitiv-ity to chemical irritants was equivalent to that of allergy [6]. 6.3% of respon-dents to a population-based survey reported a doctor's diagnosis of environmen-tal illness or MCS and 15.9% allergies or unusual sensitivity to everyday chemicals [7]. While allergic diseases can be verified by skin tests, in vitro tests and chal-lenge tests, at this time there are no methods to demonstrate sensitivity to envi-ronmental chemicals in an objective manner. As people spend most of their time indoors at work or at home, a real and frequent occurrence of hypersensitivity to chemical indoor pollution would be of major concern. We conducted a study, in which individuals complaining of hypersensitivity to indoor pollution were evaluated by a thorough allergological and psychological investigation. Further-more, measurements of common indoor air pollutants were performed in rooms of some of these patients.

Materials and Methods

Study Group

By a public campaign (newspaper, information by telephone call), a study deal-ing with hypersensitivity due to indoor pollution was announced and individu-als with respective complaints were invited to participate (24 males, 45 females, mean age 45.8±15.0 years).

Questionnaire

All individuals answered a specific questionnaire regarding their symptoms and their medical history, including family and personal history of allergies, as well as their living and work places with special regard to building materials, heat-ing, conditions of walls and floors, temperature, air humidity, interior equipment and habits (Table 1).

Allergy Diagnosis

Skin prick tests (also dermal tests, if skin prick tests were negative) with a broad spectrum of aeroallergens and food allergens (Bencard, SmithKline Beecham GmbH, Neuss, Germany) and the determination of specific IgE antibodies in the serum (Pharmacia CAP System, RAST FEIA; Pharmacia, Uppsala, Sweden) to a panel of potential indoor allergens were performed. If needed, these investiga-tions were supplemented by nasal challenge tests. Special care was taken to as-sess the relationship between hypersensitivity and their possible elicitors.

Table 1. Questionnaire

Surname: Date:
First name:
Date of birth:
Profession/Employment:
    Since when?
Previous employment:

Symptoms

Skin ☐   Respiratory tract ☐   Neurological/Psychological symptoms ☐   Others

Existence of symptoms since:
Beginning of symptoms after entrance into the room(s)
    each time ☐   sometimes ☐
End of symptoms after leaving the room(s)
    each time ☐   sometimes ☐
When (months/day/time) ?

Rooms

Which rooms? (draw a draft)
Duration of stay in rooms:
Condition at other locations (where? how long?)
Complaints of other individuals at the same locality
    No ☐   Yes ☐   What kind of complaint(s)?
How did you realize that the complaints depended on rooms?
Rooms: with much road ☐   with little road ☐   city ☐   country ☐
    Direction: to the backyard ☐   To the street ☐   Floor number: Others:
Built when:
Type of heating?
Oil tank in house: Yes ☐   No ☐
Attached garage: Yes ☐   No ☐
Flooring: Wall to wall carpeting ☐   Carpets ☐
                 Tiles ☐   Wooden floor ☐
Air humidifier: Yes ☐   No ☐
Wooden ceiling: Yes ☐   No ☐
Air conditioning: Yes ☐   No ☐   Other
Furniture:
House plants: Permanent ☐ Temporary ☐
Parasites e.g. cockroaches:
Pest control with?
How often do you or others use conventional cleaning?
Do you use exclusively alternative cleaning material?
How many individuals are usually in the rooms?
Domestic pets of these individuals?
Visitors: No ☐   Yes ☐
Smoking: ☐   No. of cigarettes/day: Non-smoking ☐   Passive smoking ☐
Already performed measures to clear up the complaints?

Results:

Table 2. Diagnostic work-up

Allergological evaluation	
History:	Complete medical and allergological history, with special emphasis on assessing the relationship of hypersensitivity to possible elicitors.
Skin tests:	Prick tests (intradermal tests, if necessary) with a broad spectrum of aeroallergens and food allergens; additional epicutaneous tests, if needed.
In vitro tests:	Determination of specific IgE antibodies to a panel of 35 potential indoor allergens.
Challenge tests:	If necessary for definite diagnosis

Psychological evaluation	
Psychological interview Questionnaires:	German Health Locus of Control Scale [8]
	Personality Test („Gießen Test") [9]
	List of complaints („Gießener Beschwerdebogen") [10]

Psychological Evaluation

An unstructured psychological interview was performed by a trained psychologist for 2 h. During this interview, particularly the following items were considered: Exact circumstances at onset of the indoor related symptoms, development, and course of the disease, conflict situations of the patient at home or at work, live events and strokes of fate, chronic distress or missing body perception and handling of the indoor related symptoms. Questions like „What advantages are derived from complaints?", „Is there a symbolic meaning relative to complaints?", „What strategies had the patient developed to overcome the complaints?" were the central points.

Furthermore individuals were investigated using the „German Health Locus of Control Scale (HLC) [8]. This questionnaire measures the attitude towards health management with three dimensions: The Internal Locus of Control Scale (ILC), the External Locus of Control Scale (ELC) and the Chance Dimension (CD). Furthermore, a personality test („Gießen Test") [9] and a questionnaire with a list of ailments („Gießener Beschwerdebogen") was used [10] (Table 2).

Analysis of Chemicals

Measurements of indoor air pollutants were performed in alleged rooms of 13 patients. These patients were selected because there were indications of actual hypersensitivity to indoor pollutants other than known allergens or because the patients themselves insisted on these measurements. Aromatic hydrocarbons (benzene, toluene, ethylbenzene, xylene) and terpenes (α-pinene, 3-caren, p-cymol, limonene) were analyzed in probes of the air collected for 12 h, lindane, pentachlorphenol (PCP) and *cis/trans*-permethrin were measured in probes of dust, which was collected by a vacuum cleaner over a time period of 2 weeks according to previous studies [11]. The results of these studies have been related to the results of the present study.

Results

In total, 95 individuals contacted us in response to the public campaign. After explaining the aim and the design of the study, 24 individuals were not further interested. A total of 71 patients attributing hypersensitivity symptoms to indoor air pollutants, especially to „chemicals", were included. 6 patients presented with disorders unrelated to indoor allergy or sensitivity (osteosarcoma, Lyme disease, multiple nevuscellnevi, pityriasis versicolor, emphysema of the lung, marital problems); these were not considered in the further study.

Subjective symptoms of the remaining 65 patients (20 males, 45 females; mean age 45.8±15.0 years) are shown in Table 3. Burning eyes, dyspnea, rhinorrhea, cough, headache and fatigue were the most common complaints.

In total, 42 patients (65%) revealed a sensitization to common allergens. Out of these 32 (49%) patients showed positive prick tests to house dust mites, often combined with positive reactions to pollen and animal epithelia (n=18, 28%). Specific antibodies against house dust mites were found in 31 (48%), against pollen in 32 (48%) and against animal epithelia in 14 (22%) patients. Total IgE was increased (>100 kU/l) in 16 (25%) patients. Nasal provocation tests to house dust mites were positive in 20 (31%) individuals (Table 4). 46 patients (71%) suffered from „classical" allergic or pseudo-allergic diseases. 38 (58%) patients suffered from psychosomatic symptoms. According to the somatic and psychological examinations, the following diagnostic criteria were applied: Presence of common (pseudo)allergic diseases (rhinoconjunctivitis, asthma, atopic eczema, urticaria, angioedema), definite association of symptoms with stay in certain rooms, somatization symptoms, psychosis, conversion disorder or psychoneurotic conflict situations. Based on these criteria, four different groups could be distinguished:

Group A 17 individuals (26.2%; 9 males, 8 females; mean age 34.8±15.7 years) suffered from „classical" allergic or pseudo-allergic diseases not treated adequately

Table 3. Subjective symptoms in 65 patients with hypersensitivity symptoms attributed to indoor pollution

Symptoms	n	Symptoms	n
Burning eyes	38	Wheals	7
Dyspnoea	26	Nausea	6
Rhinorrhoea	22	Throat irritation	3
Cough	17	Difficulty to concentrate	2
Headache	13	Diarrhoea	2
Fatigue	13	Anxiousness	2
Loss of sleep	8	Olfactory disturbance	2
Weakness	7	Paraesthesia	2
Itch	8	Hair loss	1
Tachycardia	7	Abdominal pain	1

Table 4. Numbers of patients with positive or negative results in different allergological tests

Prick testing

	House dust mites	Animal epithelia	Pollen	Negative
Group A	14	11	14	0
Group B	12	9	16	1
Group C	0	0	1	18
Group D	6	4	2	3
total	32	24	33	22

Specific IgE-antibodies

	House dust mites	Animal epithelia	Pollen	Negative
Group A	14	8	12	0
Group B	13	6	15	1
Group C	0	0	2	17
Group D	4	0	3	3
total	31	14	32	21

Total IgE

	<100kU/l	>100kU/l	Not done
Group A	8	8	1
Group B	13	6	0
Group C	19	0	0
Group D	8	2	0
Total	48	16	1

Nasal challenge

	House dust mites	Animal epithelia	Pollen	Negative	Not wanted/ done
Group A	9	2	3	0	5
Group B	7	2	1	0	11
Group C					19
Group D	4			1	5
Total	20	4	4	1	40

Group B   In 19 individuals (29.2%; 7 males, 12 females; mean age 46.3±12.6 years) there were common allergic diseases superimposed by strong psycho-somatic effects

Group C   An exclusive psychosomatic cause of the complaints was found in 19 individuals (29.2%; 4 males, 15 females; mean age 55.7±8.8 years)

Group D   In 10 individuals (15.4%, 4 males, 6 females; mean age 42.2±14.6 years) there were indications of actual hypersensitivity to indoor pollutants other than well-known allergens from biological sources, and all of these were also suffering from common allergic diseases. Details are given in Table 5.

Table 5. Diagnostic classification individuals attributing hypersensitivity symptoms to indoor air pollution

Group A: patients only with common allergic (or other hypersensitivity) diseases

Diagnosis	n
Allergic rhinoconjunctivitis	13
Allergic rhinoconjunctivitis and asthma	3
Allergic rhinoconjunctivitis and atopic eczema	1
Total	17

Group B: patients with common allergic (or other hypersensitivity) diseases superimposed by psychosomatic effects

Diagnosis	n
Allergic rhinoconjunctivitis	12
Allergic asthma	3
Urticaria/angioedema	3
Allergic rhinoconjunctivitis and atopic eczema	1
Total	19

Group C: patients without common allergic diseases

Diagnosis	n
Adjustment disorder	7
Paranoid personality disorder	5
Somatization disorder	5
Persistent delusional disorder	2
Total	19

Group D: patients with common allergic diseases in combination with indications of hypersensitivity due to indoor pollutants other than known allergens

Diagnosis	n
Allergic rhinoconjunctivitis	7
Urticaria/angioedema	3
Total	10

The results of the personality test („Gießen Test") were not statistically different between the groups. Analysis of the questionnaire with a list of complaints („Gießener Beschwerdebogen") showed a tendency to more subjective complaints in patients of group B and C. According to the results of the „German Health Locus of Control Scale" patients with „common" allergic diseases believed that their health mainly can be influenced by others, not by themselves.

Table 6. Results of the measurements in rooms of 13 patients. The highest measured value is given

Patients (group) Compounds (control values)[a]	1 (B)	2 (C)	3 (C)	4 (C)	5 (C)	6 (C)	7 (C)	8 (C)	9 (D)	10 (D)	11 (D)	12 (D)	13 (D)
Terpenes (ng/l)													
(Total) (80)	9	21	6	23	20	18	3	18	1	60	0	18	206
Alpha-Pinene (17)	0	11	4	5	7	0	0	12	0	**30**	0	0	4
3-Caren (9)	0	0	0	3	0	0	0	6	0	14	0	0	196
p-Cymol (2)	0	0	0	0	0	0	0	0	0	2	0	0	0
Limonene (45)	9	10	3	16	13	18	3	0	1	14	0	18	7
Aromatic hydrocarbons													
(ng/l) (Total) (112)	36	**207**	42	69	97	**125**	13	**370**	10	**166**	**122**	81	**230**
Benzene (11)	3	6	3	5	10	**20**	2	6	1	2	**22**	7	2
Toluene (64)	23	**121**	36	52	70	**96**	7	**358**	7	**141**	**100**	51	**167**
Ethylbenzene (6)	3	**20**	0	2	4	0	1	0	0	**13**	0	4	**11**
m,p-Xylene (19)	7	**48**	3	8	10	9	3	6	2	8	0	15-	**39**
o-Xylene (6)	0	**13**	0	2	3	0	0	0	0	2	0	4	**11**
Dust probes (ng/g)													
Lindane(416)	177	19	86	**703**	181	**945**	190	**1333**	157	256	149	382	718
PCP (1430)	261	157	592	**4154**	1067	**1962**	**4412**	**8384**	**2428**	**1120**	430	**5993**	**7146**
cis-Permethrin (0)	0	0	0	0	0	0	0	0	0	0	0	0	**1556**
trans-Permethrin (0)	0	0	0	0	0	0	0	0	0	0	0	0	**27576**

[a] The control values indicate results from measurements in n comparable local rooms.
n=131 for terpenes (total), alpha-pinene, 3-caren, cymol, limonene.
n=132 for aromatic hydrocarbons (total), benzene, toluene, ethylbenzene, m/p/o-xylene.
n=209 for lindane, PCP, cis/trans-permethrin.
Bold represents values beyond the control values.

Measurements of indoor pollutants in the dust or in the air from rooms of 13 patients (group B: $n=1$; group C: $n=7$; group D: $n=5$) revealed increased concentrations of at least one of the measured substances in rooms of 11 patients. Such increased concentrations were found in all five investigated rooms of patients from group D and in 6 of 7 investigated indoor environments from group C. Measurements done in the rooms of the patient from group B did not yield elevated concentrations of pollutants. Details are shown in Table 6.

Two selected case reports will illustrate examples from group D.

Case Reports

Patient 9

A 42-year old non-smoking male presented with a 2-week history of rhinorrhea and burning eyes, when he had bought a new sideboard for his livingroom. The symptoms usually began when he stayed for 1 h in this room and other persons reported throat irritation in this situation. The patient lived alone in his flat without pets. Specific IgE antibodies were detected in the serum against a mixture of grass pollens, natural silk, *Dermatophagoides pteronyssinus* (*D. pter.*) and *Dermatophagoides farinae* (*D. far.*). Total IgE was 291 kU/l.

Skin prick tests yielded positive reactions to grass pollen, rye pollen, corn pollen, *D. pter.*, *D. far.*, *Acarus siro* and cat epithelia. Nasal provocation with *D. far.* resulted in rhinorrhea. A psychosomatic cause for the symptoms was not found. Measurements of indoor air pollutants showed increased concentrations of PCP in the dust (Table 6).

Patient 13

A 54-year-old non-smoking housewife suffered from rhinorrhea, burning eyes, headache, hair loss, nausea, cough, tachycardia and disturbed sleep for 8 years. A relationship of her symptoms to certain rooms of her home was not evident. Her house was built in 1952 and equipped with wooden furniture. She stayed in this house for about 20 h per day. Her husband and her son who lived together with her did not have similar symptoms. There were no pets. Specific serum IgE antibodies were detected against *D. pter.* and *D. far.*, total serum IgE was not elevated. Skin prick tests yielded positive reactions also to *D. pter.* and *D. far.*. A psychosomatic disease could not be diagnosed. Measurements of indoor pollutants revealed increased concentrations of total terpenes, 3-caren, total aromatic hydrocarbons, toluene, ethylbenzene and xylenes in the air and of lindane, pentachlorphenol and permethrins in the dust (Table 6).

Discussion

The subjects evaluated in our study attributed hypersensitivity to indoor pollution, blaming „chemicals" in many cases. Part of these patients could be assigned

to different syndromes, some of which have strong similarities to the „Eco-Syndrome" [3] or also to the „multiple chemical sensitivity" syndrome [12], now named „idiopathic environmental intolerances" in order not to implicate chemical etiology or sensitivity mechanisms [13]. According to a recently published paper the consensus criteria for MCS are as follows [14]:
1. „The symptoms are reproducible with exposure."
2. „The conditions is chronic."
3. „Low levels of exposure results in manifestation of the syndrome."
4. „The symptoms improve or resolve when the incitants are removed."
5. „Responses occur to multiple chemically unrelated substances."
6. „Symptoms involve multiple organ systems."

Except for criteria 5 all other criteria can also be true for allergic reactions. In relation to that point, substances patients respond to have to be evaluated subjectively by a physician, because only the patients themselves presume that certain chemicals are responsible for their symptoms. Therefore, besides of psychosomatic investigations, carefully performed allergic tests have to be done in such patients. This was not considered by almost all other studies [15].

The importance of a thorough allergological examination is underlined by the fact, that in 71% of our patients a common allergic or other hypersensitivity disease could be diagnosed. Many of these patients showed a sensitization to house dust mites, typical indoor related allergens. Why these patients sought additional explanations for their complaints, may be explained by a lack of knowledge about this kind of allergy, underdiagnosis or undertreatment in group A or by superimposure of strong psychosomatic effects in group B. Interestingly, in a retrospective study of subjects suffering from neurologic disorders, 53% of the patients with a multiple chemical sensitivity disorder had an atopic background compared with only 20% of those without multiple chemical sensitivity [16]. In 30 patients with Eco-Syndrome 60% showed test reactions to airborne or food allergens at prick and/or intradermal tests [3]. We found indications of actual hypersensitivity to indoor pollutants other than known allergens only in patients also suffering from „common" allergic diseases (group D). The role of indoor pollutants for the development of symptoms in these patients is of interest, as concentrations of pollutants were higher than reference levels either in the air or in the dust of rooms of all five patients investigated in this group.

An exclusive psychosomatic cause of the complaints was found in 19 patients (group C). This supports one hypothesis regarding the pathogenesis of environmental illness, i.e. that such patients have a strong background of mental and emotional disorders [17–21]. However, unexpectedly also in 6 of 7 investigated cases of group C concentrations of indoor pollutants were above the reference values. The meaning of these increased levels remained unclear, because we were not able to do challenge tests. However, in studies performing provocative challenges in patients with multiple chemical sensitivity with their trigger substances manifestations of an anxiety syndrome, partly induced by hyperventilation were shown [22]. Furthermore, in double-blind, placebo-controlled studies, the pattern of responses to active agents and placebo was never found to be consistent across a series of trials [23].

It can be hypothesized that in the seven patients from group D who suffered also from allergic rhinoconjunctivitis, a combined effect of pollutants and allergens induced alteration of epithelia occurred. As measurements of indoor pollutants were not performed in rooms of individuals of group A and only in the home of one patient of group B it remains unclear, if the increased concentrations of pollutants were characteristic only for rooms of patients of group D. Mainly toluene was detected in the air, in the dust particularly pentachlorphenol was increased. Pentachlorphenol may cause irritation of the skin, conjunctiva and upper respiratory tract. From animal experiments, it is known that long-term exposure (6.5 h/day, 5 days/week) to higher concentrations of toluene (1,200 ppm) leads to signs of degeneration of olfactory and respiratory epithelia with nasal inflammation [24].

Enhancing effects of air pollutants from heavy automobile traffic on symptoms of allergic rhinitis were considered in epidemiological studies [25]. In challenge tests synergistic effects of allergens and pollutant exposure could be shown for ozone, nitrogen dioxide and sulphur dioxide in patients with mild asthma [4, 26] or rhinoconjunctivitis [5]. In animal studies, increased sensitivity to allergens could be demonstrated after pre-exposure to ozone, nitrogen dioxide and sulphur dioxide [27].

The results raise the question, if increased concentrations of indoor pollutants may alter reactions to allergens, or vice versa, possibly by inducing epithelial changes [29]. In conclusion, the attribution of hypersensitivity regarding to indoor pollution by certain individuals has to be interpreted cautiously. If a conclusive diagnosis of common allergic diseases cannot be made or seems insufficient with regard to the complaints, a psychological and/or psychiatric evaluation is indispensable. To elucidate a possible role of indoor pollutants in individual patients, measurement of such substances should be performed in their indoor areas. However, the so far unknown pathogenetic relevance of indoor pollutants below established toxic concentrations demands a meticulous and critical synopsis of all findings.

Acknowledgements. This work was supported by a grant from the Bundesministerium für Forschung und Technologie of the Federal Republic of Germany (Innenraum-Chemikalienbelastung und allergologisch-dermatologische Erkrankungen, no. 07INR 114).

References

1. Apter, A., Bracker, A., Hodgson, M., Sidman, J., Leung, W.Y.: Epidemiology of the sick building syndrome. J. Allergy Clin. Immunol. 94, 277–288 (1994).
2. Weaver, V.M.: Medical management of the multiple chemical sensitivity patients. Regul. Toxicol. Pharmacol. 24, S111-S115 (1996).
3. Ring, J., Vieluf, D., Przybilla, B., Gabriel, G., Rad von, M.: The „clinical ecology syndrome": psychology or allergy? In: New trends in allergy III (J. Ring, B. Przybilla, eds.), pp. 500–516. Springer Verlag, Berlin Heidelberg New York 1991.
4. Devalia, J.L., Rusnak, C., Herdman, M.J., Trigg, C.J., Tarraf, H., Davies, R.J.: Effect of nitrogen dioxide and sulphur dioxide on airway response of mild asthmatic patients to allergen inhalation. Lancet 334, 1668–1671 (1994).

5. Wang, J.H., Devalia, J.L., Duddle, J.M., Hamilton, S.A., Davies, R.J.: Effect of six-hour exposure to nitrogen dioxide on early-phase nasal response to allergen challenge in patients with a history of seasonal allergic rhinitis. J. Allergy Clin. Immunol. 96, 669–676 (1995).
6. Meggs, W.J., Dunn, K.A., Bloch, R.M., Goodman, P.E.: Prevalence and nature of allergy and chemical sensitivity in a general population. Arch. Environmental Health 51, 275–282 (1996).
7. Kreutzer, R., Neutra, R.R., Lashuay, N.: Prevalence of people reporting sensitivities to chemicals in a population-based survey. Am. J. Epidemiol. 150, 1–12 (1999).
8. Lohhaus, A., Schmitt, G.M.: Fragebogen zur Erhebung von Kontrollüberzeugung zu Krankheit und Gesundheit (KKG). Göttingen: Hogrefe; 1989
9. Beckmann, D., Brähler, E., Richter, H.E.: Der Gießen-Test. Bühl: Konkordia; 1991
10. Brähler, E., Scheer, J.: Der Gießener Beschwerdebogen. Berlin: Hans Huber; 1983
11. Gebefügi, I., Lörinci, G., Grassmann, M., Kettrup, A.: Occurrence of VOC´s in enclosed indoor environments in southern Bavaria. In: Indoor Air ´93 (K. Saarela, P. Kalliokoski, O. Seppänen, eds.), pp 123–128, Proceedings of the 6th International Conference. Helsinki; Vol. 2, 1993.
12. Sibbison, J.B.: Multiple chemical sensitivity. Lancet 337, 1469–1470 (1991).
13. International Programme on Chemical Safety. Conclusions and recommendations of a workshop on multiple chemical sensitivities (MCS). Regul. Toxicol. Pharmacol. 24, S188-S189 (1996).
14. Multiple Chemical Sensitivity: A 1999 Consensus. Arch. Environ. Health 54, 147–149 (1999).
15. AAAAI Board of directors. Idiopathic environmental intolerances. J. Allergy Clin. Immunol. 103, 36–40 (1999).
16. Lohmann, K, Prohl, A., Schwarz, E.: Multiple chemical sensitivity disorders in patients with neurotoxic illnesses. Gesundheitswesen 58, 322–331 (1996).
17. Black, D.W., Rathe, A., Goldstein, R.B.: Environmental illness: a controlled study of 26 subjects with „20th century disease". JAMA 264, 3166–3170 (1990).
18. Simon, G.E., Katon, W.J., Sparks, P.J.: Allergic to life: psychological factors in environmental illness. Am. J. Psychiatry 147, 901–906 (1990).
19. Salvaggio, J.E.: Psychological aspects of „environmental illness", „multiple chemical sensitivity" and building-related illness. J. Allergy Clin. Immunol. 94, 366–370 (1994).
20. Staudenmayer, H.: Multiple chemical sensitivities or idiopathic environmental intolerances: Psychophysiologic foundation of knowledge for a psychogenic explanation. J. Allergy Clin. Immunol. 99, 434–437 (1997).
21. Leznoff, A.: Provocative challenges in patients with multiple chemical sensitivity. J. Allergy Clin. Immunol. 99, 438–442 (1997).
22. Staudenmayer, H., Selner, J.C., Buhr, M.P.: Double-blind provocation chamber challenges in 20 patients presenting with „Multiple Chemical Sensitivity". Regul. Toxicol. Pharmacol. 18: 44–53 (1993).
23. Bardana, E.J. Jr. „Clinical Ecology": Critical evaluation. In: New trends in Allergy IV together with Environmental Allergy and Allergotoxicology III. (J. Ring, H. Behrendt, D Vieluf, eds.), pp 331–336 (1997).
24. Notice of intended changes – toluene, trimethylamine, and vinyl acetate. Appl. Occup. Environ. Hyg. 6, 966–977 (1991).
25. Miyamoto, T., Takafuji, S.: Environment and allergy. In: New trends in allergy III (J. Ring, B. Przybilla, eds.), pp. 459–466. Springer Verlag, Berlin Heidelberg New York 1991.
26. Sandström, T.: Respiratory effects of air pollutants: experimental studies in humans. Eur. Respir. J. 8, 976–995 (1995).
27. Matsumara, Y.: The effects of ozone, nitrogen dioxide, and sulfur dioxide on the experimentally induced allergic respiratory disorders in guinea pigs. I. The effects on sensitization with albumin through the airway. Am. Rev. Resp. Dis. 102, 430–447 (1970).
28. Montgomery, C., Reasor, M.J.: A toxicologic approach for evaluating cases of sick building syndrome or multiple chemical sensitivity. J. Allergy Clin. Immunol. 94, 371–375 (1994)
29. Meggs, W.J.: Hypothesis for induction and propagation of chemical sensitivity based on biopsy studies. Environ. Health Perspect. 105 Supp 2, 473–478 (1997).

27   Latex Allergens and Latex Allergy

K. Turjanmaa, T. Palosuo

Allergy to natural rubber latex (NRL) is currently one of the most frequently encountered occupational diseases among the health care workers. Children with spina bifida and other congenital malformations with histories of multiple surgeries form the other major risk group. Latex-allergic patients run a risk of life-threatening reactions if they are exposed to high allergenic gloves or other latex products. In the normal population, allergy to NRL is not common, frequency being under 1%. Although latex protein allergens do not seem to differ substantially from e.g. food allergens, the exposure in health care sector makes latex allergy an exceptional condition.

Proteins and Allergens

Of the more than 200 different proteins or polypeptides in NRL only about one fourth are allergens, meaning that sensitized persons have formed IgE-class antibodies to them [1]. The WHO Allergen Nomenclature Committee now lists 10 NRL allergens characterized at the molecular level [7]. Most of them have by now been cloned and sequenced and produced by recombinant-DNA-techniques which has greatly helped to assess their clinical importance. However, it should be noted that proteins produced in bacterial or yeast cells may not, e.g., fold properly and represent naturally expressed proteins. For the moment, there is evidence that at least Hev b1, Hev b3, Hev b5 and hevein (Hev b6.02) or immunologically active fragments of them can be demonstrated in latex gloves.

Since the first report suggesting allergen cross-reactivity between NRL and banana, a number of studies dealing with cross-reactivity between NRL and various food allergens have been published and it has been shown that allergic reactions to foods are common in NRL-allergic patients. However, the majority of positive skin prick test (SPT) reactions do not seem to be associated with clinically relevant symptoms. As far as the molecular specificity of these cross-reactions of NRL-allergic patients is concerned, recent studies show that reactions to banana and avocado are at least partly due to hevein-like domains in banana and avocado class I endochitinases. Exact nature of the other alleged cross-reactions in latex-fruit syndrome remains to be established [2].

Future studies will undoubtedly be focused on the analysis of immunodominant epitopes in the allergen molecules and in possibilities to modify or destroy them to decrease their allergenic potential. Knowledge of the whole spectrum of NRL allergens will help researchers to develop more specific in vivo and in vitro tests for diagnostic purposes and the production of pure allergens could

New Trends in Allergy V
J. Ring, H. Behrendt (Eds.)
© Springer-Verlag Berlin, Heidelberg 2002

provide tools for immunotherapy. For the moment there are already preliminary reports of latex-specific immunotherapy with promising results [4].

Latest Development of Latex Allergy in Europe

Organization of European Commission has asked the Scientific Committee on Medicinal Products and Medical Devices to express its opinion on risks associated with the use of medical devices manufactured from NRL and the opinion was adopted in June 2000. Sixteen given questions dealing with various aspects of allergy to NRL products were answered based on present published literature (//dg24-srv-01/common/webdev/3643.doc).

Problems with Predictive Testing

SPT and estimation of specific IgE to NRL proteins are commonly accepted as the methods of choice for diagnosing sensitization to latex allergens [9]. The sensitivity of SPT is superior to that of measuring specific IgE, but there are very few publications dealing adequately with the problem. Of the currently available serologic tests for latex-specific IgE, CAP RAST FEIA (Pharmacia UpJohn) and AlaSTAT (Diagnostic Products), and HY-TEC-EIA (HYTREC) are approved by the FDA [3].

Sensitivity and specificity can only be determined in relation to a challenge test with NRL, which verifies the presence of symptoms, i.e. allergy to NRL [5, 8]. At the present time there is only one commercial standardized SPT allergen available [10]. The challenge test is also problematic. It may be done on skin, nose or lungs but the methodologies described in the literature are not standardized. The test material used is problematic, because gloves and elutions thereof have been used, but along with the continuing decrease of allergenicity of gloves good test gloves are becoming difficult to find.

Measurement of NRL Proteins/Allergens

There is a strong need to monitor the allergenicity of gloves and other latex goods to prevent sensitization and allergy. At the moment, measurement of the total protein of gloves with the modified Lowry method seems to be the best available method for manufacturers to control the quality of their gloves because the total protein amount has been shown to correlate relatively well with the true NRL-allergen content measured by SPT or latex-specific IgE ELISA-inhibition. The measurement of total leachable proteins will remain in use until direct determination of allergens is commonly available. In Europe and especially in Germany, the amino acid analysis method is considered more reliable because it is independent of the chemicals present in gloves. Modified Lowry is considered suitable as current production control and the more complicated amino acid analysis method remains as a reference method. But at the end, protein measurement is less reliable in predicting the allergenicity of gloves, because the weight of a given allergen may be minimal in spite of a high allergic capacity.

For the detection of allergens there are two assays available, RAST-inhibition and IgE-ELISA-inhibition [6]. However, until now it has not been possible to standardize these assays because of lack of the availability of standardized human antibodies and standardized allergens. Probably monoclonal antibodies to individual NRL allergens and corresponding recombinant allergens will be available in the near future. This would solve the problems both in estimating the allergens reliably in NRL products worldwide and in the diagnosis of sensitized persons.

Prevention

The glove powder is known to be contaminated by the NRL proteins/allergens and to act as allergen carrier resulting in airborne allergens. This causes problems especially in the health care where sensitized workers can get eye symptoms, rhinitis and even asthma when exposed via airways to powder from latex gloves. Consequently, less powder could result in less airborne allergens. For the time being, low protein and no-powder gloves are becoming increasingly used in the health care although we are not aware of official recommendations for this policy in countries other than Germany. There are also anecdotal reports telling that the problems with NRL allergy are getting less frequent with this combination.

In Finland and at the Mayo Clinic in the US, there is a long tradition of assessing the allergen amount of gloves and both laboratories have their standard patient serum pools which are needed for the tests. In Finland, the National Agency for Medicines has published since1994 lists of low-, medium- and high-allergenic gloves with the recommendations to use only low-allergenic gloves in the entire health care sector (www.nam.fi). At the Tampere University Hospital, low-allergenic gloves only have been allowed since 1990. The prevalence of NRL allergy was 2.9% (15/512) in 1986 and in 1999 only 1% (6/603) among glove using hospital employees [11]. The glove powder has recently been abandoned at the University Hospital Tampere and workers have been very satisfied with this decision because they had noticed less problems with skin irritation from using powder-free gloves. On the other hand, when gloves contain insignificant levels of allergens, the amount of glove powder is not important with regard to allergy because there is less allergenic material in the gloves to become contaminated with.

References

1. Alenius H, Kurup V, Kelly K, Palosuo T, Turjanmaa K, Fink J. Latex allergy: Frequent occurrence of IgE antibodies to a cluster of 11 latex proteins in patients with spina bifida and histories of anaphylaxis. J Lab Clin Med 1994;123:712–720
2. Blanco C, Diaz-Perales A, Collada C, Sánchez-Monge R, Aragoncillo C, Castillo R, Ortega N, Alvarez M, Carrillo T, Salcedo G. Class I chitinases as potential panallergens involved in the latex-fruit syndrome. J Allergy Clin Immunol 1999;103:507–13

3. Hamilton RG, Biagini RE, Krieg EF. Diagnostic performance of Food and Drug Administration-cleared serologic assays for natural rubber latex-spepcific IgE antibody: the Multi-Center Latex Skin Testing Study Task Force. J Allergy Clin Immunol 1999;103:925–30)
4. Leynadier F, Herman D, Vervloet D, André C. Specific immunotherapy with a standardized latex extract versus placebo in allergic healthcare workers. J Allergy Clin Immunol 2000;106:585–90
5. Liss GM, Sussman GL. Latex sensitization: occupational versus general population prevalence rates. Am J Ind Med 1999;35:196–200
6. Palosuo T, Mäkinen-Kiljunen S, Alenius H, Reunala T, Yip E, Turjanmaa K. Measurement of natural rubber latex allergen levels in medical gloves by allergenspecific IgE-ELISA inhibition, RAST-inhibition, and skin prick test. Allergy 1998;53:59–67
7. Poley GE, Slater JE. Latex allergy. J Allergy Clin Immunol 2000;105:1054–62
8. Turjanmaa K, Reunala T, Räsänen L. Comparison of diagnostic methods in latex glove contact urticaria. Contact Dermatitis 1988;19:241–247
9. Turjanmaa K, Alenius H, Mäkinen-Kiljunen S et al. Natural rubber allergy. Review. Allergy 1996;51:593–602
10. Turjanmaa K, Palosuo T, Alenius H, et al. Latex allergy diagnosis: in vivo and in vitro standardization of a natural rubber latex extract. Allergy 1997;52:41–50
11. Turjanmaa K, Reinikka-Railo H, Reunala T, Palosuo T. Continued decrease in natural rubber latex (NRL) allergen levels of medical gloves in nationwide market surveys in Finland and co-occurring decrease in NRL allergy prevalence in a large university hospital. J Allergy Clin Immunol 2000;104(Part 2):S373 (abstract)

28 Long-Term Course of Natural Rubber Latex Sensitization and Allergy

E. Vocks, W. van der Leeden, J. Rakoski, J. Ring

Introduction

Immediate-type allergy to natural rubber latex (NRL) proteins has become widespread within well-defined highly exposed populations, especially health care workers [1]. The potential economic impact on workers' compensation and disability is considerable.

Since NRL represents a „new" allergen, only little is known about the long-term course of NRL sensitization and allergy [2, 3].

The present study aimed to investigate the natural course of NRL allergy and sensitization during several years, particularly the development of the intensity of sensitization resp. of the clinical symptoms in dependence on the individual exposure to NRL.

Materials and Methods

From 1993–1998, 82 subjects (63 female/19 male) sensitized to NRL consulted our department. Out of these, 23 were only sensitized (positive RAST and/or skin prick test (SPT)) without clinical symptoms, 59 were also allergic to NRL with the following symptoms: urticaria only (10), rhinoconjunctivitis and/or asthma (with or without urticaria) (38) or anaphylactic reaction (11). The total group consisted of 41 health care workers, 5 housekeepers, 31 with other occupations and 5 children. 60/82 were atopic. Most of them had IgE-sensitizations to other common (atopic) allergens.

Subjects

In the year 1999, 30/82 selected subjects were re-examined (20 f, 10 m, mean age: 33 years), 7 with an NRL sensitization but no clinical symptoms at the first ex-

Table 1. Thirty re-examined subjects and their initial symptoms [at time of diagnosis (first examination, 1993–1998)]

Sensitized (n=7)	Subjects (n=30) Allergic (n=23)			
No symptoms	Contact urticaria	Generalized urticaria	Urticaria, rhinoconjunctivitis, asthma	Anaphylaxis
7	2	4	14	3

New Trends in Allergy V
J. Ring, H. Behrendt (Eds.)
© Springer-Verlag Berlin, Heidelberg 2002

amination („sensitized group") and 23 with an initially manifest allergy to NRL („allergic group") (Table 1).

24/30 were atopic exhibiting IgE sensitizations also to other common allergens.

Examination

All patients were intensively questioned for NRL avoidance behaviour, especially occupational measures since diagnosis, and for symptoms at NRL exposition currently. A blood sample was tested for specific IgE against NRL and against NRL-related foods (CAP-RAST-FEIA, Pharmacia & Upjohn Diagnostics, Freiburg, Germany) and a skin prick test (SPT) with NRL (ALK-Scherax, Hamburg, Germany) was performed.

Parameters

I. Degree of Latex Avoidance Since Diagnosis

1. Strict: Less than 1 NRL contact per month, unintended. Health care workers: latex-free rubber gloves. Exclusively unpowdered latex gloves in the working environment (total hospital).
2. Medium: 1 to 2 NRL contacts per month on the average, unknowingly or knowingly. Health care workers: latex-free rubber gloves, but powdered latex gloves in the wider working environment.
3. Little or none: Daily or several NRL contacts per month, knowingly. Contingently avoiding stronger exposure occasionally. Health care workers: unpowdered or powdered latex gloves, and powdered latex gloves in the working environment.

II. Intensity of the NRL Allergy/Sensitization

The intensity of the NRL allergy respective NRL sensitization was assessed by an allergy/sensitization-intensity-score (ASI), which was composed by the three criterions:
1. Clinical symptoms to NRL (classes 1–4 according to the contact urticaria/anaphylaxis-classification by v. Krogh and Maibach [4])
2. SPT (positive 3, negative 0)
3. RAST class (1–6)
   ASI=symptoms (class)×2+SPT (0/3)+RAST class
   The present ASI was compared with the initial ASI (at first examination):
   ASI: decreased/constant/increased

Results

After a median of 3 years (min 1 year, max 7 year), the allergy/sensitization intensity, measured by the ASI, did not change significantly: 9 decreased, 15 were constant, 3 increased (3 missing) (Fig. 1).

12/21 allergic subjects strictly had avoided NRL contact as far as possible, in contrast to none in the sensitized (Fig. 2).

There was no significant correlation between the degree of avoidance and the development of the ASI (Figs. 3,4), although some sensitized subjects without strict avoidance became symptomatic („increased ASI") (Fig. 4).

6/17 patients with occupational NRL contact had changed the workplace in order to avoid NRL contact but out of these, only one was completely free of NRL contact and free of symptoms at the new workplace.

Cross-sensitization to NRL-related fruits (banana, kiwi and avocado) with or without clinical symptoms were found in a high number of patients by means of history, SPT and RAST (Table 2). Yet the number or intensity of these cross-sensitizations did not correlate to the intensity of the NRL allergy/sensitization (ASI).

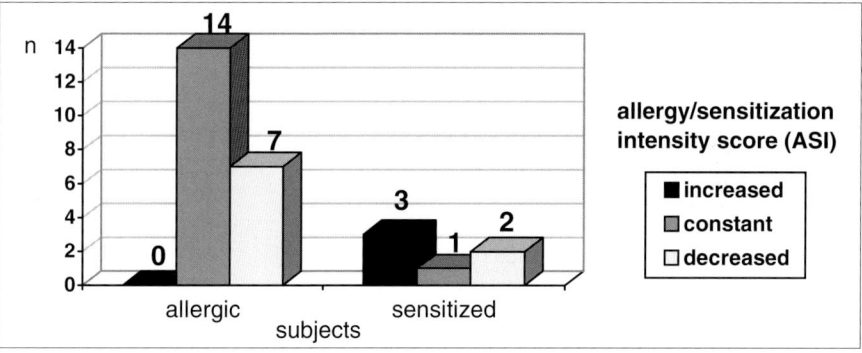

Fig. 1. Development of the allergy/sensitization intensity score (ASI) after a median of three years in NRL-allergic and -sensitized subjects ($n=27$)

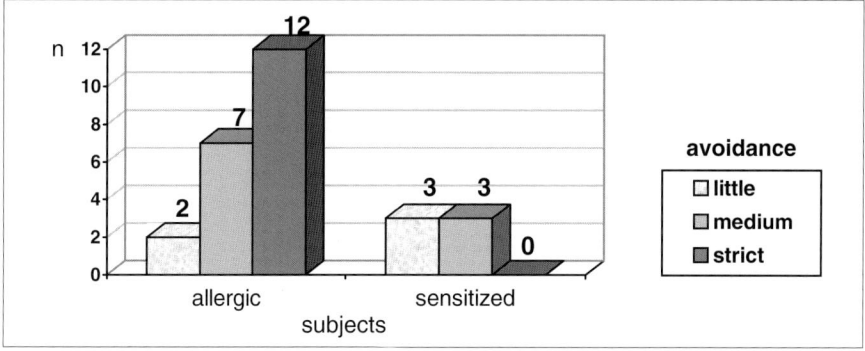

Fig. 2. Avoidance of NRL contact in NRL allergic and sensitized subjects ($n=27$)

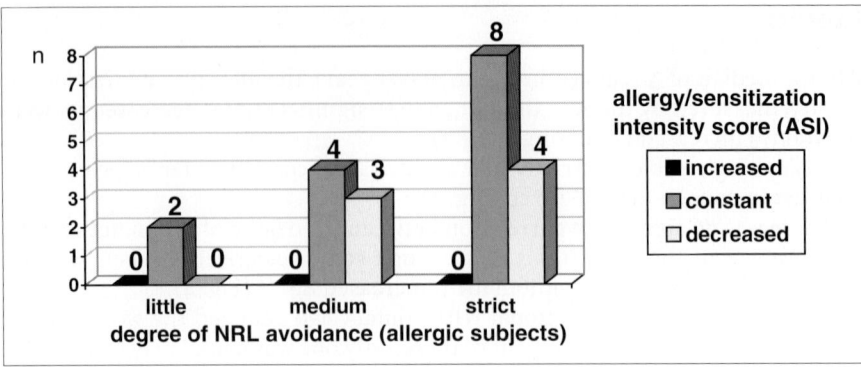

Fig. 3. Development of the allergy/sensitization intensity score (ASI) at different degrees of NRL avoidance, NRL-allergic subjects ($n=21$)

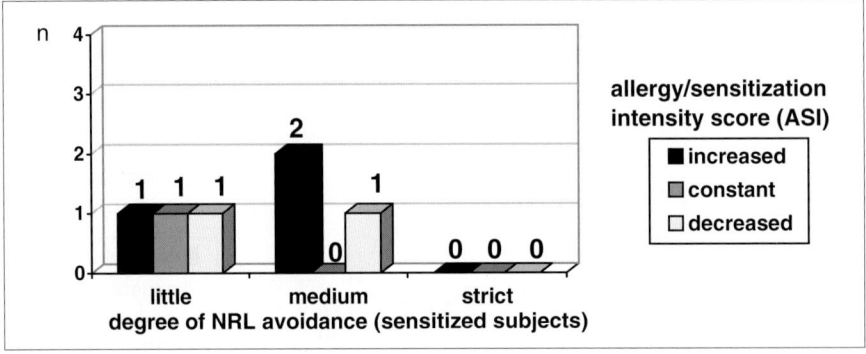

Fig. 4. Development of the allergy/sensitization intensity score (ASI) at different degrees of NRL avoidance, NRL-sensitized subjects ($n=6$)

Table 2. Cross-allergies to NRL-related fruits

| | NRL-allergic and NRL-sensitized subjects ($n=30$) | | |
	Banana	Kiwi	Avocado
Sensitization (no symptoms)	7	7	14
Allergy (oral allergy syndrome)	6	6	3

Conclusions

NRL allergic subjects should avoid NRL contact in order to minimize symptoms. However, it remains open, whether avoidance of NRL contact leads to a long-term loss or reduction of NRL allergy resp. NRL sensitization. In sensitized patients without symptoms avoidance possibly might prevent the clinical manifestation of the allergy. However, larger studies are necessary.

For subjects with occupational NRL allergy, prevention measures must be improved to provide an NRL-free working environment.

References

1. Warshaw E: Latex allergy, JAAD 39 (1998) 1–26
2. Cohen DE, Scheman A, Stewart L et al.: American Academy of Dermatology's position paper on latex allergy. JAAD 39 (1998) 98–106
3. Wakelin SH, White IR: Natural rubber latex allergy. Clin Exp Dermatol 24 (1999) 245–248
4. von Krogh G, Maibach HI: The contact urticaria syndrome –an updated review. JAAD 5 (1981) 328–342

Pharmacotherapy

29 Long-Term Continuous Antiallergic Treatment Reduces Symptoms and Controls Allergic Inflammation Better than Symptomatic Treatment

G. Ciprandi, M. Tosca, V. Ricca, G. Passalacqua, G.W. Canonica

Introduction

It is generally agreed that allergic rhinitis is sustained by an inflammatory process. Mucosal eosinophilic infiltration may be actually regarded as one of the hallmarks of allergic inflammation. Several pathophysiologic mechanisms are involved in eosinophil recruitment: release of mediators and cytokines, exerting chemoattractant, activating, and prolonging survival effects, and adhesion molecule machinery activation [1].

Eosinophils express on their surface some adhesion molecules, including the β2-integrins LFA-1 and Mac-1, which are the counter-receptors of ICAM-1, expressed on the epithelial cells of allergic subjects. Epithelial cells of allergic subjects express ICAM-1 early upon allergen challenge: thus, this phenomenon may, at least partially, account for mucosal leukocyte infiltration [2]. The relevance of these data has been confirmed by detecting ICAM-1 expression during natural exposure to the allergens [3]. Moreover, if allergen exposure persists (such as in mite allergy), allergic inflammation is in any case detectable, also when symptoms are not present. A „minimal persistent inflammation" has been demonstrated both at conjunctival and nasal level in symptom-free rhinitics with mite allergy [4]. Therefore, the constant exposure to the allergen, even though it does not always, induce symptoms is anyway able to promote and maintain inflammation, detectable for instance by monitoring ICAM-1 expression on epithelial cells or inflammatory cell presence at mucosal level.

We therefore designed a study aimed at assessing the presence of inflammation in patients with pollen allergy during a long observation period. This study was designed to evaluate patients with seasonal allergic rhinitis shortly before, during, and after the pollen season.

An inflammatory reaction was evident also during the days with low pollen count and low or absent symptoms in a significant manner and after the pollen season, inflammation persisted until 4 weeks.

It has been demonstrated that ICAM-1 expression on epithelial cells may be considered as a marker of allergic inflammation: in fact, its presence does relate with eosinophil infiltration due to the allergen exposure. Moreover, ICAM-1 expression and eosinophil recruitment may be present also without symptoms during allergen exposure, both concerning mite allergens [4] and pollen allergens, as reported in this study. In fact, the presence of a minimal persistent inflammation is detectable in those studied patients, exposed to the pollens, also during symptomless days and immediately after the pollen season (until 4 weeks). That

New Trends in Allergy V
J. Ring, H. Behrendt (Eds.)
© Springer-Verlag Berlin, Heidelberg 2002

may be considered as another piece of the complex puzzle of allergic inflammation and it underlines the importance that symptoms can not be considered anymore the unique marker of allergic disease. In fact, inflammation as well as hyperreactivity persist also without symptoms until allergen exposure occurs [4] and immediately after.

In other words, symptoms may be envisaged as an iceberg peak of the allergic reaction, where inflammation and hyperreactivity represent the submerged reality.

This evidence may represent an important knowledge from a clinical point of view.

Since pollen avoidance is not practically achievable, alternative pharmacological strategies have to be employed. The results of this study indicate that the global therapeutical strategy for allergic rhinitis should be revised and targeted to inflammatory phenomena, rather than to symptoms only. This could be achieved by using long-term treatments instead of on demand treatment as recently proposed by some clinical experiences [5].

Clinical Evidence

The nose and the eye represent an almost ideal experimental model for investigating the allergic inflammatory phenomena and their modulation, since they are target organs of the allergic reaction and they are easy to study. By means of these models, we have demonstrated the involvement of the cell adhesion molecule system (ICAM-1, in particular) in the pathophysiology of the allergic inflammation and that a minimal persistent inflammation is present in mite allergic patients also in absence of symptoms. In addition, the nasal and conjunctival models allowed to demonstrate in vivo, some of the so-called „antiallergic" actions of several new antihistamines. These actions, which were also observed in vitro, are represented by the capacity of downregulating different phenomena of the allergic inflammation, such as cellular activation, recruitment and mediator release [6]. The second generation antihistamine terfenadine was able to reduce the cellular infiltration and the expression of ICAM-1 molecules on epithelia. These effects of antihistamines could suggest a different therapeutical approach for the treatment of respiratory allergy, involving a continuous administration rather than an on demand one, in order to control not only symptoms but also the allergic inflammation. Furthermore, some studies showed that a continuous and prolonged antihistamine treatment in allergic children may have also a prophylactic action and prevent the onset of asthma [7–9]. Finally, antihistamines used for allergic rhinitis could also improve lower respiratory symptoms [10]. Based on these premises and on our clinical observations, we aimed at formally demonstrate that a continuous and prolonged antihistamine treatment could improve not only symptoms but also the occurrence of respiratory illness in children. We studied in a double blind placebo controlled fashion the effects of terfenadine in mite allergic children, by evaluating both the allergic inflammation in the nose and the clinical parameters. We observed that the actively treated group had a better control of symptoms, used less drugs and showed a reduction of cellular infiltration and ICAM-1 expression. These facts confirm the previous observations. Noteworthy, the children receiving the active treatment needed less extra visits for acute respiratory symptoms and had less school absences. These children showed, at the nasal scraping made at each extra visit, a better control of the allergic inflammation with respect of the actively treated group. Although, due to safety reasons terfenadine has been withdrawn in Italy since the end of 1996, no side effect was observed in our study.

Actually, an intriguing hypothesis for explaining the observed effects of terfenadine could be its effect on ICAM-1. In fact, the minimal persistent inflammation (with a constant weak expression of ICAM-1 on epithelia) may be responsible for the enhanced susceptibility of allergic children to rhinoviral infections [11, 12], also considering that ICAM-1 is the main receptor for human rhinoviruses [13]. The downregulation of ICAM-1 by terfenadine could be responsible for the observed effects, in addition to the fact that a good control of rhinitis is known to improve also asthma symptoms. The clinical observations herein reported, obviously need a formal scientific support such as the identification of viruses in the upper respiratory tract of patients, but may represent a suggestion for a possible new therapeutical approach.

Cetirizine is a new generation antihistamine with antiallergic properties [14]. It can down-regulate expression of ICAM-1 on epithelial cells, and it is effective in preventing inflammatory events induced by allergen-specific conjunctival challenge [15]. Cetirizine reduces both activation and migration of eosinophils from the blood-stream to the mucosa by modulating the expression and/or function of adhesion molecules on the mucosa. In fact, cetirizine reduces the eosinophil infiltrate and eosinophilic cationic protein levels in nasal lavage [16].

Here we show that continuous treatment with cetirizine is more effective in terms of reduction in symptoms and drug prescriptions than symptomatic treatment in children with allergy to dust mites.

Dust mite avoidance is an important aspect of therapy, and it has recently been shown to be useful in a low-income population of children with asthma [17]. However, the effectiveness of allergen avoidance as general preventive measure is controversial (reviewed in [18]). Overall, avoidance measures do not afford total protection and must be combined with pharmacological strategies [19].

The results of this study indicate that the entire therapeutic strategy for allergic rhinitis should be reassessed and targeted to inflammatory phenomena, rather than only to symptoms. This could be achieved by using continuous long-term treatment instead of symptomatic treatment.

Cetirizine, which reduces inflammation by affecting the recruitment and activation of inflammatory cells, seems to be suitable for the continuous treatment of allergy. Moreover, the total cost of continuous treatment for six months was significantly lower than the symptomatic treatment. A cost study should be performed on a larger patient population to verify this new strategy for continuous allergic treatment.

References

1. Bochner B.S., Schleimer R.P. The role of adhesion molecules in human eosinophil and basophil recruitment. J. Allergy Clin. Immunol. 1993;94: 427–438
2. Ciprandi G., Pronzato C., Ricca V., Passalacqua G., Bagnasco M., Canonica G.W. Allergen-specific challenge induces intracellular adhesion molecule-1 (ICAM-1 or CD54) on nasal epithelial cells in allergic subjects. Am. J. Respir. Crit. Care Med. 1994;150(6): 1653–59
3. Ciprandi G., Pronzato C., Ricca V., Bagnasco M., Canonica G.W. Evidence of intercellular adhesion molecule-1 expression on nasal epithelial cells in acute rhinoconjunctivitis caused by pollen exposure. J. Allergy Clin. Immunol. 1994;94: 738–746
4. Ciprandi G., Buscaglia S., Pesce G.P., Pronzato C., Ricca V., Parmiani S., Bagnasco M., Canonica G.W. Minimal persistent inflammation is present at mucosal level in asymptomatic rhinitic patients with allergy due to mites. J. Allergy Clin. Immunol. 1995;96:971–9
5. Ciprandi G., Ricca V., Passalacqua G., Truffelli T., Bertolini C., Fiorino N., Riccio A.M., Bagnasco M., Canonica G.W. Seasonal rhinitis and azelastine: long or short term treatment? J Allergy Clin Immunol 1997;99:301–7
6. Church M.K., Collinson A.D., Okayama Y. H1-receptor antagonists: antiallergic effects in vitro. In: Histamine and H1-receptor antagonists in allergic diseases. Simon F.E.R. Edit. Marcell Decker 1997: 117–144.
7. Iikura Y, Naspitz C.K., Mikawa H., Talaricoficho S., Baba M., Sole D., Nishima S. Prevention of asthma by ketotifen in infants with atopic dermatitis. Ann Allergy 1992;68:233–6.
8. Bustos G.J., Bustos D., Bustos G.J., Romero O. Prevention of asthma with ketotifen in pre-asthmatic children: a three-year follow-up study. Clin Exp Allergy 1995;25:568–73.
9. ETAC study group: allergic factors associated with the development of asthma and the influence of cetirizine in a double blind, randomized, placebo-controlled trial: first results of ETAC. Ped Allergy Immunol 1998;3:116–124.
10. Spector S.L., Lee M., McNut B., Kats R.M., Hustr W., Siegel S.C., Rachelefsky G.R., Rohr A. Effcet of terfenadine in asthmatic patients. Ann Allergy 1992;69:212–216.
11. Pattemore P.K., Johnston S.L., Bardin P.G. Viruses as precipitant of asthma symptoms. Clin Exp Allergy 1992;22:325–36.
12. Johnston S.L., Pattemore P.K., Sanderson G., Smith S., Campbell M.J., Josephs L.K., Cunningham A., Robinson B.S., Myint S.H., Ward M.E., Tyrrel D.A., Holgate S.T. The relationship between upper respiratory infections and hospital admissions for asthma: a time-trend analysis. Am J Resp Crit Care Med 1996;154:654–60.
13. Greve J.M., Davis G., Meyer A.M., Forte C.P., Yost S.C., Marlor C.W., Kamarck M.E., McClelland A. The major human rhinovirus receptor is ICAM-1. Cell 1989;56:839–47.
14. Spencer CM, Faulds D, Peters D. Cetirizine: a reappraisal of its pharmacological properties and therapeutic use in selected allergic disorders. Drugs. 1993;46:1055–1080.
15. Ciprandi G, Buscaglia S, Pesce GP. et al. Cetirizine reduces ICAM-1 (or CD54) expression both in early and late phase events following allergen-specific conjunctival challenge. J. Allergy Clin Immunol. 1995;95:612–2
16. Ciprandi G., Passalacqua G., Mincarini M. et al. Cetirizine continuous versus on demand treatment in allergic rhinitis. Ann Allergy Asthma Immunol. 1997; 97:507–511.
17. Shapiro G., Wighton T.G., Chinn T. et al. House dust mite avoidance for children with asthma in homes of low-income families. J Allergy Clin Immunol 1999;103:1069–74.
18. Schoberger H.J., Van Schayck C.P. Prevention of asthma in genetically predisposed children in primary care – from clinical efficacy to a feasible intervention programme. Clin Exp Allergy 1998;28:1325–1331.
19. International Consensus Report on the Diagnosis and management of Rhinitis. Allergy 1994; 49 (Supplement).

30 Rapid Onset and Sustained Efficacy of Desloratadine in Treatment of Chronic Idiopathic Urticaria

A. Gauger, R. Hein, G. Rikken, H. Staudinger, J. Ring

Abstract

Desloratadine is a nonsedating H_1-receptor antagonist with anti-inflammatory and antiallergic properties. In a multicenter, randomized, double-blind, placebo-controlled trial, desloratadine was evaluated in 190 patients with chronic idiopathic urticaria (CIU). Patients had a 6-week history of CIU symptoms prior to the study, were experiencing a current flare for 3 weeks, and had hives at least 3 days a week. Patients were given desloratadine 5 mg once daily (QD) for 6 weeks and recorded their assessment of pruritus, number of hives, and size of largest hive. Twice daily (a.m./p.m.), symptoms were evaluated over the previous 12 h (reflective) and at the time of assessment (instantaneous). The primary efficacy variable was the average a.m./p.m. reflective pruritus score for the first week of treatment. Desloratadine significantly improved pruritus compared with placebo during Week 1 (56.0% vs 21.5%; $P<0.001$) and continued to improve pruritus through Week 6 (74.0% vs 48.7%; $P<0.001$). Assessment at the end of the dosing interval (a.m. instantaneous) demonstrated that desloratadine was significantly more effective than placebo in improving pruritus scores after the first dose (45.1% vs 3.5%; $P<0.001$), demonstrating the agent's rapid onset and 24-h duration of action. Desloratadine significantly improved patient assessments of interference with sleep and interference with daily activities compared with placebo over all evaluated timepoints, including Week 6. In addition, desloratadine was significantly more effective than placebo in improving the overall condition of CIU and provided a significantly better therapeutic response as jointly evaluated by the patient and investigator.

Desloratadine 5 mg QD for 6 weeks was safe and well tolerated with a reported adverse event profile similar to that of placebo. Desloratadine demonstrated a rapid onset of action for the treatment of CIU, as shown by substantial efficacy beginning at the first dose. Desloratadine continued to be effective and well tolerated for the full 6-week treatment period, and symptom improvement resulted in significant improvements in sleep and daily activities.

Introduction

Chronic idiopathic urticaria (CIU) is a common disorder characterized by wheals and/or angioedema, symptoms that are frequently associated with severe pruritus. Patients with CIU can suffer with symptoms for greater than 6 weeks without a discernable physical or environmental allergic cause. Histamine (H_1)-recep-

New Trends in Allergy V
J. Ring, H. Behrendt (Eds.)
© Springer-Verlag Berlin, Heidelberg 2002

tor antagonists are the primary choice for treatment of CIU [1]. However, some H_1-receptor antagonists are associated with sedation and can cause serious cardiac arrhythmias.

Desloratadine is a new, nonsedating, potent H_1-receptor antagonist with antiallergic activity [2]. In clinical studies, desloratadine provided 24-h symptom relief in patients with a wide range of allergic conditions [3–7]. Desloratadine is well absorbed after oral administration, has a long elimination half-life, is not associated with cardiotoxic effects, and has no clinically significant drug interactions [8–11]. The following study evaluated the efficacy and safety of desloratadine in patients with CIU.

Methods

Study Design

This was a multicenter, randomized, double-blind, placebo-controlled, parallel-group, 6-week study. During screening of patients 3–14 days prior to treatment, inclusion and exclusion criteria and CIU severity were assessed, and patients were randomized to receive either desloratadine 5 mg QD or placebo. Visits to the study centers on Days 1 (baseline) and 4 and at Weeks 1, 2, 4, and 6 permitted joint evaluation of the efficacy and safety of treatment.

Inclusion/Exclusion Criteria

To be enrolled, patients had to be at least 12 years old and have an active flare and a minimum 6-week history of CIU. CIU had to be active for 3 weeks prior to screening, and wheals had to be visible for at least 3 days per week. The overall disease severity, pruritus, and presence of wheals had to be scored at least moderate at screening and baseline. The total reflective pruritus score had to be 14 (at least moderate) over the last 3 days and on the morning of the baseline visit. Standard laboratory biochemistry and hematology tests, and urinalysis, as well as electrocardiogram (ECG) results, were obtained at screening and had to be clinically normal.

Significant concomitant illnesses were not allowed, nor could patients be taking pharmacological agents that could interfere with the study drug or interpretation of efficacy parameters. Patients with asthma could not be using leukotriene inhibitors or chronic inhaled or systemic corticosteroid therapy unless sufficient time was allowed for the washout of these drugs.

Study Medication

The study medication was administered orally in the morning, after completion of the diary, regardless of food intake. Referral to the symptom diary, questioning of patients, and tablet counting were used to assess patient compliance.

Disease Activity and Assessment of Therapeutic Response

Patients assessed and scored their disease activity during the screening period and throughout the trial by recording their symptoms on daily diary cards. The individual CIU symptoms evaluated were pruritus, number of hives, and size of largest hive. The sum of these individual scores was the total symptom score (TSS). Patients also recorded interference with sleep and daily activities. The patients evaluated symptom severity over the previous 12 h (reflective) and at the time of assessment (instantaneous) on all study days, providing a total of 4 daily symptom severity scores (2 morning [reflective/instantaneous] and 2 evening [reflective/instantaneous]). The reflective scores for interference with sleep were assessed in the morning and interference with daily activities were assessed at night.

Joint evaluation (investigator and patient) of CIU severity occurred on Days 1 and 4 and Weeks 1, 2, 4, and 6, using another 4-point scale: 0=none to 3=severe. The investigator and patient/guardian used a 5-point scale (1=complete relief to 5=treatment failure) to jointly assess the therapeutic response to the study medication at Day 4 and Weeks 1, 2, 4, and 6.

Safety Assessments

Laboratory tests and ECGs were evaluated during screening and at the end of the study, and vital signs were recorded at each visit. Adverse events were recorded and evaluated for severity and potential relation to study medication.

Efficacy and Safety Variables

The primary efficacy variable was the change in average reflective a.m./p.m. pruritus symptom scores (recorded in the patient diaries) from baseline over the first 7 days of treatment. Secondary outcomes were changes in the following average scores: a.m./p.m. reflective, a.m./p.m. instantaneous, am instantaneous, a.m. reflective, p.m. reflective, and p.m. instantaneous scores for pruritus and TSS; interference with sleep (a.m. reflective); interference with daily activities (p.m. reflective); and joint assessment of overall condition and therapeutic response.

The incidence of treatment-emergent adverse events, discontinuations due to adverse events, and changes from baseline in vital signs, laboratory parameters, and ECG intervals were all used to evaluate safety.

Statistical Analysis

A two-way analysis of variance (ANOVA) was used to evaluate consistency between centers and 2-way ANOVA was also used to analyze the primary and secondary efficacy variables in the combined data. Analyses were performed primarily on the randomized population (intent-to-treat [ITT]), but were also confirmed in the efficacy-evaluable population (patients in whom a full set of efficacy data were available). Due to the large number of dropouts in the placebo group, the differences between active treatment and placebo were also analyzed by endpoint week, with the last available data for each subject carried forward.

Results

Demographics

The randomized patient population (ITT population) consisted of 190 patients. The baseline demographics of the two groups were similar (Table 1). Of the patients that discontinued treatment before the end of the study, 19 were in the desloratadine group and 32 were in the placebo group.

Efficacy Analysis

Reflective Pruritus Severity Scores

Desloratadine improved the mean a.m./p.m. reflective pruritus score over the first 7 days by 56.0%, compared with a 21.5% change in the placebo group ($P<0.001$). The a.m./p.m. reflective pruritus scores were also significantly improved in the

Table 1. Baseline demographic characteristics

Characteristics	Desloratadine 5 mg (n=95)	Placebo (n=95)
Mean Age (years)	38.9	42.0
Age subgroup, n (%)		
12 to <18 years	6 (6)	3 (3)
18 to <65 years	86 (91)	86 (91)
65 years	3 (3)	6 (6)
Men/Women (n)	27/68	21/74
Race, n (%)		
White	81 (85)	85 (89)
Black	5 (5)	4 (4)
Asian	3 (3)	1 (1)
Hispanic	4 (4)	5 (5)
American Indian	1 (1)	0
Other	1 (1)	0
Duration of CIU (years)		
Mean	4.3	6.4
Median	1.8	1.5
Range	0–49	0–46
Reflective a.m./p.m. pruritus score		
Least-square mean	2.24	2.22
Reflective a.m./p.m. total symptom score		
Least-square mean	6.65	6.51

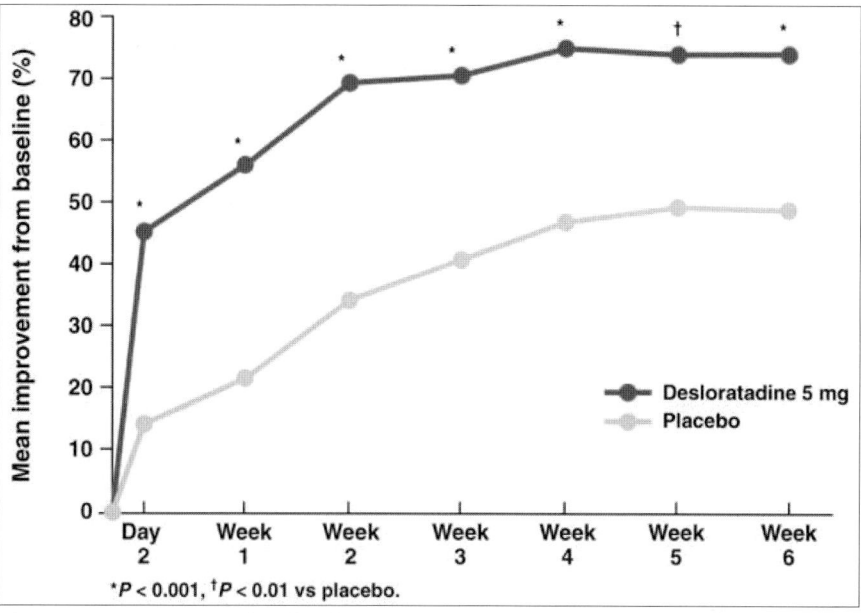

Fig. 1. Mean improvement from baseline in a.m./p.m. reflective pruritus score

desloratadine group on Day 2, when scores were improved by 45.2%, compared with a improvement of 14.0% for placebo ($P<0.001$). Desloratadine maintained improvement in pruritus throughout the trial, with a 74.0% improvement in pruritus with desloratadine at Week 6, compared with a 48.7% change with placebo ($P<0.001$) (Fig. 1).

End of Dosing Interval Pruritus Severity Scores

The a.m. instantaneous scores provide an assessment of the 24-h efficacy of the agent, and after the first dose, an assessment of the rapidity of action of the agent.

Table 2. Mean percentage improvement from baseline in end of dosing interval a.m. instantaneous pruritus score

Timepoint	Desloratadine ($n=95$)	Placebo ($n=95$)	P value
After 1 dose	45.1	3.5	<0.001
Week 1	55.1	14.5	<0.001
Week 2	64.9	26.7	0.003
Week 3	64.9	36.8	0.002
Week 4	70.8	45.1	0.004
Week 5	70.5	44.8	0.010
Week 6	68.9	46.0	0.033

Desloratadine treatment resulted in a significantly greater mean percent improvement from baseline in a.m. instantaneous pruritus score compared with placebo (45.1% vs 3.5%; $P<0.001$) 24 h after the first dose. Over the first week of therapy, desloratadine treatment also significantly improved a.m. instantaneous pruritus scores compared with placebo (55.1% vs 14.5%; $P<0.001$). At Week 6 there was a 68.9% improvement with desloratadine treatment and a 46.0% change with placebo ($P=0.033$), indicating that desloratadine treatment efficacy was maintained to the end of the trial (Table 2).

Improvements in TSS and Overall Condition of CIU

The desloratadine group had significantly greater improvements in total symptom severity scores than the placebo group. The a.m./p.m. reflective TSS was significantly improved, compared with placebo after the first dose of desloratadine (41.6% vs 10.6%; $P<0.001$) and was maintained over Week 1 (51.6% vs 19.3%; $P<0.001$). Significant improvements in TSS with desloratadine 5 mg compared with placebo were sustained when averaged over the full 6 weeks of the study ($P<0.001$). The overall condition of CIU was also significantly improved with desloratadine treatment compared with placebo ($P=0.002$) at all study visits, and the therapeutic response was significantly improved at all study visits, including the endpoint week analysis.

Interference with Sleep and Daily Activities

Desloratadine significantly improved mean a.m. reflective interference with sleep scores after the first dose ($P<0.05$), during the first week ($P<0.001$), and over all

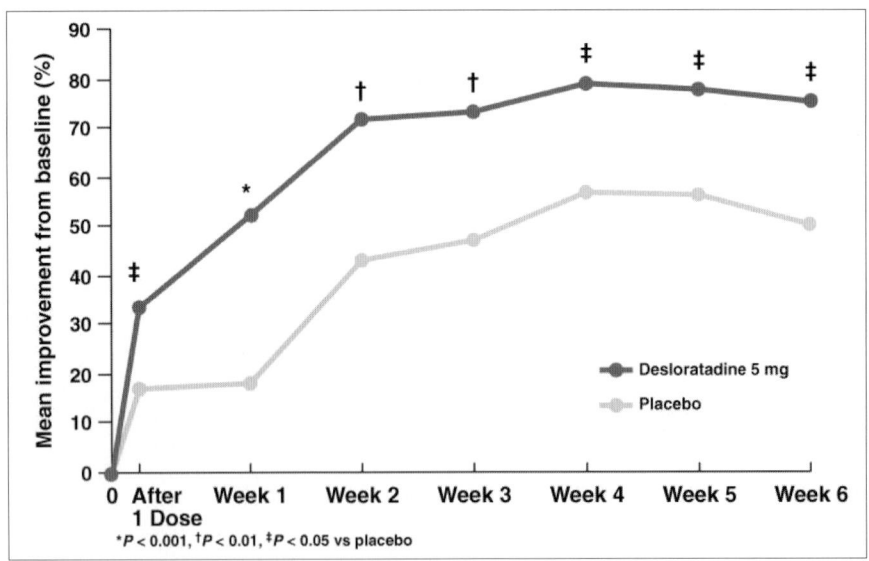

Fig. 2. Interference with sleep: mean improvement from baseline

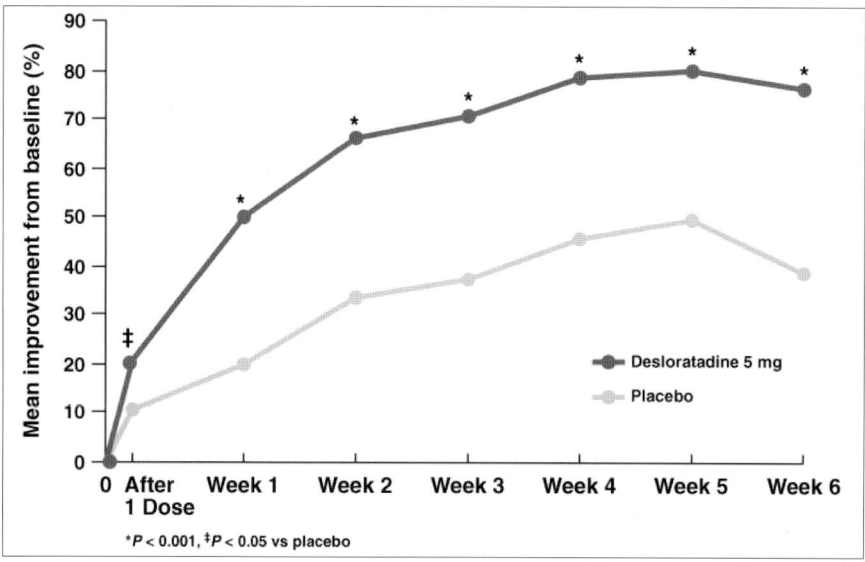

Fig. 3. Interference with daily activities: mean improvement from baseline

6 weeks of treatment ($P<0.05$) (Fig. 2). The interference with daily activity p.m. reflective scores was significantly reduced in the desloratadine group compared with the placebo group after the first dose ($P<0.05$), during the first week of treatment ($P<0.001$), and over each week of the study ($P<0.001$) (Fig. 3).

Safety

The adverse-event profile was similar in the desloratadine and placebo groups. Treatment-emergent adverse events occurred in 53 (55.8%) and 41 (43.2%) of the patients in the desloratadine and placebo groups, respectively. There were no treatment-related serious adverse events during the trial. There were no clinically significant changes in vital signs, laboratory parameters, or ECG criteria in the desloratadine or placebo groups during the study.

Discussion

CIU is a common chronic condition that is primarily treated with antihistamines. However, the sedative properties and the potential cardiotoxicity of some agents such as terfenadine and astemizole have caused patients and physicians to question the safety of these agents [12, 13]. The new antihistamine desloratadine is a potent inhibitor of the H_1 receptor, but does not have sedating effects and has no clinically relevant prolongation of the QT_c interval when coadministered with azithromycin [11], erythromycin [8], or ketoconazole [9]. These agents have been shown to promote torsades de pointes when administered with terfenadine [12]. Desloratadine therapy in this study was well tolerated and did not result in any patient discontinuations due to treatment-related adverse events. There were also no clinically significant changes in ECG parameters during the 6-week study, reinforcing the cardiovascular safety of desloratadine treatment [8–10].

This study has demonstrated that desloratadine has a rapid onset of action following the first dose, showing a significant reduction in all efficacy measures, including improvements in sleep and daily activity. Desloratadine treatment maintained improvements in efficacy measures for the duration of treatment in both the ITT and efficacy-evaluable populations.

In conclusion, the clinical benefits of desloratadine 5 mg daily for the treatment of CIU were apparent in terms of improvement in pruritus symptoms and TSS scores and better sleep and daily activity functions. These benefits were seen as early as after the first dose of desloratadine and were maintained over the full 6-week treatment period. Desloratadine 5 mg was safe and well tolerated in patients with CIU, with an adverse event profile similar to placebo.

References

1. Greaves M. Chronic urticaria. J Allergy Clin Immunol 2000; 105: 664–672.
2. Kreutner W, Hey JA, Anthes J, Barnett A, Young S, Tozzi S. Preclinical pharmacology of desloratadine, a selective and nonsedating histamine H_1 receptor antagonist: 1st communication: Receptor selectivity, antihistaminic activity, and antiallergic effects. Arzneimittelforschung 2000; 50: 345–352.
3. Agrawal DK. Pharmacology and clinical efficacy of desloratadine as an anti-allergic and anti-inflammatory drug. Exp Opin Invest Drugs 2001; 10: 547–560.
4. Bachert C. Decongestant efficacy of desloratadine in patients with seasonal allergic rhinitis. Allergy 2001; 56: 14–20.
5. Bronsky E, Desloratadine Urticaria Study Group. Desloratadine: A safe and effective therapy for chronic idiopathic urticaria. Ann Allergy Asthma Immunol 2001; 86: 109. Abstract.
6. Corren J, Desloratadine Study Group. Desloratadine has a rapid onset of action and durable response in allergic diseases. Ann Allergy Asthma Immunol 2001; 86: 110. Abstract.
7. Finn A, Rupp N, Desloratadine Study Group. Desloratadine has an early onset of action and long-term benefit for SAR symptoms. Ann Allergy Asthma Immunol 2001; 109. Abstract.
8. Glue P, Banfield C, Affrime MB, Statkevich P, Reyderman L, Padhi D et al. Lack of electrocardiographic interaction between desloratadine and erythromycin. Allergy 2000; 55 (Suppl 63): 276. Abstract.
9. Affrime MB, Banfield C, Glue P, Ngo LY, Keung A, Herron JM et al. Lack of electrocardiographic effects when desloratadine and ketoconazole are coadministered. Allergy 2000; 55 (Suppl 63): 277. Abstract.
10. Marino M, Glue P, Herron JM, Statkevich P, Affrime MB, Lim J. Lack of electrocardiographic effects of multiple high doses of desloratadine. Allergy 2000; 55(Suppl 63): 279. Abstract.
11. Gupta S, Banfield C, Kantesaria B, Marino M, Clement R, Affrime M et al. Pharmacokinetic and safety profile of desloratadine and fexofenadine when coadministered with azithromycin: a randomized, placebo-controlled, parallel-group study. Clin Ther 2001; 23: 451–466.
12. Paris DG, Parente TF, Bruschetta HR, Guzman E, Niarchos AP. Torsades de pointes induced by erythromycin and terfenadine. Am J Emerg Med 1994; 12: 636–638.
13. DuBuske LM. Clinical comparison of histamine H_1-receptor antagonist drugs. J Allergy Clin Immunol 1996; 98: S307-S318.

31 Preclinical Efficacy and Antiallergic Profile of Desloratadine, a Potent Histamine H$_1$-Receptor Antagonist

W. Kreutner, J.A. Hey, J.C. Anthes, A. Barnett

Abstract

Desloratadine is a novel antiallergic therapy for allergic rhinitis, chronic idiopathic urticaria and other allergic conditions. The studies reported here demonstrate the potent antihistaminic and antiallergic effects as well as the exceptional safety profile of desloratadine.

In vivo studies of antihistamine activity showed that orally administered desloratadine (median effective dose [ED$_{50}$] = 0.15 mg/kg) was 2.5 to 4-fold more potent than loratadine in inhibiting histamine-induced lethality in guinea pigs and histamine-induced paw edema in mice. Applied topically into the nose of guinea pigs, desloratadine (ED$_{50}$=0.9 µg) was tenfold more potent than loratadine in blocking histamine-induced increases in nasal microvascular permeability. The antiallergic profile of desloratadine has been expanded by two recent studies. In vivo, orally administered desloratadine inhibited the increase in airway resistance and decrease in compliance in allergic cynomolgus monkeys challenged by inhaling the *Ascaris suum* antigen. Also, in allergic guinea pigs that cough in response to inhaled ovalbumin, desloratadine exhibited antitussive activity with an ED$_{50}$=0.3 mg/kg. The safety of desloratadine has been demonstrated by numerous preclinical studies that have focused mainly on examining potential central nervous system or cardiovascular effects of desloratadine. In mice, desloratadine produced no behavioral, neurologic, or autonomic effects at doses up to 300 mg/kg. Furthermore, desloratadine did not protect mice from electroconvulsive shock, acetic-acid–induced writhing, or physostigmine-induced death. It is likely that desloratadine does not have access to histamine H$_1$ receptors in the brain that are linked to sedation because the in vivo administration of desloratadine to guinea pigs did not interfere with the subsequent binding of ^{3}H-mepyramine to brain H$_1$ receptors in vitro. In cardiovascular studies, desloratadine at concentrations up to 10 µM did not inhibit the human ether-a-go-go (HERG) K$^+$ channel. Furthermore, studies in numerous animal species, including monkeys, indicated that desloratadine, even at large doses, did not alter heart rate, blood pressure, or the electrocardiogram, including QT$_c$ or QRS intervals. In radioligand receptor-binding assays utilizing cloned human H$_1$-receptor expressed in Chinese hamster ovary (CHO) cells, desloratadine binding affinity was at least 25 times and up to 200 times more potent than terfenadine, fexofenadine, cetirizine, loratadine, ebastine, and mizolastine. Similar results were obtained from Ca^2 flux assays in CHO cells.

Preclinical studies support clinical data that desloratadine is a potent antihistamine with multiple antiallergic effects and an excellent safety profile.

Introduction

Desloratadine is a novel, potent, next-generation H_1-receptor antagonist with antiallergic properties (Kreutner et al. 2000a). Clinical studies have demonstrated that desloratadine provides full 24-h symptomatic relief of various allergic conditions, including seasonal allergic rhinitis (SAR) and chronic idiopathic urticaria (Agrawal 2001; Ring et al. 2001).

Histamine is a major mediator in the pathophysiology of the allergic response and, as such, is a primary target for therapeutic intervention. H_1-receptor antagonists constitute the therapy of choice for inhibiting the inflammatory effects of histamine release and the inhibition of other proinflammatory activities that occur subsequent to histamine release. Some of the H_1-receptor antagonists also have antiallergic effects that do not appear to be mediated through the H_1 receptor; these include inhibition of histamine release and the inhibition of the release of such other proinflammatory agents as cytokines, chemokines, and adhesion proteins (Lippert et al. 2000).

Two issues of importance for antihistamine therapy are potential central nervous system (CNS) and cardiovascular effects. First-generation antihistamines were noted for their sedative effects, which limited their use to situations in which mental alertness was not critical. Most second-generation antihistamines lack the CNS sedating effects since they are largely restricted from passing through the blood-brain barrier (Kay 2000). An exception to this is cetirizine which has been shown to cause sedation (Product information). Some second-generation antihistamines such as astemizole and terfenadine, however, pose a serious threat to cardiovascular safety through inhibition of the cardiac human-ether-a-go-go (HERG) K^+ channel. These agents may cause lengthening of the QT_c interval, especially when coadministered with agents such as ketoconazole, erythromycin, and azithromycin that affect their metabolism and absorption (Barbey et al. 1999).

The following preclinical studies demonstrate the potent antihistaminic and antiallergic effects of desloratadine. These studies also present the potential of a superior safety profile of desloratadine through demonstration of minimal CNS and cardiovascular effects.

Methods

In Vivo Antihistaminic Activity

Measurement of Histamine-Induced Paw Edema in Mice

Fasting mice (25–30 g) were injected with 13 µg of histamine (right foot) or saline vehicle (left foot) 1 h after receiving desloratadine 0.03–1.0 mg/kg, loratadine 0.3–3.0 mg/kg, or methylcellulose vehicle. After 30 min, the mice were sacrificed and both paws were removed and weighed. The dose that resulted in 50% inhibition of edema (ED_{50}) was calculated, and 95% confidence intervals were determined by the linear least-square dose-response method.

Evaluation of Effects on Lethal Doses of Histamine in Guinea Pigs

Guinea pigs (250–350 g) were given a lethal intravenous (IV) injection of histamine dihydrochloride (1.1 mg/kg) 1 h after administration of 3 to 4 log-spaced doses of desloratadine or loratadine. PD_{50} (determined by probit analysis) was the calculated dose that would prevent death in 50% of the guinea pigs for at least 30 min.

Inhibition of Histamine-Induced Increases in Nasal Microvascular Permeability in Guinea Pigs

Guinea pigs (400–500 g) were anesthetized and nares (50 µl/nostril) were instilled with vehicle (1% v/v DMSO in 10 mmol/l PBS, pH 7.2), desloratadine (0.1–3.0 µg), loratadine (1.0–10 µg), or levocabastine (0.01–1.0 µg). Animals had a tracheal cannula inserted in a cephalic direction 10 min after treatment and were challenged with 1 mmol/l of histamine at a rate of 0.2 ml/min for 30 min. The animals were given an IV injection of Evans blue dye (30 mg/kg) 15 min before the histamine challenge. Microvascular permeability was measured by collecting and spectrophotometrically analyzing perfusate that exited the nares.

Antiallergic Profile

Measurement of Pulmonary Function in Allergic Monkeys Challenged with Inhalation of *Ascaris suum* Antigen

In this crossover, placebo-controlled experiment, cynomolgus monkeys received desloratadine 5 mg/kg or placebo administered through a stomach tube. After 90 min, monkeys were challenged with 15 inhaled breaths of nebulized *Ascaris suum* antigen. Pulmonary mechanics were monitored for 5 min immediately after inhalation of antigen. After 24 h, the monkeys were anesthetized and bronchoal-veolar lavage fluid was collected from the right lung.

Assessment of Allergic Cough in Ovalbumin-Sensitized Guinea Pigs

Fasting guinea pigs (350–450 g) were orally administered vehicle (0.4% methylcellulose), desloratadine 0.003–1 mg/kg, or loratadine 0.003–1 mg/kg 2 h before they were exposed to aerosolized ovalbumin (0.3%) for 4 min in a transparent chamber. A microphone and a trained observer monitored the number of coughs experienced by the animals. ANOVA, in conjunction with a Dunnett's t-test, was used to evaluate statistical significance.

Central Nervous System Safety

Changes in Behavioral, Neurologic, and Autonomic Activity

Mice (20–24 g) were administered oral desloratadine (30, 100, or 300 mg/kg) or astemizole, and then tested for changes in behavioral, neurologic, and autonomic activity 1 h after each dose. At baseline, CNS symptoms were given a score of 0 for normal spontaneous activity, alertness, and pupil size. After medication, decreases (–) or increases (+) in these parameters or any other abnormal effects (e.g., convulsions or tremors) were given a score of ± 1–3 for slight, moderate, or marked changes from baseline. Animals were monitored for 24 h to determine if there were any delayed reactions to the study drug.

Electroconvulsive Shock (ECS) and Acetic Acid-Induced Writhing

Mice (20–24 g) were administered log-spaced doses of desloratadine or azatadine. ED_{50} was estimated using the percentage of protection at each dose. For ECS, mice were corneally administered a 13-mA, 60-cycle alternating-current shock for 0.2 s. For acetic-acid–induced writhing, mice were injected intraperitoneally with 10 ml/kg of a 0.6% solution of acetic acid 15 min after dosing with the test drug. The number of writhes (arching of back, pelvic rotation, and hind-limb extension) were recorded for each animal during a 10-min period beginning 3 min after acetic acid administration.

Physostigmine Lethality

Mice were orally administered desloratadine or azatadine 30 min before subcutaneous administration of physostigmine salicylate (1 mg/kg). Assessment of the number of survivors occurred 20 min after administration of physostigmine.

Inhibition of ^{3}H-mepyramine binding In the Brain

Guinea pigs (500–600 g) were intraperitoneally administered desloratadine (6 mg/kg), loratadine (6 mg/kg), chlorpheniramine (2 mg/kg), or vehicle. After 30 min the animals were sacrificed, and the cerebral cortexes (right hemispheres) were dissected out and homogenized in 1:10 (weight/volume) of 50 mmol/l sodium potassium phosphate buffer, pH 7.5. The homogenate (0.5 ml) was incubated with 2 nmol/l of ^{3}H-mepyramine at 25°C for 15 min, and then the bound ^{3}H-mepyramine was separated from the unbound ^{3}H-mepyramine. The study drug was compared with placebo for receptor-bound ^{3}H-mepyramine counts using Duncan's multiple-range statistics.

Cardiovascular Safety

In Vitro Effects on the HERG Channel

The cloned HERG K^+ channel was expressed in prepared *Xenopus* oocytes, after which oocytes were placed in a 0.150-ml recording chamber and superperfused with desloratadine, loratadine, terfenadine, or quinidine (positive control). Two standard glass microelectrodes filled with 3 mol/l KCl (1–10 MO) were used to probe the oocytes at the animal pole by applying a conditioning pulse (up to 40 mV) followed by a pulse to –80 mV. The percent inhibition of the K^+ channel was recorded.

Changes in Blood Pressure, Heart Rate, and ECGs in Rats, Guinea Pigs, and Monkeys

Fasting rats (225–350 g) were administered desloratadine 4 mg/kg or 12 mg/kg orally. Heart rate and blood pressure were measured immediately before drug administration and at 1-min intervals at each half hour up to 8 h postdose. ECGs were measured in the same rats with leads implanted in the right and left forelegs and the left rear leg. Wires were subcutaneously anchored from the implant to the point of emergence at the nape of the neck. ECGs were used to determine the PR, QRS, QT, and RR intervals of the lead-II ECG. The ECG assessment timepoints were the same as those used to determine the heart rate and blood pressure.

Fasting guinea pigs (450–600 g) were administered desloratadine (25 mg/kg) or vehicle (methylcellulose) via infusion of the jugular vein. Baseline lead-II ECGs were determined before drug infusion and 30 min postinfusion. ECGs were used to determine the QT, QT_c, PR, and QRS intervals and heart rate. Data were analyzed by 1-way ANOVA and Dunnett's t-test.

Fasting monkeys (5–7 kg) were administered desloratadine (12 mg/kg) or vehicle (methylcellulose). The same monkeys were administered the reverse treatment 1 week later in this crossover study. Four hours after administration of study drug or vehicle, 6-limb-lead ECGs were obtained using a lead-II rhythm strip. ECG intervals were determined as the average of 5 consecutive cardiac cycles. The data were analyzed by ANOVA and Scheffe's f-test.

Results

In Vivo Antihistaminic Activity

Desloratadine had 4 times more antihistaminic potency than loratadine in inhibiting paw edema in mice after injection of histamine. The ED_{50} value was 0.15 (0.09–0.24) mg/kg for desloratadine and 0.60 (0.29–0.99) mg/kg for loratadine. Desloratadine was also potent for inhibiting lethality after injection of histamine in guinea pigs. Desloratadine was 2.5 times more potent than loratadine in pro-

Table 1. Activity of topical antihistamines (1 µg) in guinea pig nasal challenge model

Antihistamine	Inhibition of permeability (%)*	ED_{50} (µg)
Desloratadine	$50 \pm 12^+$	0.9
Loratadine	13 ± 13	8.7
Levocabastine	$85 \pm 8^+$	0.025

* Mean$\pm$SEM; $^+P<0.05$ compared with vehicle.

tecting against lethal doses of histamine. The ED_{50} for desloratadine was 0.15 mg/kg, compared with an ED_{50} of 0.37 mg/kg for loratadine. After 1 h, desloratadine protected 100% of the animals, compared with 80% for loratadine. At 4 and 8 h desloratadine and loratadine protected 100% of the animals, and at 24 h the protection was 40% and 60%, respectively (5 guinea pigs in each group).

The topical application of the antihistamines to guinea pig nasal passages was used to test the topical antihistaminic activity of desloratadine (0.1–3.0 µg), loratadine (1.0–10 µg), and levocabastine (0.01–1.0 µg). After challenge with histamine, the order of antihistaminic potency in the upper airways of guinea pigs was levocabastine >desloratadine >loratadine (Table 1).

Antiallergic Profile

The antiallergic profile of desloratadine and loratadine was compared with placebo in the guinea pig cough model. After controlled exposure to ovalbumin in ovalbumin-sensitized guinea pigs, desloratadine and loratadine exhibited a dose-dependent decrease in the number of coughs (Fig. 1). Compared with placebo, desloratadine 0.3 mg/kg, desloratadine 1.0 mg/kg, and loratadine 1.0 mg/kg all significantly reduced the number of coughs compared with placebo ($P<0.05$). In another antiallergic model, monkeys naturally allergic to *Ascaris suum* were given desloratadine 5 mg/kg and then challenged with nebulized *Ascaris suum*. Compared with placebo, desloratadine significantly inhibited the increase in airway resistance (44% vs 103%) ($P<0.0025$) and decrease in compliance (–33% vs –52%) ($P<0.0025$) following inhalation of *Ascaris suum* in allergic monkeys.

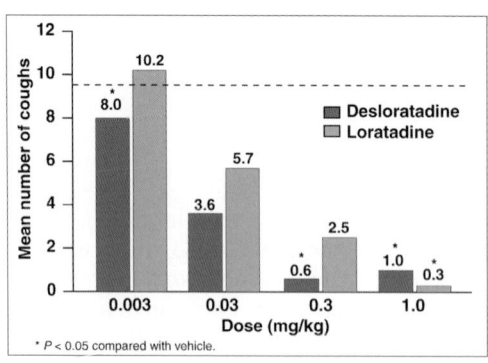

Fig. 1. Desloratadine reduces cough in the guinea pig model (*dashed line* indicates vehicle effect)

Central Nervous System Safety

A summary of the results of preclinical CNS studies is presented in Table 2. There were minimal effects on behavioral, neurologic, and autonomic responses in mice treated with doses of desloratadine up to 300 mg/kg. There were minimal decreases in motor activity or muscle tone; no evidence of tremors/convulsions, ataxia, or reactivity; and the treatment did not result in any lethality. The only effects at this high dose of desloratadine were mydriasis and ptosis. In contrast, astemizole 100 mg/kg and 300 mg/kg showed ptosis and decreased motor activity, respectively (see Table 2).

High doses of desloratadine (160 mg/kg) and azatadine at the highest nonlethal dose (80 mg/kg) did not protect against ECS-induced tonic convulsions, indicating reduced access to the CNS. However, there was a large difference in the ED_{50} of desloratadine and azatadine in the acetic-acid–induced writing test. Desloratadine and azatadine inhibited acetic-acid–induced writing at an ED_{50} of 147 mg/kg and 4.8 mg/kg, respectively (see Table 2).

The potential anticholinergic effects of desloratadine were tested by administration of desloratadine or azatadine followed by challenge with a lethal dose of the potent cholinergic agonist, physostigmine. Desloratadine did not alter the physostigmine-induced lethality in mice at doses up to 300 mg/kg, however, azatadine, which is more accessible to the CNS, protected 50% of the mice at a dose of 2.2 mg/kg (see Table 2). In addition, neither desloratadine nor loratadine altered ^{3}H-mepyramine binding to brain H_1 receptors at intraperitoneal doses of desloratadine 6 mg/kg or loratadine 6 mg/kg in guinea pigs (Table 2). ^{3}H-mepyramine-bound counts/minute were 3,208, 1,694, and 3,313 for desloratadine, chlorpheniramine, and vehicle, respectively. These studies show that unlike

Table 2. Summary of preclinical CNS studies

Model	Desloratadine	Comparator
General (mice)	No significant behavioral, neurologic, or autonomic effects at doses up to 300 mg/kg	Astemizole 100 mg/kg– ptosis; astemizole 300 mg/kg– motor activity; mydriasis
ECS (mice)	Did not alter ECS response at 160 mg/kg	Azatadine did not alter ECS response at its highest nonlethal dose (80 mg/kg)
Acetic-acid-induced writhing (mice)	Inhibited writhing with an ED_{50} value of 147 mg/kg	Azatadine inhibited writhing with an ED_{50} value of 4.8 mg/kg
Physostigmine lethality (mice)	Did not alter lethality at doses up to 300 mg/kg	Azatadine protected 50% of mice at dose of 2.2 mg/kg
^{3}H-mepyramine (guinea pigs)	Did not alter binding to brain H_1 receptors at 6 mg/kg	Chlorpheniramine 2 mg/kg–49% inhibition (P <0.05)

ECS, electroconvulsive shock; ED_{50}, median effective dose.

chlorpheniramine, desloratadine has limited access to H_1 receptors in the brain after systemic administration.

Cardiovascular Safety

Perturbation of the HERG K^+ channel is associated with increasing QT and QT_c intervals. Desloratadine, terfenadine, and quinidine were tested for inhibition of HERG-induced current in vitro using *Xenopus* oocytes expressing the cloned HERG gene. Desloratadine had no effect on the HERG channel at concentrations between 10 nmol/l and 10 µmol/l. Quinidine and terfenadine, however, inhibited the HERG channel at low concentrations (30 nmol/l); the IC_{50} values were 82 and 167 nmol/l, respectively.

In animal models, desloratadine, even at high doses, did not alter heart rate, blood pressure, or the ECG, including QT_c and QRS intervals. Rats, guinea pigs, and monkeys were administered desloratadine or vehicle and monitored for changes in blood pressure, heart rate, QRS, QT, and PR. In rats, at doses of 4 mg/kg and 12 mg/kg desloratadine there were no significant differences from placebo in mean blood pressure. In guinea pigs, there were no significant differences from vehicle in blood pressure, heart rate, QT, QT_c, PR, or QRS intervals at doses of desloratadine that were 500 times the ED_{50} for IV antihistaminic activity. In monkeys, desloratadine 12 mg/kg did not induce any significant changes in PR, QRS, or QT_c compared with vehicle.

Discussion

These preclinical in vitro and in vivo animal studies demonstrate that desloratadine, an active metabolite of loratadine, has potent H_1-receptor binding and excellent antihistaminic and antiallergic activity, while lacking adverse CNS and cardiovascular effects. This profile epitomizes the best aspects of the new H_1-receptor antagonists such as desloratadine. As previously reported, desloratadine has been shown to be a potent H_1-receptor antagonist with a high affinity for the receptor, even higher than the high-affinity agent pyrilamine (Anthes 2001). In that study, Chinese hamster ovary (CHO) cells expressing the cloned human H_1-receptor were used to assess receptor-binding ([^{3}H]-pyrilamine displacement) and histamine-induced Ca^{2+} flux. Desloratadine had a higher affinity for the human H_1 receptor than other antagonists used to treat allergic rhinitis such as loratadine, mizolastine, cetirizine, ebastine, and fexofenadine. In addition, other studies have shown that at doses needed for antihistaminic activity, desloratadine is highly selective for the H_1 receptor (Kreutner et al. 2000b).

The in vivo antihistaminic activity of desloratadine was demonstrated in mice by prevention of histamine-induced paw edema and in guinea pigs by prevention of death from a lethal dose of histamine. Desloratadine was 4 times more potent than loratadine in inhibiting histamine-induced paw edema and 2.5 times more potent than loratadine in protecting against lethal doses of histamine, with protection lasting up to 24 h. Other studies have shown that desloratadine is 2 to

3 times more potent than loratadine in inhibiting dermal wheal and flare reactions in guinea pigs (Handley et al. 1997). Topical application of desloratadine also resulted in antihistaminic activity. When applied to the nasal passages of guinea pigs, desloratadine was 10 times more potent than loratadine in inhibiting histamine-induced microvascular permeability.

In animal models that tested the antiallergic profile of desloratadine, ovalbumin-induced cough in guinea pigs and *Ascaris suum* challenge in allergic monkeys resulted in a reduction of allergic cough and acute bronchospasm, respectively (Fig. 1). Other reported in vitro studies complement these in vivo studies (Berthon et al. 1994; Letari et al. 1994; Genovese et al. 1997; Vignola et al. 1995; Schoenwetter 2000; Cagnoni and Mincarini 1998). Desloratadine has been shown to inhibit IgE and non-IgE-induced release of histamine from basophils (Kleine-Tebbe et al. 1994) and the release of other proinflammatory agents such as cytokines, chemokines, and adhesion proteins (Berthon et al. 1994; Letari et al. 1994; Genovese et al. 1997; Vignola et al. 1995; Schoenwetter 2000; Cagnoni and Mincarini 1998).

A primary drawback of first-generation antihistamines is their sedating effects. The older antihistamines are lipophilic and easily cross the blood-brain barrier. Many of the newer generation antihistamines, such as loratadine and desloratadine, are nonsedating and have relatively few effects on the CNS. The preclinical studies reported here demonstrate the nonsedating properties of desloratadine. Up to 300 mg/kg of desloratadine did not cause any behavioral, neurologic, or autonomic effects in mice. In addition, desloratadine was tested for protection against the CNS effects in mouse models using convulsion-induced ECS and acetic acetic-acid–induced writhing. Desloratadine was tested against agents known to protect the CNS from these effects. High doses of desloratadine were required to protect against acetic-acid–induced writhing (approximately 30 times the ED_{50} of azatadine), and desloratadine did not protect against physostigmine-induced lethality at doses up to 300 mg/kg in mice. These results are further supported by guinea pig ex vivo studies that demonstrate that desloratadine does not prevent the binding of ^{3}H-mepyramine in vitro after in vivo exposure to desloratadine. In addition, other preclinical studies of CNS effects in animals have resulted in findings similar to those reported here (Barnett et al. 1984; Hey et al. 1995).

Although most second-generation antihistamines have improved or placebo-like effects on the incidence of sedation, some have resulted in serious, significant cardiac arrhythmias. Both terfenadine and astemizole have been subject to scrutiny due to association with lengthening of the QT and QT_c, which can result in torsades de pointes and other ventricular arrhythmias (Woosley et al. 1993; Honig et al. 1992; Monahan et al. 1990; Craft 1986). The cause of these adverse cardiovascular events appears to be through inhibition of the HERG K^+ channel. The results from the studies presented here show that desloratadine has no significant effect on the HERG K^+ channel. At concentrations of 10 nmol/l to 10 µg/l, desloratadine did not affect the K^+ current in *Xenopus* oocytes expressing the HERG gene. In contrast, known inhibitors of the HERG channel such as quinidine and terfenadine inhibited the channel at low concentrations of agent (30 nmol/l). In addition, the in vivo studies reported here show that desloratadine has no significant effect on blood pressure, heart rate or ECG data, including lengthening of the QT_c interval. The cardiovascular studies are supported by other in vivo studies that showed no effects on cardiac K^+ channels at 10–100 times the therapeutic dose of desloratadine (Ducic et al. 1997).

Conclusions

Desloratadine potently displaces [^{3}H]-pyrilamine from the human H_1 receptor in CHO cell assays and has greater binding affinity than mizolastine, terfenadine, cetirizine, ebastine, loratadine, and fexofenadine. In addition, desloratadine is more potent than commercially available second-generation antihistamines in the Ca^{2+} flux assay at the human H_1 receptor. In addition, as demonstrated in allergen-challenge models, desloratadine has antiallergic properties. Desloratadine has an excellent CNS and cardiovascular safety profile, even at high doses, with no known effects on cardiac ion channels and no alteration of ECG parameters, including the QT_c interval.

References

1. Agrawal DK (2001) Pharmacology and clinical efficacy of desloratadine as an anti-allergic and anti-inflammatory drug. Exp Opin Invest Drugs 10(3): 547–560.
2. Anthes JC, Eckel S, Richard C, West R, Greenfeder S, Saluja S et al. Characterization of [3H]desloratadine at the human H1 receptor. J Allergy Clin Immunol 2001; 107: S160. Abstract.
3. Barbey JT, Anderson M, Ciprandi G, Frew AJ, Morad M, Priori SG, Ongini E, Affrime MB (1999) Cardiovascular safety of second-generation antihistamines. Am J Rhinol 13: 235–243.
4. Barnett A, Iorio LC, Kreutner W, Tozzi S, Ahn HS, Gulbenkian A (1984) Evaluation of the CNS properties of SCH 29851, a potential non-sedating antihistamine. Agents Actions 14: 590–597.
5. Berthon B, Taudou G, Combettes L, Czarlewski W, Carmi-Leroy A, Marchand F, Weyer A (1994) In vitro inhibition, by loratadine and descarboxyethoxyloratadine, of histamine release from human basophils, and of histamine release and intracellular calcium fluxes in rat basophilic leukemia cells. Biochem Pharmacol 47 No. 5: 789–794.
6. Cagnoni F, Mincarini M. In vitro effects of loratadine and its active metabolite on T lymphocytes [abstract]. J Allergy Clin Immunol 101[Number 1 (Pt.2)], 578–579. 1998.
7. Craft TM. Torsade de pointes after astemizole overdose [abstract].. Br.Med J (Clin Res Ed) 292[6521], 660. 3-8-1986.
8. Ducic I, Ko CM, Shuba Y, Morad M (1997) Comparative effects of loratadine and terfenadine on cardiac K+ channels. J Cardiovasc Pharmacol 30: 42–54.
9. Genovese A, Patella V, De Crescenzo G, De P, Spadaro G, Marone G (1997) Loratadine and desethoxylcarbonyl-loratadine inhibit the immunological release of mediators from human FcɛRI+ cells. Clin Exp Allergy 27: 559–567.
10. Handley DA, McCullough JR, Fang Y, Wright SE, Smith ER. Descarboethoxyloratadine, a metabolite of loratadine is a superior antihistamine [abstract]. Ann Allergy, Asthma, Immunol 78, 143. 1997.
11. Hey JA, del Prado M, Cuss FM, Egan RW, Sherwood J, Lin CC, Kreutner W (1995) Antihistamine activity, central nervous system and cardiovascular profiles of histamine H1 antagonists: comparative studies with loratadine, terfenadine and sedating antihistamines in guinea-pigs. Clin Exp Allergy 25: 974–984.
12. Honig PK, Woosley RL, Zamani K, Conner DP, Cantilena LR, Jr. (1992) Changes in the pharmacokinetics and electrocardiographic pharmacodynamics of terfenadine with concomitant administration of erythromycin. Clin Pharmacol Ther 52: 231–238.

13. Kay GG (2000) The effects of antihistamines on cognition and performance. J Allergy Clin Immunol 105: S622-S627.
14. Kleine-Tebbe J, Josties C, Frank G, Stalleicken D, Buschauer A, Schunack W, Kunkel G, Czarnetzki B (1994) Inhibition of IgE- and non-IgE-mediated histamine release from human basophil leukocytes in vitro by a histamine H1-antagonist, desethoxycarbonyl-loratadine. J Allergy Clin Immunol 93: 494-500.
15. Kreutner W, Hey JA, Anthes J, Barnett A, Tozzi S (2000) Preclinical efficacy and antiallergic profile of desloratadine, a selective and nonsedating histamine H_1-receptor antagonist [abstract]. J Allergy Clin Immunol 104[Number 1, Part 2], S382-S383. 2000a.
16. Kreutner W, Hey JA, Anthes J, Barnett A, Young S, Tozzi S (2000) Preclinical pharmacology of desloratadine, a selective and nonsedating histamine H_1 receptor antagonist: 1st communication: receptor selectivity, antihistaminic activity, and antiallergenic effects. Arzneimittelforschung 50: 345-352.
17. Letari O, Miozzo A, Folco G, Belloni PA, Sala A, Rovati GE, Nicosia S (1994) Effects of loratadine on cytosolic Ca2+ levels and leukotriene release: novel mechanisms of action independent of the anti-histamine activity. Eur J Pharmacol 266: 219-227.
18. Lippert U, Moller A, Welker P, Artuc M, Henz BM (2000) Inhibition of cytokine secretion from human leukemic mast cells and basophils by H1- and H2-receptor antagonists. Exp Dermatol 9: 118-124.
19. Monahan BP, Ferguson CL, Killeavy ES, Lloyd BK, Troy J, Cantilena LR, Jr. (1990) Torsades de pointes occurring in association with terfenadine use. JAMA 264: 2788-2790.
20. Ring J, Hein R, Gauger A, Bronsky E, Miller B, Desloratadine Study Group (2001) Once-daily desloratadine improves the signs and symptoms of chronic idiopathic urticaria: a randomized, double-blind, placebo-controlled study. Int J Dermatol 40: 1-5.
21. Schoenwetter WF (2000) Allergic rhinitis: Epidemiology and natural history. Allergy Asthma Proc 21: 1-6.
22. Vignola AM, Crampette L, Mondain M, Sauvere G, Czarlewski W, Bousquet J, Campbell AM (1995) Inhibitory activity of loratadine and descarboethoxyloratadine on expression of ICAM-1 and HLA-DR by nasal epithelial cells. Allergy 50: 200-203.
23. Woosley RL, Chen Y, Freiman JP, Gillis RA (1993) Mechanism of the cardiotoxic actions of terfenadine [see comments]. JAMA 269: 1532-1536.
24. Zyrtec (cetirizine) prescribing information. In: Physician's; Desk Reference. Montevale (NJ); Medical Economics; 2000. p.2404-6.

32 Desloratadine Is Effective at Relieving Nasal Congestion, as Demonstrated in Three Placebo-Controlled Trials in Patients with Seasonal Allergic Rhinitis

R. Lorber, L.M. Salmun, M.R. Danzig

Abstract

Desloratadine is a new antiallergic agent that has inherent decongestant properties. It has been shown to provide full 24-h symptom relief in patients with seasonal allergic rhinitis (SAR) and other allergic conditions. Nasal congestion/stuffiness is a common symptom of SAR and is related to the late-phase allergic response. Currently available oral histamine H_1-receptor antagonists are not effective for treating nasal congestion. The effect of desloratadine 5 mg once daily on nasal congestion was evaluated in three separate, randomized, double-blind, placebo-controlled, parallel-group, multicenter studies in patients with at least a 2-year history of SAR and moderate or severe symptoms at baseline.

Studies 1 and 2 were 4-week studies of patients with SAR and concurrent asthma. Study 3 was a 2-week study of patients with SAR. These three studies enrolled a total of 948 patients.

In all three studies, the severity of nasal congestion over the previous 12 h was graded twice daily using the following grading scale: 0=none, 1=mild, 2=moderate, 3=severe. The average reflective (as assessed over the previous 12 h) a.m. and p.m. nasal congestion severity scores at baseline were between 2.4 and 2.1 for the three studies. The reductions from baseline in these scores over a 2-week period were significantly greater with desloratadine than with placebo for all three studies (P values were <0.05 for all studies).

In both of the longer studies, the reduction in nasal congestion continued throughout the 4-week evaluation. The reduction from baseline over the 4-week treatment period was significantly greater in the desloratadine groups than in the placebo groups (P<0.05 for both studies).

Desloratadine was well tolerated in all three studies, with a side effect profile similar to placebo. These findings demonstrate that desloratadine relieves nasal congestion in patients with SAR over a period of at least 4 weeks without significant side effects.

Introduction

Nasal congestion/stuffiness is a common and especially troublesome symptom of allergic rhinitis (AR). Multiple complications can arise from nasal congestion, including sleep disturbances, facial changes, headache, halitosis, and allergic shiners (Dykewicz et al. 1998; Rachelefsky 1999; Hadley 1999; Settipane 1999; Beckman

New Trends in Allergy V
J. Ring, H. Behrendt (Eds.)
© Springer-Verlag Berlin, Heidelberg 2002

and Grammer 1999). In addition, AR predisposes patients to asthma, as demonstrated by the high association between patients with allergic rhinitis and asthma. Up to 58% of patients with allergic rhinitis also have asthma and up to 78% of patients with asthma also have allergic rhinitis.(Rachelefsky, 1999)

Nasal congestion is one of the common links between AR and asthma and is associated with mouth breathing. When patients breathe through the nose, inspired air is humidified and warmed, but when breathed through the mouth this does not occur as efficiently and, therefore, may increase the risk of exercise-induced asthma. Furthermore, nasal congestion increases lower airway access of aeroallergens and can activate the neural reflex, resulting in a decrease in forced expiratory volume at 1 s (FEV_1). Postnasal drainage of inflammatory material and absorption of mediators from the inflammatory process in the nose or sinuses into the lower airways may also contribute to the mechanism that links allergic rhinitis with asthma (Rachelefsky 1999; DuBuske 1999).

Because most antihistamines are ineffective for relieving congestion, antihistamines are frequently coadministered with decongestants. However, the concomitant use of decongestants with antihistamines increases the likelihood of adverse events (Beierle et al. 1999), which can include increased blood pressure, palpitations, tremor, loss of appetite, nervousness, and insomnia. Thus, the use of these medications in combination can increase the risk of serious complications through a synergistic increase and exacerbation of adverse events (Dykewicz et al. 1998).

Desloratadine is a nonsedating, potent, next-generation H_1-receptor antagonist with antiallergic activity (Kreutner et al. 2000). Once-daily dosing has been shown to provide full 24-h symptom relief in patients with various allergic disorders, including seasonal allergic rhinitis (SAR) (Agrawal 2001) and chronic idiopathic urticaria (Ring et al. 2001). Desloratadine is well absorbed after oral administration and has a long elimination half-life (Henz 2001), No clinically relevant drug interactions have been demonstrated (Gupta et al. 2001; Affrime et al. 2000; Glue et al. 2000), and no evidence of cardiotoxicity has been observed, even at doses 9 times above the dose used clinically (Banfield et al. 2000a). Furthermore, in clinical trials, the adverse event profile of desloratadine has been shown to be similar to placebo (Ring et al. 2001; Gupta et al. 2001; Agrawal 2001).

The three studies reported here evaluated the safety and efficacy of desloratadine compared with placebo for relieving nasal congestion/stuffiness. Two studies included patients with both SAR and asthma. One study included patients with SAR alone.

Methods

Study Design

Studies 1 and 2 were identically designed, randomized, double-blind, placebo-controlled, parallel-group multicenter studies, performed during the autumn/winter season at medical centers throughout the United States. During screening (3 to 14 days), subjects were evaluated with respect to disease severity and inclusion/exclusion criteria. Eligible patients were randomized by computer to 4 weeks of treatment with desloratadine 5 mg once daily or placebo. Visits occurred at screening and on Days 1 (baseline), 8, 15, 22, and 29 (endpoint). All subjects or their parents/guardians provided written informed consent and the protocol was approved by the institutional review boards of the participating study centers.

Inclusion/Exclusion Criteria

Subjects had at least a 2-year history of SAR (Studies 1, 2, and 3) and increased asthma signs and symptoms during the autumn/winter allergy season (Studies 1 and 2). A positive skin test response to appropriate seasonal allergens within the previous 24 months was required for all subjects. All subjects were clinically symptomatic with at least moderate rhinorrhea, a total nasal symptom score of at least 6 (see below), and a total nonnasal symptom score=5 (see below) (Studies 1, 2, and 3). In Studies 1 and 2, subjects required an FEV_1 ≥70% of the predicted value at screening, and a total frequency of asthma score and/or bronchodilator use score of =2 (see below). The total of the reflective scores for the 3 days prior to baseline and the a.m. diary score of the baseline visit were =42 for the total SAR nasal score and =35 for the total nonnasal score (see below). Subjects with asthma and SAR required a demonstrated reversibility, which was defined as an increase in absolute FEV_1 of at least 12% over baseline, and an absolute volume increase =200 ml within 30 min after inhalation of albuterol. All subjects were free of any clinically significant disease other than asthma and SAR (Study 1 and 2) or SAR alone (Study 3) based on routine clinical and laboratory testing. A negative serum pregnancy test (HCG) was required at screening for all women of childbearing potential and a medically accepted method of birth control was required throughout the study (no pregnant women or nursing mothers were allowed).

Chronic use of inhaled or systemic corticosteroids or dependence on nasal, oral, or ocular decongestants, nasal topical antihistamines, or nasal corticosteroids were grounds for exclusion. Prohibited medications included cromolyn sodium, nedocromil, decongestants, corticosteroids, antihistamines, montelukast, zafirlukast, zileuton, ipratropium bromide, nasal atropine, ocular or nasal saline, theophylline, and sympathomimetic bronchodilators. If prohibited medications had been in use, sufficient washout time was required before the start of the study. Desensitization was not permitted during the study, but subjects could continue a regular maintenance schedule of immunotherapy as long as it was not administered within 24 h before a scheduled visit. The following conditions resulted in subject exclusion: clinically significant sinusitis, chronic purulent postnasal drip, nasal structural abnormalities, rhinitis medicamentosa, a history of allergies to more than two classes of medication, allergies or intolerance of antihistamines, hypersensitivity to the study drugs, or recent upper respiratory tract or sinus infections.

Study Medication

After completion of the diary in the morning, study medication was administered orally; the first dose was administered on Day 1 in the clinic. Compliance was assessed by questioning subjects and counting their remaining tablet supply. Inhaled albuterol (90 µg/inhalation) was given to all subjects in Studies 1 and 2, but they were instructed to administer only 2 inhalations as needed to control asthma symptoms and not to exceed 12 inhalations per day. SAR and asthma symptoms were evaluated prior to use of albuterol, and each use of albuterol was recorded in the subjects' diaries. Schering-Plough Corporation (Kenilworth, NJ) provided all study drugs.

Evaluations

Disease activity was assessed by the subjects during the screening period and throughout the course of the trial using a scoring system for signs and symptoms. Scores for all signs and symptoms were recorded on daily diary cards. The signs and symptoms of SAR included congestion, rhinorrhea, nasal itching, sneezing, itchy/burning eyes, tearing/watering eyes, redness of eyes, and itching of ears or palate. These were assessed using a 4-point scale with 0=none to 3=severe. The total SAR symptom score (TSS) was the sum of these individual symptom scores. Using the same scale as described for SAR, individual asthma symptoms (cough, wheeze, and difficulty breathing) were assessed. In Studies 1 and 2, the total asthma score was the sum of the three individual asthma symptom scores. Twice daily subjects scored the severity of both SAR and asthma symptoms (Studies 1 and 2 only) based upon their status over the previous 12 h (reflective) and how they felt at the time of assessment (instantaneous). The symptoms were assessed and recorded 2 times each day, immediately after awakening (predose) and approximately 12 h later.

Efficacy Variables

The primary efficacy outcome for congestion was the mean change from baseline in the Weeks 1–2 average a.m./p.m. reflective congestion scores (Studies 1, 2, and 3). Secondary outcomes included mean changes from baseline in Day 1 (Studies 1, 2, and 3) and Weeks 1–4 (Studies 1 and 2) average a.m./p.m. reflective congestion scores; and mean changes from baseline in Day 2, Weeks 1–2, and Weeks 1–4 (Studies 1 and 2) a.m. instantaneous congestion scores.

Safety Evaluations

Vital signs, clinical laboratory tests (blood chemistry, hematology, and urinalysis), and a standard 12-lead electrocardiogram (ECG) (ventricular rate, PR, QRS, QT, and QT_c intervals) were determined at screening and at study end (3 h after the last dose). Adverse events were assessed at each study visit.

If subjects were noncompliant or had intolerable symptoms, significant adverse events, laboratory abnormalities, or an FEV_1 below 40% of the predicted normal value (Studies 1 and 2), they were removed from the study. If patients had an exacerbation of SAR or asthma (Studies 1 and 2) that was associated with intolerable symptoms or the need for intensive treatment, they were considered for discontinuation from the study. In addition, subjects were considered for discontinuation if they required medical emergency treatment, used 12 or more puffs of albuterol per day on 2 or more consecutive days, or had a decrease in FEV_1 of 20% or more from baseline, a decrease in morning or evening peak expiratory flow rate (PEFR) of 20% or more on 2 or more consecutive days relative to the mean PEFR value 3 days prior to baseline, or nighttime awakenings requiring albuterol on 2 or more nights during any consecutive 7-day period (Studies 1 and 2).

Statistical Analysis

If randomized subjects received at least 1 dose of study medication, they were included in the data analysis. General descriptive statistics and two-way analyses of variance (ANOVA) with terms for treatment and center were applied for the efficacy variables. Comparisons were made at the two-sided 5% level of significance using t-tests of the least square means from ANOVA.

Results

Demographics and baseline disease severity were similar between placebo and the treatment group in each study (Table 1). Patients generally had moderate-to-severe nasal congestion at baseline; baseline average a.m./p.m. nasal congestion/stuffiness severity scores (maximum=3) were between 2.4 and 2.1 for the three studies.

Table 1. Baseline demographics

Characteristic	Study 1 DL 5 mg	Placebo	Study 2 DL 5 mg	Placebo	Study 3 DL 5 mg	Placebo
Mean age (years)	33	32	32	32	34	35
Sex, %						
Men	38	30	36	36	40	47
Women	62	70	64	64	60	53
Race, n (%)						
White	77	79	87	84	75	75
Black	9	10	8	8	12	14
Asian	2	0	1	<1	3	3
Hispanic	12	10	2	6	7	5
Other	0	<1	1	<1	3	2
Mean duration of SAR (years)	21	20	19	20	18	17
Mean duration of asthma (years)	17	16	16	16	—	—
Mean predicted FEV_1 (%)	87	85	86	87	—	—

The reductions from baseline in the 2-week average a.m./p.m. reflective nasal congestion/stuffiness scores were significantly greater with desloratadine 5 mg than with placebo in all 3 studies (Fig. 1). For patients with SAR and asthma in studies 1 and 2, the mean percent reduction from baseline was greater for the desloratadine 5 mg group compared with placebo ($P<0.05$). In patients with SAR alone, desloratadine 5 mg reduced congestion scores from baseline significantly more than placebo ($P<0.05$) (Fig. 1).

Analysis of the 4-week data in Studies 1 and 2 revealed similar treatment benefits with desloratadine 5 mg compared with placebo. The reductions in the average a.m./p.m. reflective nasal congestion/stuffiness scores from baseline were greater for desloratadine than placebo ($P<0.05$) (Fig. 2).

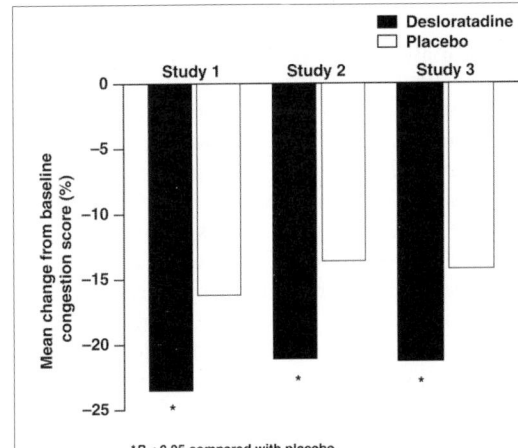

Fig. 1. Mean reduction from baseline in average a.m./p.m. reflective nasal congestion/stuffiness scores for weeks 1 and 2

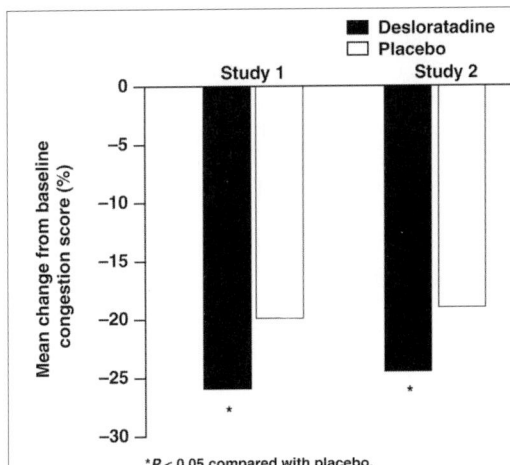

Fig. 2. Mean reduction from baseline in average a.m./p.m. reflective nasal congestion/stuffiness scores for weeks 1–4

Safety

For all studies, the adverse event profile was similar for the desloratadine and placebo groups. In addition, there were no clinically relevant changes in mean clinical laboratory tests, vital signs, or ECGs.

Discussion

These three studies have demonstrated that the potent H_1-receptor antagonist, desloratadine, provides rapid relief of the nasal congestion/stuffiness associated with SAR in patients with SAR only and in those with SAR and concurrent asthma. The results of these studies are consistent with the findings of other studies involving patients with SAR that have shown that desloratadine is effective for relieving congestion and total SAR symptoms (Meltzer et al. 2001). Since desloratadine is effective for treating SAR symptoms and nasal congestion, the use of this antihistamine may obviate the need for simultaneous treatment with a decongestant. This is beneficial for patients, since eliminating a decongestant from antihistamine therapy can reduce the incidence of such adverse events as increased blood pressure, insomnia, and tachycardia (Dykewicz et al. 1998).

Desloratadine was well tolerated in these three studies, with an adverse event profile similar to placebo. As in other desloratadine trials (Nayak et al. 2000; Banfield et al. 2000b; Gupta et al. 2001; Banfield et al. 2001; Padhi et al. 2000), adverse events were mild or moderate in severity, and there was no evidence of cardiovascular effects such as QT_c interval prolongation. In other studies, patients given 9 times the recommended dose of desloratadine did not experience cardiovascular effects, including no clinically relevant lengthening of the QT_c interval (Banfield et al. 2000a).

Conclusions

Desloratadine was effective for relieving nasal congestion/stuffiness associated with SAR for the full length of the studies in patients with SAR and asthma (4-week studies) and in patients with SAR alone (2-week study). There were no clinically relevant changes in clinical laboratory test results or mean ECG intervals, including QT_c intervals. Desloratadine was well tolerated and had an adverse event profile similar to that of placebo in all studies.

References

1. Affrime, M. B., Banfield, C., Glue, P., Ngo, L. Y., Keung, A., Herron, J. M., Padhi, D., Maxwell, S., and Clement, R. P. Lack of electrocardiographic effects when desloratadine and ketoconazole are coadministered. Allergy 55 (Suppl 63), 277. 2000. Abstract: 992
2. Agrawal DK (2001) Pharmacology and clinical efficacy of desloratadine as an anti-allergic and anti-inflammatory drug. Exp Opin Invest Drugs 10: 547–560.

3. Banfield, C., Cayen, M., Gupta, S., and Affrime, M. Grapefruit juice has no effect on the bioavailability of desloratadine, but reduces the C_{max} and AUC of fexofenadine by 30%. Annals of Allergy, Asthma, and Immunology 86, 108. 2001. Abstract: P60

4. Banfield, C., Padhi, D., Glue, P., Herron, J. M., Statkevich, P., and Affrime, M. B. Electrocardiographic effects of multiple high doses of desloratadine. Journal of Allergy and Clinical Immunology 104 (1 part 2), S383. 2000a. Abstract: 1119

5. Banfield, C., Rosenberg, M., Cohen, A., Padhi, D., Gupta, N., Affrime, M. B., Boutros, T., Thonoor, M., and Cayen, M. N. Race and gender do not affect the multiple-dose pharmacokinetics and safety of desloratadine. Allergy 55 (Suppl 63), 277. 2000b. Abstract: 991

6. Beckman DB, Grammer LC (1999) Pharmacotherapy to prevent the complications of allergic rhinitis. Allergy Asthma Proc 20: 215–223.

7. Beierle I, Meibohm B, Derendorf H (1999) Gender differences in pharmacokinetics and pharmacodynamics. Int J Clin Pharmacol Ther 37: 529–547.

8. DuBuske LM (1999) The link between allergy and asthma. Allergy Asthma Proc 20: 341–345.

9. Dykewicz MS, Fineman S, Skoner DP, Nicklas R, Lee R, Blessing-Moore J, Li JT, Bernstein IL, Berger W, Spector S, Schuller D (1998) Diagnosis and management of rhinitis: complete guidelines of the Joint Task Force on Practice Parameters in Allergy, Asthma and Immunology. Ann Allergy Asthma Immunol 81: 478–518.

10. Glue, P., Banfield, C., Affrime, M. B., Statkevich, P., Reyderman, L., Padhi, D., Maxwell, S., and Clement, R. P. Lack of electrocardiographic interaction between desloratadine and erythromycin. Allergy 55 (Suppl 63), 276. 2000. Abstract: 989

11. Gupta S, Banfield C, Kantesaria B, Marino M, Clement R, Affrime M, Batra V (2001) Pharmacokinetic and safety profile of desloratadine and fexofenadine when coadministered with azithromycin: a randomized, placebo-controlled, parallel-group study. Clin Ther 23: 451–466.

12. Hadley JA (1999) Evaluation and management of allergic rhinitis. Med Clin North Am 83: 13–25.

13. Henz BM (2001) The pharmacological profile of desloratadine: a review. Allergy 56: 7–13.

14. Kreutner W, Hey JA, Anthes J, Barnett A, Young S, Tozzi S (2000) Preclinical pharmacology of desloratadine, a selective and nonsedating histamine H_1 receptor antagonist: 1st communication: Receptor selectivity, antihistaminic activity, and antiallergic effects. Arzneimittelforschung 50: 345–352.

15. Meltzer E, Prenner B, Nayak A, Desloratadine Study Group (2001) Efficacy and safety of once-daily 5 mg desloratadine, a potent histamine H_1-receptor antagonist, in patients with seasonal allergic rhinitis. Assessment during the spring and fall allergy seasons. Clin Drug Invest 21: 25–32.

16. Nayak, A., Salmun, L. M., and Lorber, R. R. Desloratadine relieves nasal congestion in patients with seasonal allergic rhinitis. Allergy 55 (Suppl 63), 193–194. 2000. Abstract: 686

17. Padhi, D., Banfield, C., Gupta, S., Herron, J. M., and Affrime, M. B. Multiple-dose pharmacokinetics, safety, and tolerance of desloratadine in healthy volunteers. Journal of Allergy and Clinical Immunology 104(1 Pt 2), S385. 2000. Abstract: 1124

18. Rachelefsky GS (1999) National guidelines needed to manage rhinitis and prevent complications. Ann Allergy Asthma Immunol 82: 296–305.

19. Ring J, Hein R, Gauger A, Bronsky E, Miller B, The Desloratadine Study Group (2001) Once-daily desloratadine improves the signs and symptoms of chronic idiopathic urticaria: a randomized, double-blind, placebo-controlled study. Int J Dermatol 40: 1–5.

20. Settipane RA (1999) Complications of allergic rhinitis. Allergy Asthma Proc 20: 209–213.

33 Novel Concepts on Allergic Rhinitis: From Pathogenesis to Treatment

R. Pawankar, S. Yamagishi, R. Takizawa, C. Ozu, T. Yagi

Abstract

Atopic diseases like allergic rhinitis, atopic asthma, and atopic dermatitis are prevalent and on the rise. The need to understand the pathogenesis better is central to the development of newer therapeutic strategies. Conventional knowledge tells us that mast cells are only important in the immediate phase allergic reaction and that T cells orchestrate the late phase allergic reaction. Yet, in recent years, much evidence has accumulated on the versatile role of mast cells in allergic inflammation. Here, we describe the novel roles of mast cells and T cells in allergic inflammation. Like T cells, mast cells in the allergic nasal mucosa are a profound source of Th2 type cytokines and can induce IgE synthesis. Mast cells can also enhance self activation in an autocrine manner via the IL-4 and IgE-induced upregulation of the high affinity IgE receptor (FcεRI) and interaction with the extracellular matrix proteins. Mast cells are also capable of modulating the function of other cells, like epithelial cells. Hence, it is increasingly evident that mast cells contribute to various arms of allergic inflammation. Of the T cells, those of the γδ phenotype are increased at sites of allergic inflammation, and potentially play a role at various steps of the allergic inflammation. Thus mast cells and γδ T cells may play crucial roles as both effector and immunoregulatory cells in perpetuating allergic inflammation.

The strategy of management of allergic rhinitis includes optimal allergen avoidance followed by pharmacotherapy or immunotherapy. This is complemented with patient education, and surgery in selected cases. However, a significant proportion of patients with rhinitis also have associated asthma or minimal persistent inflammation in the lower airways. Since the IgE-IgE receptor network, a central component of the allergic inflammation, novel therapies like the humanized Anti-IgE monoclonal antibodies which target this component of the allergic inflammation may play an important role in the treatment of allergic diseases.

Introduction

Allergic rhinitis is an IgE-mediated allergic inflammation of the nose occurring due to the interaction of allergen with IgE and resulting in the release of a variety of mediators that induce the typical symptoms of rhinorrhea, sneezing, itching and nasal blockage. It is a global health problem affecting approximately 10 to 50% of the population world-wide, altering the quality of life of patients, affecting school learning performance, and work productivity.

New Trends in Allergy V
J. Ring, H. Behrendt (Eds.)
© Springer-Verlag Berlin, Heidelberg 2002

The chain of events that lead to an allergic reaction includes recognition of the allergen by the APC, antigen presentation to T cells, activation of T cells resulting in the production and release of cytokines like IL-4 and IL-13, class switch of IgM+ B cells to IgE+ plasma cells, the production of IgE, binding of IgE to the high affinity IgE receptor (FcεRI) on the surface of mast cells, and the cross linking of the bound IgE-FcεRI complex with multivalent allergen on subsequent exposure to the allergen, resulting in the release of inflammatory mediators like histamine, leukotrienes and prostaglandins. Yet, the allergic reaction comprises of two phases, the immediate phase and the late phase allergic reaction. Mast cells are known to play an important role in the immediate phase of the allergic reaction. On the other hand, T cells, eosinophils and basophils are considered to play important roles in the late phase of the allergic reaction. Yet, the question is what exactly do these cells do to perpetuate the allergic inflammation, and in situations where their functions overlap what is the relative contribution of each cell type to allergic inflammatory responses. Recent knowledge on the pathophysiological mechanisms underlying allergic rhinitis has led to a better understanding of the disease process itself as well as to the development of newer therapeutic strategies.

The purpose of this review is to discuss the pathogenesis of allergic rhinitis in the light of the novel roles of effector cells like mast cells and T cells in allergic inflammation, thereby bringing a link between the biology of these cells and their relative significance in clinical disease.

Clinically, perennial allergic rhinitis is characterized by repeated attacks of sneezing, runny nose (rhinorrhea) and blockage of the nose (nasal obstruction). These typical symptoms are observed throughout the year and the most common cause of PAR is the house dust mite. This disease is observed even in childhood and is more common in those with a family history of atopic disease. Clinically, these patients are diagnosed on the basis of the above mentioned typical symptoms, clinical findings of a pale, boggy nasal mucosa often with hypertrophy of the turbinates and watery nasal discharge, positive RAST, positive skin and nasal provocation tests, as well as nasal eosinophilia (by nasal smear examination).

The immediate phase allergic reaction occurs within several seconds to few minutes upon encounter with antigen and lasts for 2–3 h, as a result of crosslinking of the IgE receptor on the surface of mast cells by allergen and allergen specific IgE resulting in the release of chemical mediators like histamine, leukotreines and prostaglandin and is characterized by sneezing, rhinorrhea and nasal obstruction. It is conventionally believed that mast cells when activated via the high affinity IgE receptor react by undergoing several morphological changes including swelling of the cytoplasmic granules and subsequent solubilization of its granule contents. Histamine, tryptase, PGD_2 and LTC_4 are among the mast cell products that can be detected immediately after exposure to allergens [1, 2]. Histamine induces vasodilatation, increased vascular permeability and increased glandular secretion in the ipsilateral as well as contralateral sides through neural reflexes. Sneezing results from the action of histamine on H_1 receptors present on the sensory nerve endings of the trigeminal nerve. Of particular importance is the action of histamine on the subepithelial blood vessels, causing, vasodilatation, hyperaemia and mucosal edema. Prostaglandins like PGD_2 also cause edema by vasodilatation, and increased vascular permeability. These facts provide definite evidence that the mast cell is the central cell involved in the type I allergic reaction.

By contrast, the late phase allergic reaction occurs after several hours (4–6 h) with a recurrence of symptoms and lasts for about 24 h. Several in vivo studies have shown that the late phase allergic reaction occurs as a result of cytokines released from T lymphocytes which induce the upregulation of adhesion molecules like VCAM-1 and ICAM-1 on endothelial cells, resulting in the infiltration of eosinophils, basophils and T cells and the subsequent release of a number of soluble products like prostaglandins, leukotrienes, PAF, ECP, MBP and so on [3–5]. The physiological effects of the newly synthesized leukotrienes like LTC_4, LTD_4 and LTE_4 are mediated by increasing vascular permeability, vasodilatation and inducing mucous secretion. Moreover, studies on the levels of mediators like histamine, PGD2 and tryptase in nasal lavage fluid after allergen challenge have implicated that basophils but not mast cells are the main histamine containing cells involved in the late phase (based on results that the levels of histamine but not PGD2 increased in LPR, since only mast cells but not basophils contain PGD2) [4–5]. Yet, recent studies have implicated that mast cells are also an important source of Th2 type cytokines and that mast cells may play more important and as yet unknown roles in allergic inflammation [6–9].

Results and Discussion

Mast cells are known to play a central role in the immediate phase allergic reaction through the allergen and IgE-dependent release of a variety of inflammatory mediators. In humans, mast cells in can be divided into phenotypically distinct subpopulations based on the neutral proteases they express, namely $MC_{(T)}$ mast cells that express only tryptase, and the $MC_{(TC)}$ mast cells that express chymase, cathepsin G, carboxypeptidase and tryptase [10]. In allergic rhinitics, an increase in the number of $MC_{(T)}$ mast cells in the nasal epithelium has been well documented [11]. Recent studies have shown that the mast cell is an important source of a variety of cytokines. Thus the mast cell cannot be simplistically assigned a role in the immediate phase allergic response and recent studies suggest a more versatile role for the mast cell in regulating on-going allergic inflammation.

Characteristics of Mast Cells in Allergic Inflammation

Cytokines

Mast cells can synthesis and release a variety of cytokines via IgE-dependent mechanisms [6–9, 12]. In humans, mast cells are a potential source of IL-4, IL-5, IL-6, IL-7, IL-8, IL-10, IL-13, TNF-α, and basic fibroblast growth factor [13, 14]. Bradding et al. first reported the expression of IL-4, IL-5, IL-6 in bronchial mast cells of atopic asthmatics and it is well known now that bronchial and nasal mast cells from atopic asthmatics and allergic rhinitics are an important source of Th2 type cytokines IL-4, IL-5, IL-6, and IL-13 [6–9]. In fact, nasal mast cells from patients with perennial allergic rhinitis to house dust mite can release the protein of IL-4, IL-6 and IL-13 when stimulated by mite antigen [9, 15].

IgE Synthesis

Recent studies have shown that not only T cells but also mast cells can induce IgE synthesis in B cells [9, 16]. In fact, nasal mast cells from PAR patients not only released sufficient amounts of IL-4 or IL-13 on stimulation with specific mite antigen, but also expressed the CD40L and induced IgE synthesis in B cells [9]. Interestingly, the nasal mast cell-induced IgE synthesis was more IL-13 dependent [9] bringing us to our earlier observations of a strong correlation between the levels of IL-13 expression in the nasal mucosa of PAR patients and the levels of serum IgE [7]. Again, while it is well known that allergen activated Th2 cells can produce IL-4 / IL-13 and induce IgE synthesis in B cells, the findings that mast cells can induce IgE synthesis led us to investigate the possibility of local IgE synthesis. We demonstrated that nasal mast cells in PAR patients produced higher levels of IL-4 and IL-13 than T cells and that IgE was synthesized locally in the nasal mucosa [17]. Similar observations have been reported after in patients with seasonal allergic rhinitis [18].

Cell–Cell Interactions

Lymphocytes and mast cells in the tissues are surrounded by other cells like fibroblasts and mucosal cells as well as extracellular matrix (ECM) proteins (e.g. collagen, fibronectin and laminin). Therefore, the interaction of these inflammatory cells with fibroblasts and ECM may be important in the perpetuation of chronic inflammation. Recently, we demonstrated an upregulation of the expression of VLA-4 and VLA-5 in nasal mast cells from PAR patients, and that IgE-mediated activation of mast cells induced the release of greater levels of IL-4, IL-13 and TNF-α when cultured on fibronectin [19]. Thus mast cell-ECM interactions may contribute to the enhancement of mast cell activation especially when the levels of IgE and Ag in the microenvironment are rather low. This in fact may explain in part the phenomenon of hypersensitivity seen in patients with allergic rhinitis.

In addition, mast cell activation may directly or indirectly promote the release of cytokines from other resident cells in the respiratory tract, such as epithelial cells, endothelial cells, fibroblasts, and nerves. In fact, cytokines released in these responses then contribute to the vascular and epithelial changes and to the angiogenesis. Our most recent studies show that mast cell mediators like histamine and tryptase can upregulate the production of RANTES and GM-CSF in cultured nasal epithelial cells (CNEC) whereas IL-4 and IL-13 in co-operation with TNF-α can upregulate the production of Eotaxin and TARC.

Update on the Roles of Mast Cells in IgE-Mediated Allergy

Immediate Phase Response

It is conventionally believed that mast cells when activated via the high affinity IgE receptor react by undergoing several morphological changes including swelling of the cytoplasmic granules and subsequent solubilization of its granule contents. Histamine, tryptase, PGD_2 and LTC_4 are among the mast cell products that can be detected immediately after exposure to allergens. Histamine induces vasodilatation, increased vascular permeability and increased glandular secretion in the ipsilateral as well as contralateral sides through neural reflexes. Prostaglandins like PGD_2 also cause edema by vasodilatation, and increased vascular permeability.

Late Phase Response

The late phase allergic reaction occurs as a result of the infiltration of a variety of inflammatory cells like eosinophils, basophils and T cells and the subsequent release of a number of soluble products like prostaglandins, leukotrienes, PAF, ECP, MBP and so on. Tissue eosinophilia is an important aspect of the late phase allergic reaction. Mast cells can orchestrate the late phase reaction by inducing the infiltration of eosinophils not only through the upregulation of VCAM-1 (TNF-α, IL-4, IL-13) on endothelial cells but also through release of eosinophil-chemotactic factors like platelet activating factor and Leukotriene B4. In addition, mast cells can also enhance eosinophil survival through the release of granulocyte-macrophage colony-stimulating factor and IL-5. Interestingly, strong correlations were reported to exist between the numbers of IL-4+, IL-5+ and TNF-α+ mast cells and the number of tissue eosinophils in atopic asthma and allergic rhinitis [6] These recruited eosinophils (also basophils and T cells) then promote the further progression of the inflammatory response by providing additional sources of certain cytokines [that can also be produced by mast cells stimulated by ongoing exposure to allergen), as well as new sources of cytokines and other mediators that may not be produced by mast cells. In fact, time-kinetics of cytokine secretion from purified lung or nasal mast cells from PAR patients have shown that upon IgE-mediated stimulation induces the secretion of IL-13, TNF-α and IL-4 as early as from 2–6 h and peaked at 24–48 h [20, 21] Again, TNF-α is constitutively expressed in mast cells and can be released within 2 h of IgE-mediated stimulation. In fact, Klien et al. [22] have shown that activation of mast cell products in fragments of human skin in vitro, resulted in the upregulation of E-selectin expression in adjacent vascular endothelial cells and this was attributed to the release of TNF-α. Moreover, interaction of mast cells with extracellular matrix further enhances the IgE-mediated cytokine release from mast cells [19]. Mast cells can contribute to the eosinophil/T cell infiltration in the late phase allergic reaction through the histamine-induced upregulation of Eotaxin, RANTES, and GM-CSF production from nasal epithelial cells [20]. Taken together, these studies strongly suggest that the mast cell is a key effector cell in the late phase reaction.

Chronic Allergic Inflammation

Under allergic inflammatory conditions, „primed" mast cells express high levels of the high affinity receptor for IgE and the ligand for the surface antigen CD40, involved in T-B cell interactions leading to immunoglobulin production, as well as Th2-type cytokines, IL-4 and IL-13 [9]. Mast cells also have the potential to function as antigen presenting cells with the ability to shift T cells into Th2 subtypes.

Characteristics and Roles of $\gamma\delta$ T Cells in Allergic Rhinitis

Phenotypic and Functional Characteristics

$\gamma\delta$ T cells are increased in the nasal mucosa of patients with allergic rhinitis (25–30% of the total CD3+ T cell population in the allergic nasal mucosa, but <than 5–10% in the normal nasal mucosa). Moreover, the phenotypes, proportion, and stages of activation of the nasal $\gamma\delta$ T cells differed from those of the peripheral blood [23]. In fact, the expanded population of nasal $\gamma\delta$ T cells in PAR patients comprised mainly of CD4$^+$ and CD4$^-$8$^-$ $\gamma\delta$ T cells with no parallel alteration of the respective $\gamma\delta$ T cell subsets in the peripheral blood of the same patients [30]. Moreover, these nasal $\gamma\delta$ T cells were Vγ1/Vδ1-Jδ1 TCR+ and expressed the CD45RO surface antigen (for memory T cells), whereas their counterparts in the peripheral blood were Vγ2/Vδ2 TCR+. More importantly, nasal (but not peripheral blood) $\gamma\delta$ T cells from mite allergic patients proliferated well in vitro, in response to the mite specific antigen (Der f II), but not to an unrelated antigen Cry j 1 (major allergen of Japanese cedar pollen) [24]. These findings strongly suggest that $\gamma\delta$ T cells in allergic rhinitics are organ specific, and are oligoclonally expanded under specific antigenic stimulation.

Yet, what exactly these cells do in the development or perpetuation of allergic inflammation remains to be elucidated. One possible role of these antigen specific $\gamma\delta$ T cells is that they may function as a constant source of Th2 type cytokines providing the necessary environment for the perpetuation of an allergic inflammation through the shift of T cells to Th2 type cells, upregulation of the FcϵRI in mast cells, and infiltration of basophils and eosinophils. Again, CD4+ nasal $\gamma\delta$ T cells can induce IgE synthesis in B cells in an MHC-restricted manner [24]. Although there are controversial reports on the capacity of $\gamma\delta$ T cells to induce IgE synthesis, recently, in OVA-sensitized mice, C. Zuany-Amorin demonstrated that $\gamma\delta$ T cells are essential for inducing IL-4-dependent IgE synthesis [25]. This is of importance since the level of IgE produced by interaction of the same numbers of $\alpha\beta$ T cells with B cells was relatively less. Furthermore, although mast cells can induced IgE production in B cells, the mast cell-induced IgE synthesis is MHC-unrestricted manner. These observations suggest important aspects of the allergic inflammation in that even though several cells may share similar functions each may have comparable importance depending on the stage of disease, the phase of reaction or their specific manner of action. Furthermore, since intraepithelial $\gamma\delta$ T cells are potent producers of Th2 type cytokines these cells may also be involved in regulating their differentiation of $\alpha\beta$ T cells into Th1 or

Th2 type cells early in the primary immune response. Also nasal CD3+4-8- γδ T cells were capable of inducing the proliferation of αβ T cells [26].

Novel Therapy of Allergic Rhinitis Targeting the IgE–IgE Receptor Network

The key to the treatment of allergic diseases like allergic rhinitis or asthma lies in the capacity of the specific treatment to reduce the severity of symptoms either by interfering with or modulating the allergic inflammatory cascade. Preference would always be given to therapeutic measures that can immuno-modulate the allergic inflammation. Over the years, much effort has been focussed on regulating IgE production. The knowledge that Th2 cells secrete IL-4 and IL-13, and are key regulators of IgE synthesis has led to the development of therapeutic measures, that can suppress the synthesis of these cytokines. Glucocorticoids and cyclosporine are known to inhibit cytokine production in many cell types. Again IL-4 antagonists, anti-CD23 antibodies can down regulate IgE synthesis. Immunotherapy has also been shown to be effective via its capacity to induce an immune deviation from Th2 to a Th1 cytokine profile thus suppressing IgE synthesis after continued use. Yet, in polysensitized patients, and in those who have both rhinitis and asthma, the identification of key cells and molecules involved in the initiation and maintenance of allergic inflammation is likely to become an important target in the treatment of allergic diseases.

The current evidence-based concept on the management of allergic rhinitis as suggested by the latest international consensus (ARIA document) includes a step wise approach based on a new classification of 'intermittant' and 'persistent' rhinitis. It comprises of optimal allergen avoidance followed by pharmacotherapy and immunotherapy and is complemented with patient education and surgery in selected cases [27]. However, a significant proportion of rhinitis patients have associated asthma or at least minimal persistent inflammation [28]. Although anti-IgE mAbs have always been used to trigger mediator release from basophils or mast cells, nonanaphylactogenic anti-human IgE Abs are now in clinical evaluation as a therapeutic agent hat can target a central component of the allergic disease as well as IgE. One type of this new mAb that is nonanaphylactogenic recognizes receptor-bound IgE and prevents the association of IgE with its receptor if immune complexes were formed between IgE and anti-IgE mAb [29] This can explain the phenomenon that addition of anti-IgE Ab to receptor-bound IgE resulted in a decrease of receptor-bound IgE, because IgE dissociating from the receptor was complexed, altering the thermodynamic balance of receptor-bound vs free IgE. Other properties are by neutralizing IgE, inhibiting IgE synthesis, and reducing the IgE receptor expression on mast cells/basophils.

Specific Humanized Monoclonal Antibodies Against IgE Used in Clinical Trials

Three biotech companies, namely Genentech, South San Francisco, CA, Novartis Pharma AG, Basel, Switzerland, and Tanox Biologicals Inc Houston, TX have been focussing on the development of anti-IgE therapy and monoclonal antibodies against human IgE have been raised (e.g. rhu-Mab-E25 and CGP 51901, respectively). However, only the former of these two anti-IgE mAbs is currently developed for the treatment of allergic rhinitis or asthma.

Efficacy and Side Effects

The administration of rhuE25 Mab reduced plasma IgE levels, down-regulated FceRI expression in basophils, and altered the skin test reactivity by reducing the sensitivity of mast cells / basophils to specific allergen in patients with perennial allergic rhinitis. Although one study mentioned no significant difference in the symptom scores between placebo and rhuE25 Mab treated groups, in patients with ragweed-induced allergic rhinitis [30], another double blind placebo controlled multi-centre (Phase II/III) study performed later clearly showed an improvement in symptoms like sneezing, itchy nose, runny nose and stuffiness of the nose and less use of rescue medication in the rhuE25 Mab treated group as compared to the placebo treated group [31]. No serious side effects except one case with mild asthma was reported [31]. No evidence of antibodies to rhuE25 Mab was detected in the patients serum. In another more recent randomized double-blind placebo controlled study in 317 patients with moderate to severe allergic asthma, More patients in the rhuE25 Mab treated group were able to discontinue the use of corticosteroids [32].

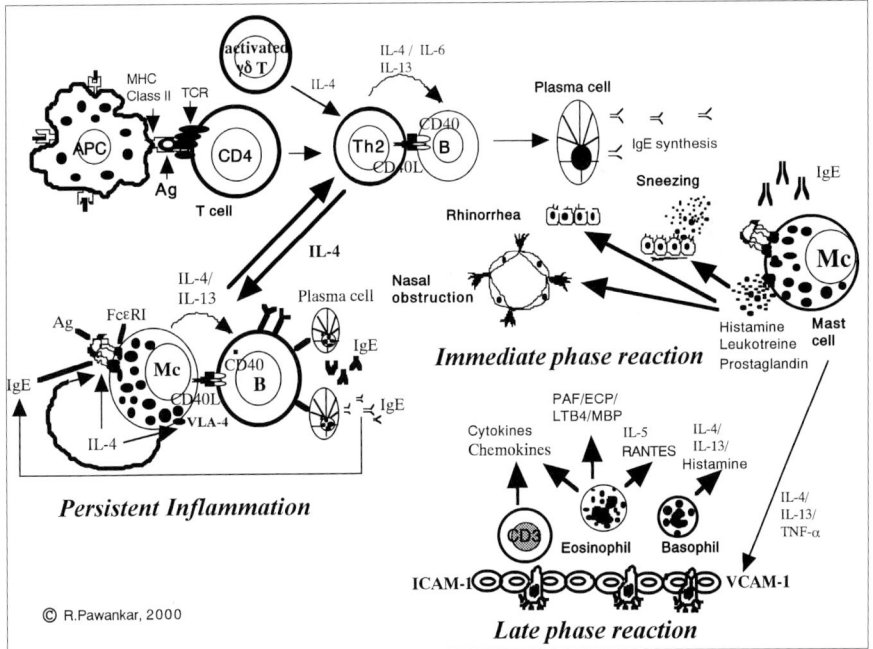

Fig. 1. Novel concepts on the pathogenesis of allergic rhinitis

Future of this Therapy

In many patients, drug treatment is insufficient to control symptoms and patient's satisfaction was shown to be poor [33]. Moreover, some patients experience side effects to treatment with drugs. Using the humanized non-anaphylactogenic Anti-IgE mAb in the treatment of allergic disease especially in patients who suffer from both rhinitis and asthma, may modulate allergic inflammation by inducing a decrease in the levels of serum free IgE. Anti-IgE therapy interferes with its binding to both high and low-affinity receptors, should inhibit on-going allergic inflammation, as well as reduce the early and late phase airway responses through inhibition of mast cell degranulation. Anti-IgE therapy may improve inflammatory reactions independently of the shock organ. Consequently, the allergen-IgE-mediated disease should be seen as a multi-organ disease [34, 35]. Such a therapy would therefore be specifically directed against a central component of the inflammatory response in contrast to currently available treatments. Furthermore, the potential use of combining anti-IgE therapy as an adjunct to other forms of existing therapies like immunotherapy (especially preceding rush immunotherapy) need to be assessed.

Thus, allergic rhinitis can be perceived as an on-going inflammation, with mast cells and T cells playing novel and versatile roles in the pathogenesis of allergic rhinitis (Fig. 1). Because of their favorable risk/benefit ratio, and their effect on on-going allergic inflammation in both the upper and lower airways, satisfactory pharmacological and clinical efficacy, the anti-IgE is emerging as an important therapy targeting a central component of allergic inflammatory response.

References

1. Proud D, Bailey G, Naclerio RM, et al. Tryptase and histamine as markers to evaluate mast cell activation during the responses to nasal challenge with allergen, cold dry air, and hyperosmolar solutions. J Allergy Clin Immunol 1992; 89: 1098–1110.
2. Castells M, Schwartz L. Tryptase levels in nasal lavage fluid as an indicator of immediate allergic response. J Allergy Clin Immunol 1988; 82: 348–55.
3. Naclerio RM, Proud D, Togias AG. Inflammatory mediators in late antigen induced rhinitis. N. Engl. J. Med. 1985; 313: 65–70.
4. Naclerio RM, Meier HL, Kagey-Sobotka A, et al. Mediator release after nasal airway challenge with allergen. Am. Rev. Resp. Dis. 1983; 128: 597–602.
5. Bascom R, Pipkorn U, Lichtenstein L, Naclerio R. the influx of inflammatory cells into nasal washings during the last response to antigen challenge. Effect of systemic steroid pretreatment. Am Rev Resp Dis 1988; 138: 405–412.
6. Bradding P, Feather IH, Wilson S, et al. Immunolocalization of cytokines in the nasal mucosa of normal and perennial rhinitic subjects. J. Immunol. 1993; 151: 3853–3865.
7. Pawankar R, Okuda M, Hasegawa S, et al. Interleukin-13 expression in the nasal mucosa of perennial allergic rhintics. Am. J. Resp. Crit. Care Med. 1995; 152: 2059–67.
8. Pawankar R, and Ra C. Heterogeneity of mast cells and T cells in the nasal mucosa. J. Allergy Clin. Immunol. 1996; 98 : 249–62.
9. Pawankar R, Okuda M, Yssel H, Okumura K, Ra C. Nasal mast cells in perennial allergic rhiniics exhibit increased expression of the FcεRI, CD40L, IL-4 and IL-13, and can induce IgE synthesis in B cells. J. Clin Invest 1997; 99 : 1492–9.
10. Irani AMA, Schecter NM, Craig SS, DeBlois G, and Schwartz LB. Two types of human mast cells that have distinct neutral protease compositions. Proc. Natl .Acad. Sci.. USA. 1986; 83 : 4464–4469.

11. Enerback L, Pipkorn U, Olofsson A. Intraepithelial migration of mucosal mast cells in hay fever. Int. Arch. Allergy Appl. Immunol 1986; 80 : 44–51.

12. Bradding P, Feather IH, Wilson S, et al. Immunolocalization of cytokines in the nasal mucosa of normal and perennial rhinitic subjects. J. Immunol 1993 ; 151: 3853–3865.

13. Gordon JR, Burd PR, Galli SJ. Mast cells as a source of multifunctional cytokines. Immunol. Today 1990; 11: 458–464.

14. Costa JJ, Church MK, Galli SJ. Mast cell cytokines in allergic inflammation. In: Holgate ST, Busse W, eds. Inflammatory Mechanisms in Asthma. New York, NY: Marcel Dekker Inc; 1997; pp 111–127.

15. Pawankar R, and Ra C. IgE-IgE receptor mast cells axis in allergy. Clin. Exp. Allergy 1998; 28: 6–11.

16. Gauchet JF, Henchoz S, Mazzei G, Aubry JP, Brunner T, Blasey H, Life H, Talabot T, Flores-Romo L, Thompson J, Kishi K, Butterfield J, Dahiden C, Bonnefoy J-F. Induction of human IgE synthesis in B cells by mast cells and basophils. Nature 1993; 365: 340–343

17. Pawankar R, Yamagishi S, Yagi T. Revisiting the roles of mast cells in allergic rhinitis and its relation to local IgE synthesis. Am J Rhinol 2000; 14: 309–317.

18. Durham SR. Gould HJ. Thienes CP, et al. Expression of epsilon germ-line gene transcripts and mRNA for the epsilon heavy chain of IgE in nasal B cells and the effects of topical corticosteroid. European J. Immunol. 1997; 27 (11): 2899–906.

19. Pawankar R, Yamagishi S, Nipapan D, Yagita H, Ra C, Okumura K. Nasal mast cells in perennial allergic rhinitics express increased levels of b1 integrins. Arerugi (Japanese) 1999; 49: 134 (abstract)

20. Pawankar R, Yamagishi S, Takizawa R, et al. Roles of mast cells in the late phase allergic reaction. Arerugi (Japanese) 2000; 50 : 144 (abstract)

21. Kobayashi, H., Y. Okayama Y, T. Ishizuka, Pawankar R et al. Production of IL-13 by human lung mast cells in response to FceR crosslinkage. Clin Exp Allergy 1998; 28 (10) 1219–27.

22. Klien LM, Lavker RM, Mais WL, Murphy GF. Degranulation of human mast cells induces an endothelial antigen central to leukocyte adhesion. Proc. Natl. Acad Sci. USA. 1989; 86 : 8972–8976.

23. Pawankar R, Okuda M, Suzuki K, Okumura K, Ra C. Phenotypic and molecular characteristics of nasal mucosal gd T cells in allergic and infectious rhinitis. Amer J Resp Crit Care Med 1996; 153 : 1655–65.

24. Pawankar R, Okuda M, Azuma M, et al Characterization of nasal gamma delta T cells in perennial allergic rhinitis. J Allergy Clin Immunol. 1995; 95:190 (abstract).

25. Zuany-Amorin C, Ruffie C, Haile S, et al. Requirement for gd T cells in allergic airway inflammation. Science 1996; 280; 1265–67

26. Pawankar R. gd T cells in airway allergic diseases. Clin Exp Allergy 130 : 318–23, 2000.

27. WHO Position Paper. ARIA: Allergic Rhinitis and its Impact on Asthma. Bousquet J, Kalthaev N and van Cauwenberge P. edts. J Allergy Clin Immunol 2000 (in press)

28. Ciprandi G, Buscaglia S, Pesce G, et al. Minimal persistent inflammation is present at mucosal level in patients with asymptomatic rhinitis and mite allergy. J Allergy Clin Immunol 1995; 96:971–9.

29. Kolbinger F, Saldanha J, Hardman N, Mendig MM. Humanization of a mouse anti-human IgE antibody: a potential therapeutic for IgE-mediated allergies. Protein Eng 1993; 6: 971–80.

30. Casale TB, Bernstein LI, Busse WW et al. Use of anti-IgE humanized monoclonal antibody in ragweed-induced allergic rhinitis. J Allergy Clin Immunol 1997; 100: 110–21.

31. Casale T, Condemi J, Miller SD, Fick R, McAlary M, Taylor AF, Gupta N, Rohane PW. rhuMabE25 in the treatment of seasonal allergic rhinitis. Ann Allergy Asthma & Immunol 1999 (abstract).

32. Milgrom H, Fick RB, Su JQ, Reimann JD, Bush RK, Waltrous ML, Metzger WJ. Treatment of allergic asthma with monoclonal anti-IgE antibody. New Engl. J. Med 1999; 341 :1966–73

33. White P, Smith H, Baker N, Davis W, Frew A. Symptom control in patients with hay fever in UK general practice: how well are we doing and is there a need for allergen immunotherapy? Clin Exp Allergy 1998; 28: 266–70.

34. Bousquet J, Lockey R, Malling H. WHO Position Paper. Allergen Immunotherapy: Therapeutic Vaccines for allergic diseases. Allergy 1998; 53, suppl 54: 558–62

35. Vignola AM. Chanez P. Godard P. Bousquet J. Relationships between rhinitis and asthma. Allergy 1998; 53 (9): 833–9.

Immunotherapy

34 CpG Oligodeoxynucleotides and Their Potential Role in the Immunotherapy of Allergic Diseases

A.M. KRIEG

The incidence of asthma and allergic diseases has been steadily increasing over the past few decades in industrialized countries. The „hygiene hypothesis" provides one possible explanation for this increase. Briefly, it posits that improvements in hygiene and reduced infections during childhood years lead to incomplete maturation of the immune system, resulting in a default Th2-type of response to environmental allergens. This hypothesis is supported by a variety of epidemiologic studies, as reviewed recently [1–3]. An assumption of the hygiene hypothesis is that the Th1-inducing effect of many infections prevents the emergence of Th2 responses to allergen exposure. This hypothesis does not address the question of why Th1 responses are made to certain infections in the first place.

The fundamental question of how the immune system „decides" to make a Th1 or Th2 response to a particular infectious agent or antigen has been the subject of great interest in immunology. In recent years, there has been increasing evidence that activation of the innate immune system during the early response to the infectious agent determines the subsequent Th1 or Th2 pattern of the adaptive immune response. Innate immune cells such as macrophages, dendritic cells, neutrophils, and monocytes use pattern recognition receptors (PRRs) to determine the type of pathogen that is present. Evolution has selected for the immune system to induce different types of immune responses to different pathogens. For example, Th1-like responses need to be induced against intracellular pathogens such as viruses or intracellular bacteria. On the other hand, Th2-like responses are better optimized for defense against extracellular infections such as gram-negative bacteria. The immune system has evolved the ability to specifically detect gram-negative bacteria using the toll-like receptor, TLR-4 [4]. Since endotoxins are not present on other types of organisms nor on host cells, activation of the TLR-4 receptor would indicate to the immune system that a gramnegative bacterium had breached the body's primary defenses, such as the skin or mucous membranes. This would then presumably trigger a predominantly Th2-like response to the associated antigens.

Recent studies have identified a molecular pattern that may be used by the immune system to identify intracellular pathogens. This molecular pattern, CpG DNA, is based on a subtle but important difference between vertebrate and microbial DNA. „CpG" refers to a cytosine followed by guanine and linked by a phosphodiester bond that forms the backbone of DNA. In vertebrate DNA, it has long been known that this base combination occurs less frequently than would be predicted if base usage was random, with only about one quarter of the expected CpG dinucleotides [5]. Furthermore, approximately 80% of the CpG di-

New Trends in Allergy V
J. Ring, H. Behrendt (Eds.)
© Springer-Verlag Berlin, Heidelberg 2002

nucleotides that are present in vertebrate genomes are methylated. Since prokaryotes typically do not methylate their CpGs, this creates a structural difference that could indicate to the immune system the presence of foreign nucleic acids. Indeed, B cells, natural killer cells, and dendritic cells are strongly and specifically activated by unmethylated CpG dinucleotides in particular base contexts („CpG motifs") [6]. CpG motifs induce these immune cells to synthesize large amounts of cytokines, especially Th1-like cytokines such as IL-12 and IFN-γ [7,8]. A recent exciting advance in our understanding of the molecular mechanism through which immune cells detect CpG DNA has come with a demonstration that another member of the TLR family, TLR-9, is essential for immune activation by synthetic oligodeoxynucleotides (ODN) containing CpG motifs [9].

If immune recognition of CpG motifs is an effective defense, then it may be expected that pathogens would evolve ways to avoid triggering this. Indeed, the genomic DNA of all small DNA viruses and retroviruses is severely CpG suppressed, with only 6–20% of the CpG dinucleotides that would be expected if base utilization was actually random [10, 11]. Immune recognition of CpG DNA appears to have evolved most particularly as a defense against intracellular pathogens, as suggested by several lines of evidence. First, cellular uptake of the DNA is required, since conjugation of the DNA to a solid support that prevents uptake eliminates the immune activation [6, 12]. Second, lipofection of ODN into cells enhances their immune stimulatory effect [13]. Finally, endosomal maturation and/or acidification is required for immune activation by CpG DNA since this is completely blocked by inhibitors such as chloroquine [14–16]. These studies suggest the unifying hypothesis that immune detection of CpG DNA represents a signal to the immune system of the presence of intracellular pathogens. Since effective defense against pathogens requires strong Th1-like immune responses, evolution has linked CpG DNA to the induction of Th1 immune activation. In theory, CpG DNA could restore the missing Th1 stimuli in modern society as posited by the hygiene hypothesis. This model predicts utility of CpG DNA in the immunotherapy of Th2-mediated diseases such as allergy and asthma.

This hypothesis that CpG DNA could prevent the development of Th2 responses or even overcome established Th2 responses has been tested and confirmed in a series of mouse models. First, we tested the effect of CpG DNA in the immature immune system, where there is known to be a bias toward the development of Th2 responses upon antigen exposure. In the hygiene hypothesis, it is thought that this bias leads to the development of allergic responses to pollens and other allergens, unless there has been a counteracting Th1 stimulus, which is normally provided by infections in early life. To test whether CpG DNA could provide such a Th1 stimulus, mice were exposed to several different antigens in the presence or absence of CpG DNA during the first week of life [17, 18]. The results conclusively demonstrated that CpG induced a more mature Th1-type of antigen-specific response. In fact, even when neonatal mice were primed to have a Th2 response in the absence of CpG, addition of CpG DNA to the booster dose of the vaccine led to the production of some Th1-like IgG2a antibody [17]. In adult mice, administration of CpG ODN to the booster dose of a vaccine had a far more dramatic effect at overcoming the initial Th2 immune response, and inducing a strong Th1-like antibody profile [17]. Together, these studies in neonatal and adult mice show the ability of CpG ODN to prevent or reverse Th2-like immune responses. These data suggest the hypothesis that CpG DNA exposure would prevent the development of allergic disease. To test this hypothesis, mice were sensitized to schistosome eggs, which provide a very strong Th2-like stimulus, by intraperitoneal (IP) injection in the presence or absence of CpG DNA [19]. In mice that were sensitized to schistosome eggs without CpG, an inhalation challenge with schistosome egg antigen (SEA) caused an acute eosinophilic airways disease with markedly increased airway eosinophils, Th2-like cytokines in the airways, and indirect evidence of broncho-constriction [19]. However, if the mice were initially exposed to the schistosome eggs in the presence of CpG, they did not become sensitized and did not produce IgE against the allergen nor develop disease or airway release of Th2 cytokines upon SEA inhalation. More importantly, even if CpG was not administered until the time of SEA inhalation, CpG could still block the development of the eosinophilic airways disease [19]. This confirmed that CpG DNA could still have therapeutic activity even after sensitization to allergen. CpG immunotherapy in this model was associated with the development of an airway SEA-specific Th1-like immune response, but this did not appear to cause any pathologic effects.

The mechanism of action of CpG-induced immunotherapy in this mouse model was further investigated using mice that were genetically deficient in IL-12 and/or IFN-γ. Surprisingly, these studies demonstrated that neither cytokine was absolutely required for CpG immunotherapy. Even mice deficient in both IL-12 and IFN-γ could still be protected against the development of airways eosinophilia by CpG [20]. However, these cytokines did appear to contribute somewhat to the protective effects of CpG, since higher doses of CpG immunotherapy were required in Th1 cytokine-deficient mice.

Since these studies, several other groups have extended and confirmed the utility of CpG DNA in allergy immunotherapy. It has been effective in preventing sensitization of mice to ovalbumin, and could be administered through either the IP or mucosal routes [21]. Of note, a single dose of CpG DNA inhibited airway eosinophilia at least as effectively as 7 days of daily steroid injections [21]. Unlike CpG DNA, steroid therapy was not associated with the induction of a Th1-like immune response, demonstrating a difference in the mechanisms of action of these two agents.

The protective effect of CpG DNA against allergen sensitization has also been demonstrated in a ragweed allergy model [22]. In this model, the protective effect of CpG DNA was shown to last for 6 weeks after administration. This result confirms and extends previous reports demonstrating that the Th1-like effect of CpG is prolonged and can protect against infectious challenge for approximately 1 month [23]. Further studies have extended the protective effects of CpG DNA to models of cedar pollen and birch pollen allergies [24–26].

It remained to be demonstrated whether CpG DNA would still have a protective effect even after airway challenges with allergen. The first evidence that CpG could be effective in such a model was reported by Serebrisky et al., who sensitized mice to conalbumin IP, and then reinforced this with two airway challenges at 1-week intervals [27]. Mice that were given a CpG ODN 24 h after the first airway challenge had a reduced airway inflammatory response. In collaboration with

Joel Kline, we have been investigating the therapeutic effects of CpG in mice sensitized to ovalbumin who were given one or more airway challenges of ovalbumin prior to the initiation of CpG immunotherapy. In these experiments, CpG immunotherapy has been highly effective in reversing established airway hypereosinophila, especially if the CpG is given together with the allergen and if the immunotherapy is continued for several doses [20a].

Remarkably, this immunotherapy was effective whether given subcutaneously, intranasally, or orally. The effectiveness of CpG DNA as a mucosal adjuvant has become well established in recent years, with studies confirming its ability to induce Th1-like systemic and mucosal responses after intranasal, oral, or intrarectal immunization [28–33]. Oral administration of CpG ODN for immunotherapy of allergic humans may require formulation to protect the DNA against hydrolysis since the human stomach has a lower pH than that of the mouse.

Although mouse models provide encouraging support for the concept of CpG immunotherapy in humans, there is no substitute for actual human data. Although early studies suggested that human cells may not be specifically stimulated by CpG motifs [34], subsequent studies have clearly established that particular CpG motifs are highly effective at activating human cells, but that the optimal motifs differ from those that had previously been identified in mice [35–39]. Recent studies have demonstrated the efficacy of CpG DNA in enhancing antigen specific responses in non-human primates [40–42]. More than ten human clinical trials are currently underway in the fields of infectious disease, allergy, and cancer. Preliminary results from these trials indicate that CpG DNA is reasonably well tolerated in humans with little toxicity at doses that cause immune activation. Whether CpG DNA will live up to the exciting promise suggested by mouse experimental models will soon become clear.

Acknowledgements. I thank Vickie Akers for outstanding secretarial assistance. Financial support was provided through a Career Development Award from the Department of Veterans Affairs and grants from the National Institutes of Health, and the Coley Pharmaceutical Group.

References

1. Erb, K. J. 1999. Atopic disorders: a default pathway in the absence of infection? *Immunol. Today* 20:317–322.
2. Folkerts, G., G. Walzl, and P. J. Openshaw. 2000. Do common childhood infections 'teach' the immune system not to be allergic? *Immunol. Today* 21:118–120.
3. Illi, S., E. von Mutius, S. Lau, R. Bergmann, B. Niggemann, C. Sommerfeld, and U. Wahn. 2001. Early childhood infectious diseases and the development of asthma up to school age: a birth cohort study. *BMJ* 322:390–395.
4. Poltorak, A., X. He, I. Smirnova, M. Y. Liu, C. V. Huffel, X. Du, D. Birdwell, E. Alejos, M. Silva, C. Galanos, M. Freudenberg, P. Ricciardi-Castagnoli, B. Layton, and B. Beutler. 1998. Defective LPS signaling in C3H/HeJ and C57BL/10ScCr mice: mutations in Tlr4 gene. *Science* 282:2085–2088.
5. Bird, A. P. 1987. CpG islands as gene markers in the vertebrate nucleus. *Trends in Genetics* 3:342–347.

6. Krieg, A. M., A. K. Yi, S. Matson, T. J. Waldschmidt, G. A. Bishop, R. Teasdale, G. A. Koretzky, and D. M. Klinman. 1995. CpG motifs in bacterial DNA trigger direct B-cell activation. *Nature* 374:546–549.

7. Klinman, D. M., A. K. Yi, S. L. Beaucage, J. Conover, and A. M. Krieg. 1996. CpG motifs present in bacteria DNA rapidly induce lymphocytes to secrete interleukin 6, interleukin 12, and interferon g. *Proc. Natl. Acad. Sci. U S. A* 93:2879–2883.

8. Jakob, T., P. S. Walker, A. M. Krieg, M. C. Udey, and J. C. Vogel. 1998. Activation of cutaneous dendritic cells by CpG-containing oligodeoxynucleotides: a role for dendritic cells in the augmentation of Th1 responses by immunostimulatory DNA. *J Immunol.* 161:3042–3049.

9. Hemmi, H., O. Takeuchi, T. Kawai, T. Kaisho, S. Sato, H. Sanjo, M. Matsumoto, K. Hoshino, H. Wagner, K. Takeda, and S. Akira. 2000. A Toll-like receptor recognizes bacterial DNA. *Nature* 408:740–745.

10. Shpaer, E. G. and J. I. Mullins. 1990. Selection against CpG dinucleotides in lentiviral genes: a possible role of methylation in regulation of viral expression. *Nucleic Acids Res.* 18:5793–5797.

11. Karlin, S., W. Doerfler, and L. R. Cardon. 1994. Why is CpG suppressed in the genomes of virtually all small eukaryotic viruses but not in those of large eukaryotic viruses? *J Virol.* 68:2889–2897.

12. Manzel, L. and D. E. MacFarlane. 1999. Lack of immune stimulation by immobilized CpG-oligodeoxynucleotide. *Antisense Nucleic Acid Drug Dev.* 9:459–464.

13. Yamamoto, T., S. Yamamoto, T. Kataoka, and T. Tokunaga. 1994. Lipofection of synthetic oligodeoxyribonucleotide having a palindromic sequence of AACWT to murine splenocytes enhances interferon production and natural killer activity. *Microbiol. Immunol.* 38:831–836.

14. Yi, A. K., R. Tuetken, T. Redford, M. Waldschmidt, J. Kirsch, and A. M. Krieg. 1998. CpG motifs in bacterial DNA activate leukocytes through the pH-dependent generation of reactive oxygen species. *J Immunol.* 160:4755–4761.

15. Macfarlane, D. E. and L. Manzel. 1998. Antagonism of immunostimulatory CpG-oligodioxynucleotides by quinacrine, chloroquine, and structurally related compounds. *J Immunol.* 160:1122–113

16. Hacker, H., H. Mischak, T. Miethke, S. Liptay, R. Schmid, T. Sparwasser, K. Heeg, G. B. Lipford, and H. Wagner. 1998. CpG-DNA-specific activation of antigen-presenting cells requires stress kinase activity and is preceded by non-specific endocytosis and endosomal maturation. *EMBO J* 17:6230–6240.

17. Kovarik, L, P. Bozzotti, L. Love-Homan, M. Pihlgren, H. L. Davis, P. H. Lambert, A. M. Krieg, and C. A. Siegrist. 1999. CpG oligodeoxynucleotides can circumvent the Th2 polarization of neonatal responses to vaccines but may fail to fully redirect Th2 responses established by neonatal priming. *J Immunol.* 162:1611–1617.

18. Brazolot Millan, C. L., R. Weeratna, A. M. Krieg, C. A. Siegrist, and H. L. Davis. 1998. CpG DNA can induce strong Th1 humoral and cell-mediated immune responses against hepatitis B surface antigen in young mice. *Proc. Natl. Acad. Sci. U. S. A* 95:15553–15558.

19. Kline, J. N., T. J. Waldschmidt, T. R. Businga, J. E. Lemish, J. V. Weinstock, P. S. Thorne, and A. M. Krieg. 1998. Modulation of airway inflammation by CpG oligodeoxynucleotides in a murine model of asthma. *J Immunol.* 160:2555–2559.

20. Kline, J. N., A. M. Krieg, T. J. Waldschmidt, Z. K. Ballas, V. Jain, and T. R. Businga. 1999. CpG oligodeoxynucleotides do not require TH I cytokines to prevent eosinophilic airway inflammation in a murine model of asthma. *J Allergy Clin. Immunol.* 104:12581264.

20a. Kline, J. N., Kitagaki, K., Businga T. R., and Jain V. V. 2002. Treatment of established asthma in a murine model using CpG oligodeoxynucleotides Am. J. Physiol. Lung Cell Mol. Physiol. 283:170–179

21. Broide, D., J. Schwarze, H. Tighe, T. Gifford, M. D. Nguyen, S. Malek, J. Van Uden, E. Martin-Orozco, E. W. Gelfand, and E. Raz. 1998. Immunostimulatory DNA sequences inhibit IL-5, eosinophilic inflammation, and airway hyperresponsiveness in mice. *J Immunol.* 161:7054–7062.

22. Sur, S., J. S. Wild, B. K. Choudhury, N. Sur, R. Alam, and D. M. Klinman. 1999. Long term prevention of allergic lung inflammation in a mouse model of asthma by CpG oligodeoxynucleotides. *J Immunol.* 162:6284–6293.

23. Krieg, A. M., L. Love-Homan, A. K. Yi, and J. T. Harty. 1998. CpG DNA induces sustained IL-12 expression in vivo and resistance to Listeria monocytogenes challenge. *J Immunol.* 161:2428–2434.
24. Kohama, Y., O. Akizuki, K. Hagihara, E. Yamada, and H. Yamamoto. 1999. Immunostimulatory oligodeoxynucleotide induces THI immune response and inhibition of IgE antibody production to cedar pollen allergens in mice. *J Allergy Clin. Immunol.* 104:1231–1238.
25. Hard, A., J. Kiesslich, R. Weiss, A. Bernhaupt, S. Mostbock, S. Scheiblhofer, C. Ebner, F. Ferreira, and J. Thalhamer. 1999. Immune responses after immunization with plasmid DNA encoding Bet v 1, the major allergen of birch pollen. *J Allergy Clin. Immunol.* 103:107–113.
26. Jahn-Schmid, B., U. Wiedermann, B. Bohle, A. Repa, D. Kraft, and C. Ebner. 1999. Oligodeoxynucleotides containing CpG motifs modulate the allergic TH2 response of BALB/c mice to Bet v 1, the major birch pollen allergen. *J Allergy Clin. Immunol.* 104:1015–1023.
27. Serebrisky, D., A. A. Teper, C. K. Huang, S. Y. Lee, T. F. Zhang, B. H. Schofield, M. Kattan, H. A. Sampson, and X. M. Li. 2000. CpG oligodeoxynucleotides can reverse Th2-associated allergic airway responses and alter the B7.1/B7.2 expression in a murine model of asthma. *J Immunol.* 165:5906–5912.
28. Moldoveanu, Z., L. Love-Homan, W. Q. Huang, and A. M. Krieg. 1998. CpG DNA, a novel immune enhancer for systemic and mucosal immunization with influenza virus. *Vaccine* 16:1216–1224.
29. Horner, A. A., A. Ronaghy, P. M. Cheng, M. D. Nguyen, H. J. Cho, D. Broide, and E. Raz. 1998. Immunostimulatory DNA is a potent mucosal adjuvant. *Cell Immunol.* 190:77–82.
30. McCluskie, M. J. and H. L. Davis. 2000. Oral, intrarectal and intranasal immunizations using CpG and non-CpG oligodeoxynucleotides as adjuvants. *Vaccine* 19:413–422.
31. McCluskie, M. J. and H. L. Davis. 1998. CpG DNA is a potent enhancer of systemic and mucosal immune responses against hepatitis B surface antigen with intranasal administration to mice. *J Immunol.* 161:4463–4466.
32. McCluskie, M. L, R. D. Weeratna, A. M. Krieg, and H. L. Davis. 2000. CpG DNA is an effective oral adjuvant to protein antigens in mice. *Vaccine* 19:950–957.
33. McCluskie, M. L, Weeratna, R. D., and Davis, H. L. Intranasal immunization of mice with CpG DNA induces strong systemic and mucosal responses that are influenced by other mucosal adjuvants and antigen distribution. Mol. Med. 2000.
34. Liang, H., Y. Nishioka, C. F. Reich, D. S. Pisetsky, and P. E. Lipsky. 1996. Activation of human B cells by phosphorothioate oligodeoxynucleotides. *J Clin. Invest* 98:1119–1129.
35. Hartmann, G. and A. M. Krieg. 1999. CpG DNA and LPS induce distinct patterns of activation in human monocytes. *Gene Ther.* 6:893–903.
36. Hartmann, G., G. J. Weiner, and A. M. Krieg. 1999. CpG DNA: a potent signal for growth, activation, and maturation of human dendritic cells. *Proc. Natl. Acad Sci. U.S.A* 96:9305–9310.
37. Hartmann, G. and A. M. Krieg. 2000. Mechanism and function of a newly identified CpG DNA motif in human primary B cells. *J Immunol.* 164:944–953.
38. Hartmann, G., R. D. Weeratna, Z. K. Ballas, P. Payette, S. Blackwell, I. Suparto, W. L. Rasmussen, M. Waldschmidt, D. Sajuthi, R. H. Purcell, H. L. Davis, and A. M. Krieg. 2000. Delineation of a CpG phosphorothioate oligodeoxynucleotide for activating primate immune responses in vitro and in vivo. *J Immunol.* 164:1617–1624.
39. Bohle, B., B. Jahn-Schmid, D. Maurer, D. Kraft, and C. Ebner. 1999. Oligodeoxynucleotides containing CpG motifs induce IL-12, IL-18 and IFN-g production in cells from allergic individuals and inhibit lgE synthesis in vitro. *Eur. J Immunol.* 29:2344–2353.
40. Jones, T. R., N. Obaldia, Ill, R. A. Gramzinski, Y. Charoenvit, N. Kolodny, S. Kitov, H. L. Davis, A. M. Krieg, and S. L. Hoffman. 1999. Synthetic oligodeoxynucleotides containing CpG motifs enhance immunogenicity of a peptide malaria vaccine in Aotus monkeys. *Vaccine* 17:3065–3071.
41. Gramzinski, R. A., C. L. Millan, N. Obaldia, S. L. Hoffman, and H. L. Davis. 1998. Immune response to a hepatitis B DNA vaccine in Aotus monkeys: a comparison of vaccine formulation, route, and method of administration. *Mol. Med.* 4:109–118.
42. Davis, H. L., I. I. Suparto, R. R. Weeratna, Jumintarto, D. D. Iskandriati, S. S. Chamzah, A. A. Ma'ruf, C. C. Nente, D. D. Pawitri, A. M. Krieg, Heriyanto, W. Smits, and D. D. Sajuthi. 2000. CpG DNA overcomes hyporesponsiveness to hepatitis B vaccine in orangutans. *Vaccine* 18:1920–1924

35 Allergen 3-D Structure-Based Design of Future Vaccines for Specific Allergy Vaccination

H. Løwenstein, H. Ipsen, M.D. Spangfort, J.N. Larsen

The history of specific allergy vaccination is long, and through all these years opinions and attitudes towards the treatment have been changeable. Likewise changeable has been the terms describing the treatment: allergen hyposentisisation, specific immunotherapy, specific allergy vaccination. The inconsistency is reflected also in the models concerning the underlying immunological mechanisms. Serum antibody analyses were performed as early as 1960, even before the discovery of IgE, searching for markers of successful therapy. Few years later the 'blocking IgG' hypothesis was forwarded [1] and for the following twenty years the immunological mechanism of successful immunotherapy was thought to include the induction of circulating allergen specific immunoglobulins capable of blocking the interaction between IgE and allergen. A disturbing problem, however, was the time delay of 4 to 6 months between the appearance of relatively high concentrations of allergen specific immunoglobulin, mainly of the IgG_4 type, and the clinical improvement of the patient.

In the eighties and nineties the scene was dominated by the theories of the rapidly growing field of immunology positioning the allergen specific T cells as a central player in the general regulation of immune responses. The introduction of the Th1/Th2 paradigm by Romagnani in 1991 [2] led to a very fruitful period during which the allergic immune response was characterised in detail and several cell types and interleukins were placed in a common framework. Combined with studies of the very early human immune response the model evolved that early in life every human has allergen specific T cells of both the Th1 and Th2 type. In early years the balance between Th1 and Th2 may shift towards Th1 leading to a protective immune response, or towards the Th2 type leading to the allergic immune response. Thus, if therapy was designed to address the allergen specific T cells it might be possible to influence the balance between Th1 and Th2 towards Th1 leading to a reduction in disease [3]. Denatured allergens [4] and more recently synthetic peptides [5–8] were thought to represent the optimal medicament, since being derived from the allergen they would act specifically while at the same having no spatial structure resembling the allergen they would not bind IgE and hence would not cause anaphylactic side reactions. Clinical trials, however, were not encouraging [9, 10].

One of the points that was raised arguing against the concept of using synthetic peptides or recombinant allergens for allergy vaccination was based on the vast complexity of allergen composition as well as of immune responses of individual patients. Detailed knowledge of allergen structure and function has evolved in parallel with the discovery of the allergic immune response. Accordingly no common structure has been identified that would enable distinguish-

New Trends in Allergy V
J. Ring, H. Behrendt (Eds.)
© Springer-Verlag Berlin, Heidelberg 2002

ing of an allergen simply by looking at proteins. Any protein is a potential allergen, and an allergen is defined by the immunological reactivity of allergic patients. Thus, if several patients are analysed a limited number of major allergens, to which a majority of the patients react, will be found as well as a large number of minor allergens, to which only a limited number of patients react. Analysing more patients it is found that the total number of allergens converge towards the total number of proteins in the allergen source. Further complexity is added by the phenomenon of isoallergenic variation. Most, if not all, allergens are heterogeneous mixtures of molecules having different amino acid sequences. The difference may be only one amino acid or it may approach 30% of the amino acids, thereby exceeding the difference between homologous allergens from different species [11]. Laboratory experiments have shown that even a single amino acid difference may be recognised by monoclonal antibodies or individual T cell clones. Thus, each individual allergic patient has her own individual reactivity pattern defined by the joint specificity profile of all individual allergen specific B and T cells.

Another argument that may explain the limited success of the peptide treatment is the ignoring of the significance of allergen specific IgG antibodies induced by successful allergy vaccination using conventional vaccines. The appearance of these antibodies is actually a good indication of a T helper cell shift towards the Th1 type. In theory, a shift towards Th1 may be brought about by a reduction in Th2 (induction of anergy), a shift from Th1 to Th2 (immune deviation), or by the recruitment of new Th1 cells. In carefully designed quantitative immuno-assays we have measured the concentration and affinity of allergen specific IgE antibodies before and after allergy vaccination treatment using conventional vaccines. In spite of the fact that patients improve clinically, there seems to be no difference in their IgE. In our interpretation this means that allergen specific IgG antibodies are important in the causal effect of allergy vaccination, and that the mechanism is likely to be based upon the recruitment of new cells of the Th1 type. This conclusion is supported by experiments performed by the Durham group [12], analysing interleukin production of cells in nasal and skin biopsies following allergen provocation. In these experiments there seems to be no reduction in cells producing interleukins characteristic of the Th2 type, whereas there is an increase in cells producing Th1 type interleukins as an effect of allergy vaccination.

If the induction of a new immune response of the Th1 type were indeed an important aspect of the causal effect of allergy vaccination, this would in addition provide an explanation for the time lag observed between the appearance of allergen specific IgG and the clinical improvement of the patient. We would like to propose that the relatively slow process of antibody affinity maturation cause the time lag. Initially, soon after commencement of treatment, a substantial increase in the concentration of allergen specific IgG is observed, however, since newly recruited B cells produce the IgG it is of low affinity. The IgE, on the other hand, though present in low concentration, is of high affinity since B cells influenced by allergen exposure for extended time periods produce it. Repeated injections cause increasing affinity of the allergen specific IgG by somatic mutation in the variable domains of the gene encoding the complementary determining regions (CDRs) of the antibody molecule. This process is known to take place in the so-called germinal centres. The capacity of the allergen specific IgG to compete for binding to the allergen is determined by the concentration multiplied by the average affinity, not solely by the concentration. Thus, it is essential that the vaccine contain B cell epitopes capable of inducing an allergen specific IgG response. A further indication of the significance of competing IgG antibodies is the negative regulation of FcεRI signalling by FcγRII co-stimulation observed in human blood basophils [13].

Recently we determined the first crystal structure of an important inhalant allergen, the major birch allergen, Bet v 1 [14]. The structure of Bet v 1 is formed by a seven-stranded β-sheet that wraps around a long carboxy-terminal α-helix. The structure is peculiar in that it has a large internal cavity with three openings on the molecular surface. Determination of the molecular structure unambiguously identifies which amino acids are located on the molecular surface accessible for antibody binding. Combining this information with a computer search of conserved amino acid residues comparing a total of 57 sequences representing homologous major allergens within the birch family, reveals patterns of conserved surface areas that are large enough to accommodate antibody binding. These conserved surface areas not only provide a molecular explanation for the clinically observed cross-reactivity of birch pollen allergic patients towards the related trees alder, hazel and hornbeam, they are also likely to constitute dominating IgE-binding epitopes. In Scandinavia, exposure to hazel occurs in January and February, exposure to alder in March and April, and exposure to birch in April and May. Thus, exposure to the conserved surface areas takes place over a period of four months each year. The topologies of other molecular surface areas are specific to the major allergens from individual species and thus, exposure to these structures is comparably lower. This means that based on antibody affinity maturation considerations, high affinity IgE is likely to be directed towards the conserved patches.

The concept of dominant IgE epitopes represented by conserved surface areas outlined above has important implications for the prospect of using recombinant allergens for allergy vaccination. Laboratory studies have shown that individual isoallergens and variants show differential reactivity with individual T cell clones derived from allergic patients and with individual monoclonal antibodies. However, if a majority of high affinity specificities in a polyclonal IgE antiserum is directed towards epitopes that are conserved, even among homologous allergens from different species, treatment based on recombinant vaccines may very well be feasible. At least with respect to IgE-binding the vast complexity literally collapses into a few shared epitopes. Experimental support for this assumption may be found in IgE-inhibition studies demonstrating that one homogenous recombinant allergen inhibit the binding of IgE to Bet v 1 almost 100%.

Another piece of experimental support for the dominant IgE-binding epitopes comes from the study of mutated recombinant allergens produced by site directed mutagenesis. We have produced a crystal structure of a Bet v 1-antibody complex [15]. In the crystal the antibody is represented by the Fab fragment of a murine monoclonal antibody cross-reactive between the homologous major allergens of the *Fagales*, alder, birch, hazel, and hornbeam. As expected, the antibody

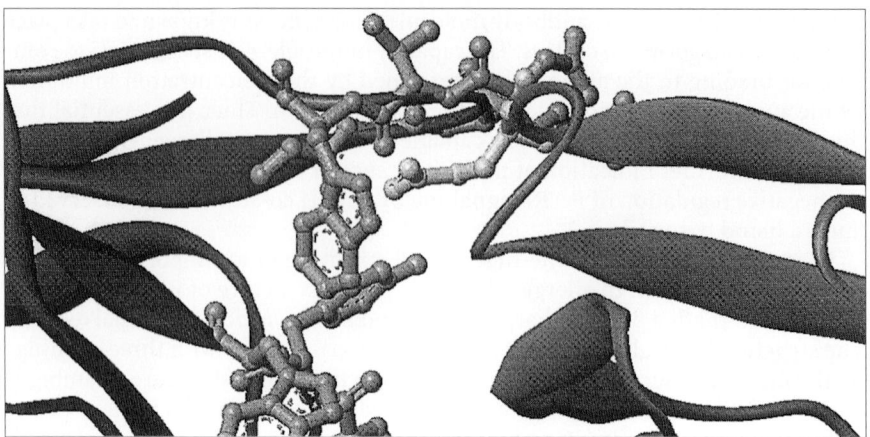

Fig. 1. Crystal structure of an antibody Fab-Bet v 1 complex. Near the centre of the epitope a long side chain of a glutamic acid amino acid residue stretches outwards from the molecular surface of the allergen (*right*) and fits into a pocket in the antibody-combining site (*left*)

occupies one of the conserved surface areas identified previously. Near the centre of the epitope a long side chain of a glutamic acid amino acid residue stretches outwards from the molecular surface of the allergen and fits into a pocket in the antibody-combining site (see Fig. 1). Substitution of this amino acid is likely to affect the binding of all antibodies having specificity for this conserved surface area. By site directed mutagenesis we substituted this glutamic acid-45 into serine, which only has a very short side chain. The substitution not only completely abolished binding of the monoclonal antibody, it also reduced the binding of serum IgE from birch pollen allergic individuals 20–50% when analysing different patients. When performing amino acid substitutions by site directed mutagenesis unpredictable alterations in the overall molecular structure often occur. To experimentally assess the effect of the mutation on the overall molecular structure we therefore crystallised the mutant. Comparing the crystal structures of the two molecules it was apparent that only local perturbations of the surface topology surrounding the mutation had occurred. The surface area of the Bet v 1 allergen is calculated from the crystal structure to be approximately 9000 $Å^2$. The surface area affected by the mutation covers less than 0.5% of the surface. The observation that such a minute alteration of the surface topology affects the binding of serum IgE by up to a factor of 2 supports the concept of dominant IgE binding epitopes.

The vast complexity of allergen molecules and responses of individual patients previously hampered the prospect of using recombinant allergens for specific allergy vaccination. Recent findings based on bio-molecular structure determination revealed the existence of conserved surface areas representing candidates for dominant IgE binding epitopes. The introduction of minute changes in surface topology by amino acid substitution in the conserved surface areas has a dramatic effect on IgE binding. The approach described may lead to safer and more efficient mutated recombinant vaccines for specific allergy treatment. An important aspect, however, is retaining of the overall structure of the molecular surface preserving the capacity to generate allergen specific IgG antibodies characteristic of successful intervention.

References

1. Lichtenstein LM, Holtzman NA, Burnett LS: A quantitative in vitro study of the chromatographic distribution and immunoglobulin characteristics of human blocking antibody. J Immunol 101: 317–324, 1968.
2. Romagnani S: Human TH1 and TH2 subsets: doubt no more. Immunol Today 12: 256–257, 1991.
3. Holt PG: Immunoregulation of the allergic reaction in the respiratory tract. Eur Respir J Suppl 22: 85s–89s, 1996.
4. Ishizaka K, Okudaira H, King TP: Immunogenic properties of modified antigen E. II. Ability of urea-denatured antigen and alpha-polypeptide chain to prime T cells specific for antigen E. J Immunol 114: 110–115, 1975.
5. Briner TJ, Kuo MC, Keating KM, Rogers BL, Greenstein JL: Peripheral T-cell tolerance induced in naive and primed mice by subcutaneous injection of peptides from the major cat allergen Fel d I. Proc Natl Acad Sci USA 90: 7608–7612, 1993.
6. Müller U, Akdis CA, Fricker M, Akdis M, Blesken T, Bettens F, Blaser K: Successful immunotherapy with T-cell epitope peptides of bee venom phospholipase A2 induces specific T-cell anergy in patients allergic to bee venom. J Allergy Clin Immunol 101: 747–754, 1998.
7. Haselden BM, Kay AB, Larche M: Immunoglobulin E-independent major histocompatibility complex-restricted T cell peptide epitope-induced late asthmatic reactions. J Exp Med 189: 1885–1894, 1999.
8. Haselden BM, Kay AB, Larche M: Peptide-mediated immune responses in specific immunotherapy. Int Arch Allergy Immunol 122: 229–237, 2000.
9. Norman PS, Ishizaka K, Lichtenstein LM, Adkinson NF Jr: Treatment of ragweed hay fever with urea-denatured antigen E. J Allergy Clin Immunol 66: 336–341, 1980.
10. Norman PS, Ohman JL Jr, Long AA, Creticos PS, Gefter MA, Shaked Z, Wood RA, Eggleston PA, Hafner KB, Rao P, Lichtenstein LM, Jones NH, Nicodemus CF: Treatment of cat allergy with T-cell reactive peptides. Am J Respir Crit Care Med 154: 1623–1628, 1996.
11. Larsen JN: Isoallergens – significance in allergen exposure and response. ACI News 7: 141–146, 1995.
12. Durham SR, Ying S, Varney VA, Jacobson MR, Sudderick RM, Mackay IS, Kay AB, Hamid QA: Grass pollen immunotherapy inhibits allergen-induced infiltration of CD4+ T lymphocytes and eosinophils in the nasal mucosa and increases the number of cells expressing messenger RNA for interferon-gamma. J Allergy Clin Immunol 97: 1356–1365, 1996.
13. Kepley CL, Cambier JC, Morel PA, Lujan D, Ortega E, Wilson BS, Oliver JM: Negative regulation of FceRI signaling by FcgRII costimulation in human blood basophils. J Allergy Clin Immunol 106: 337–348, 2000.
14. Gajhede M, Osmark P, Poulsen FM, Ipsen H, Larsen JN, van Neerven RJJ, Schou C, Løwenstein H, Spangfort MD: X-ray and NMR structure of Bet v 1, the origin of birch pollen allergy. Nature Structural Biology 3: 1040–1045, 1996.
15. Mirza O, Henriksen A, Ipsen H, Larsen JN, Wissenbach M, Spangfort MD, Gajhede M: Dominant epitopes and allergic cross-reactivity: complex formation between a Fab fragment of a monoclonal murine IgG antibody and the major allergen from birch pollen Bet v 1. J Immunol 165: 331–338, 2000.

36 Immunological Mechanisms of Anti-IgE Treatment

R.J.J. van Neerven, C.P.A.A. van Roomen, E.F. Knol

Summary

Non-anaphylactogenic anti-IgE mAb have been developed over the past decade to treat atopic allergies. These antibodies neutralize circulating IgE molecules, and thus prevent IgE from binding to its receptors, FcεRI and CD23. Efficacy of anti-IgE treatment has been shown in several clinical trials, and new, unanticipated, mechanisms by which anti-IgE exerts its clinical effect are being discovered. Here we summarize a number of studies on the immunological mechanisms underlying anti-IgE treatment.

Introduction

Type I allergy is now recognized as a disease that is at least in part based on immune deviation. Allergic patients respond strongly to innocuous proteins, to which they should be tolerant, as these proteins pose no threat. In allergic responses, an allergen enters the body, binds to allergen-specific IgE that in turn binds to the high affinity IgE receptor (FcεRI) present on mast cells and basophils. Upon receptor crosslinking, these cells release inflammatory mediators such as histamine, leukotrienes and prostaglandins, resulting in an immediate hypersensitivity reaction. By allergen avoidance, serum IgE levels can be decreased in allergic patients. Another, much more efficient, way of decreasing serum IgE levels is the promising new approach of treatment with non-anaphylactogenic anti-IgE antibodies.

Non-Anaphylactogenic Anti-IgE Antibodies: Clinical Experience

The rationale of anti-IgE treatment as a therapeutic approach is to neutralize circulating IgE, without binding to FcεRI already occupied by IgE. Two different anti-IgE mAb, rhuMAb E25 and CGP-51901, are currently being developed for the treatment of atopic allergies [1, 2]. Both mAb bind to the Cε3 domain of the IgE molecule and do not bind to IgE already bound to FcεRI and thus do not induce histamine release from IgE coated basophils or mast cells and are therefore termed 'non-anaphylactogenic'. Both antibodies have been chimerized (CGP 51901) or humanized (rhuMAb-E25, and Hu-901, the humanized version of CGP 51901) to prevent the occurrence of neutralizing anti-mouse antibody responses. To date, over 3,000 patients have been treated with these anti-IgE mAb. Anti-IgE treatment is very well tolerated [3, 4], and anti-IgE mAbs have been found not to be very antigenic; neutralizing antibodies have only been demonstrated in a single patient [3].

New Trends in Allergy V
J. Ring, H. Behrendt (Eds.)
© Springer-Verlag Berlin, Heidelberg 2002

Clinical results of the anti-IgE treatment have been promising. Anti-IgE has been administered intravenously, subcutaneously, and as an aerosol. Whereas aerosolized anti-IgE was not effective in neutralizing IgE levels [5], serum concentrations of free IgE drop dramatically within minutes after IV administration of the antibody [3, 6, 7]. Similarly, subcutaneous administration also reduces serum IgE levels [4, 8]. The half life of this neutralization of free serum IgE when given in adequate doses is in the range of several days, and when given repeatedly free serum IgE levels can be neutralized for prolonged periods of time. When total serum IgE levels were measured, increased levels were found because of circulating small IgE-anti-IgE complexes [7, 9].

As expected in a passive immunization, the serum IgE levels rise again after discontinuation of treatment [3, 10]. However, a remarkable finding after repeated administration of the anti-IgE antibody was that serum IgE levels did not reach pretreatment levels in a 90 day follow up study [6]. It has been suggested that this effect was due to selective removal of IgE-producing plasma cells, but this has not been proven.

In the first allergic rhinitis trial no clinical efficacy was shown because IgE levels were not reduced by more than 70% due to low dose treatment [4]. Another dose finding trial in allergic rhinitis patients demonstrated that when a 85% reduction in IgE levels was achieved, nasal symptoms were improved during the mountain cedar pollen season [11]. The most recent allergic rhinitis trial with anti-IgE demonstrated significant improvement in nasal and ocular symptom severity scores, as well as decreased anti-histamine usage [8].

In clinical trials of moderate to severe allergic asthma patients, treatment with anti-IgE resulted in increased allergen thresholds to induce immediate asthmatic reactions upon allergen challenge [7, 12]. In addition, a reduced fall in FEV-1 in early as well as late phase asthmatic reactions was noted in one study, accompanied by decreased numbers of eosinophils in induced sputum and peripheral blood [7]. Another study also demonstrated decreased airway hyperreactivity upon metacholine challenge [12]. However, no clear clinical effect and no decrease in SPT and bronchodilator use was reported in this study. A recent phase III study in allergic asthma patients showed that the administration of anti-IgE resulted in decreased disease severity scores, decreased corticosteroid use, as well as an increased quality of life [9].

All trials described here had a duration between 9 and 12 weeks. A 3-month treatment regime with anti-IgE mAb may not be sufficient to resolve the allergic inflammation which is more sustained in asthma patients, indicating that clinical efficacy may even be better upon extended treatment.

Regulation of FcεRI and CD23 by IgE Levels: Effects of Anti-IgE Treatment

FcεRI on Mast Cells and Basophils

It has been known for several decades that serum IgE levels and IgE receptor expression on mast cells and basophils are positively correlated [13]. Recently, it has become clear that IgE itself regulates the expression of FcεRI on basophils and mast cells [14–16] The supposed mechanism of this is through decreased FcεRI turnover after IgE binding. After IgE treatment free serum IgE levels are decreased by 90–99%.

This may, however, not completely explain the clinical effects seen as the resulting IgE levels could still be sufficient to saturate FcεRI in some of the patients. Together with the demonstration that anti-IgE treatment results in a drastically reduced allergen-induced basophil histamine release [6], this may suggest that FcεRI downregulation may be an important feature in achieving clinical efficacy. Indeed, it was demonstrated in several studies that anti-IgE downregulates the expression of FcεRI on basophils and mast cells [6, 17], and that expression levels are restored upon discontinuation of anti-IgE treatment [10]. This indicates that on the one hand IgE is prevented from binding to its receptor as a result of anti-IgE treatment, but on the other hand, IgE effector functions are also inhibited because of the downregulated expression of FcεRI.

Interestingly, IgE knock out mice still have a baseline expression of FcεRI (and CD23), indicating that IgE is not the sole regulator of FcεRI expression [15, 28]. The observed baseline FcεRI expression is likely to be under the control of cytokines [18]. Transcription levels of the α-chain in mast cells are increased by IL-4 [19], whereas the transcription of the γ-chain is enhanced by IFN-γ. The transcription factors GATA-1 and ELF-1 bind to enhancer elements in the FcεRIα-chain gene, and are thought to be involved in the upregulation of FcεRIα mRNA production [20]. No factors that modulate the expression of the β-chain have been published to date.

Monocytes and Dendritic Cells

In addition to expression on basophils and mast cells, expression of FcεRI on antigen presenting cells such as monocytes and dendritic cells has been demonstrated [21, 22]. The receptor complex exists of an αβγ2 complex on basophils/mast cells and as an αγ2 complex on APC [23]. The membrane expression of the IgE binding α-chain critically depends on the expression of the other chain(s).

Even though FcεRI expression on Langerhans cells is correlated to serum IgE concentration [24], a recent study demonstrated that IgE did not increase FcεRI expression of antigen-presenting cells [25]. In another study however, the presence of IgE was shown to inhibit the disappearance of FcεRI from monocytes upon overnight culture [26]. So far, the only other factor that has been shown to regulate FcεRI expression in APC is IL-4, that was shown to increase the intracellular, but not cell surface, expression of the FcεRI α-chain [27]. In contrast to humans, rodents display no FcεRI on antigen-presenting cells, possibly explaining some differences between animal models and the situation in humans.

In addition to cytokines and CD40 signaling, the expression of the low affinity receptor for IgE, CD23, is regulated by IgE levels [28]. Moreover, in mice that had been treated with anti-IgE mAb, CD23 expression was downregulated [29]. These studies all suggest that anti-IgE treatment of humans may also affect the expression of CD23 on activated B cells and FcεRI on monocytes/dendritic cells.

IgE-Mediated Presentation of Allergens to CD4+ T Cells: Inhibition by Anti-IgE mAb

T lymphocytes have been shown to be key players in the induction of both the immediate allergic response and the late phase reaction. Allergen-specific T cells of allergic patients, but not control donors, display a Th2-like pattern of cytokine production upon activation. This Th2-like cytokine production profile includes cytokines such as IL-4, and IL-5, cytokines that play an important role in the induction of class switching of B lymphocytes towards the production of IgE, and differentiation and survival of eosinophilic granulocytes, respectively [30, 31].

In addition to type 2 dominated immune responses to allergens, atopic allergic patients have been shown to have an increased expression of FcεRI on monocytes and dendritic cells [21–23], and of CD23 on B cells and macrophages [32]. The expression of these IgE Fc receptors on APC suggests that they may play a functional role in the presentation of allergens to specific T cells, and possibly in the activation of these APC as well. Indeed, both IgE receptors have been shown to facilitate the presentation of allergens in the presence of specific serum-IgE, resulting in T-cell activation at 100–1,000 fold lower allergen concentrations than which are required when control sera are used [33–35]. Similarly, the occurrence of a positive atopy patch test after epicutaneous application of allergens in atopic dermatitis patients correlates with the presence of IgE-coated Langerhans cells, suggesting that also in this model IgE mediated allergen presentation occurs [36].

As the cumulative exposure to major allergens is in the range of several µg/year this is a crucial step in the activation and persistence of allergen-specific Th2-like cells (illustrated in Fig. 1).

As discussed above, results from clinical trials with neutralizing anti-IgE mAb rhuMAb-E25 have shown that anti-IgE mAb treatment not only has an effect on early phase allergic responses, but also inhibits bronchial late phase responses and the number of eosinophils in sputum of allergic asthma patients [7]. These data strongly suggest that IgE is important for the development of late phase responses, either directly via an effect on T-cell activation or indirectly via an effect on the influx of effector cells. As late phase reactions are mainly T-cell dependent [37, 38], these data indicate that anti-IgE treatment may also inhibit T-cell activation in vivo. Serum IgE-facilitated allergen presentation (S-FAP) can be inhibited by polyclonal anti-IgE antibodies [34], and by allergen-specific IgG molecules induced by specific allergy vaccination [39]. It is therefore very likely that anti-IgE treatment has a similar effect.

Recently we have shown that the activation of a T cell line reacting to Der p 1, the major allergen of Dermatophagoides pteronyssinus, is about 100-fold more efficient in the presence of house dust mite-specific IgE. Preincubation of the mite-specific IgE with anti–IgE mAb Hu-901, a humanized version of CGP 51901, completely inhibited IgE-facilitated antigen presentation to Der p 1-specific T cells [40], preventing their proliferation as well as cytokine production. Hu-901 prevented the binding of IgE-allergen complexes to CD23 on the membrane of the EBV-B cells used as antigen presenting cells. This finding would indicate that anti-IgE mAb treatment inhibits Th2-activation at physiologically relevant allergen exposure, thus explaining its effects on late phase reactions. A prolonged pre-

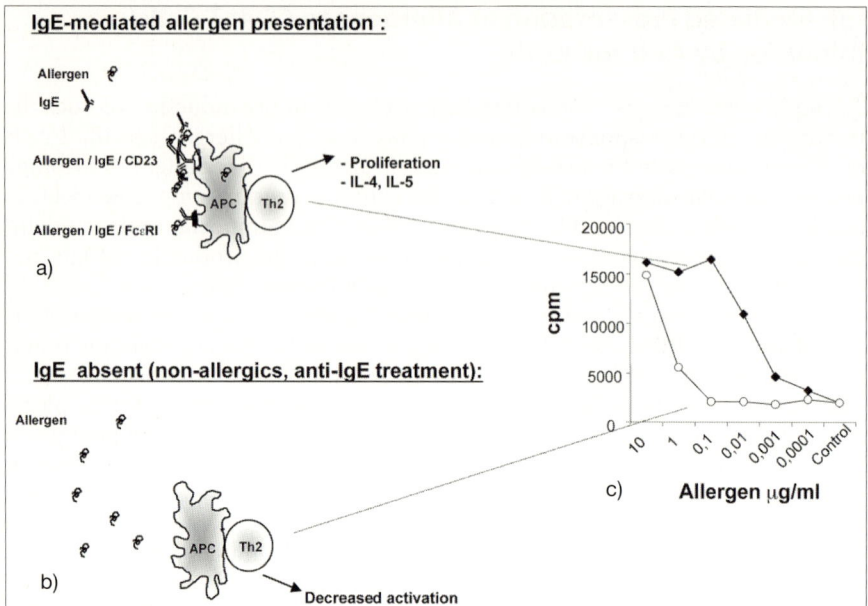

Fig. 1a–c. IgE-mediated allergen presentation. An allergen that enters the body is bound by IgE. Allergen-IgE complexes bind to CD23 or FcεRI on antigen presenting cells, and specific-T cells are activated at low allergen doses (**a**). If no free IgE molecules are present much higher allergen doses are required to activate allergen-specific T cells because the allergen is not targeted to the antigen presenting cell (**b**). The resulting proliferative T-cell responses from an actual experiment for the presence of IgE (*closed lozenges*) or absence of IgE (*open circles*) are shown in (**c**)

vention of Th2 activation by long-term anti-IgE treatment could lead to a decreased frequency of allergen specific Th2 cells. As a result the production of cytokines may shift from the production of Th2 to Th0 cytokines because newly formed allergen-specific T cells will not mature in a Th2-biasing environment. If this is the case, long-term treatment of patients with anti-IgE may turn out to be a causal treatment of the disease with long-term efficacy.

Conclusions

It is becoming more and more clear that anti-IgE treatment exerts its effects on several levels (Fig. 2). First, Anti-IgE treatment strongly decreases free serum IgE levels. Second, as a result of these decreased serum IgE levels the expression of FcεRI on basophils and mast cells is downregulated, thus preventing mast cell and basophil degranulation. We now hypothesize that thirdly, as IgE-mediated allergen presentation may be crucial for the perpetual activation of allergen-specific Th2 cells at low allergen doses, anti-IgE treatment has the quite unanticipated effect of inhibiting T-cell responses and therefore also late phase allergic responses.

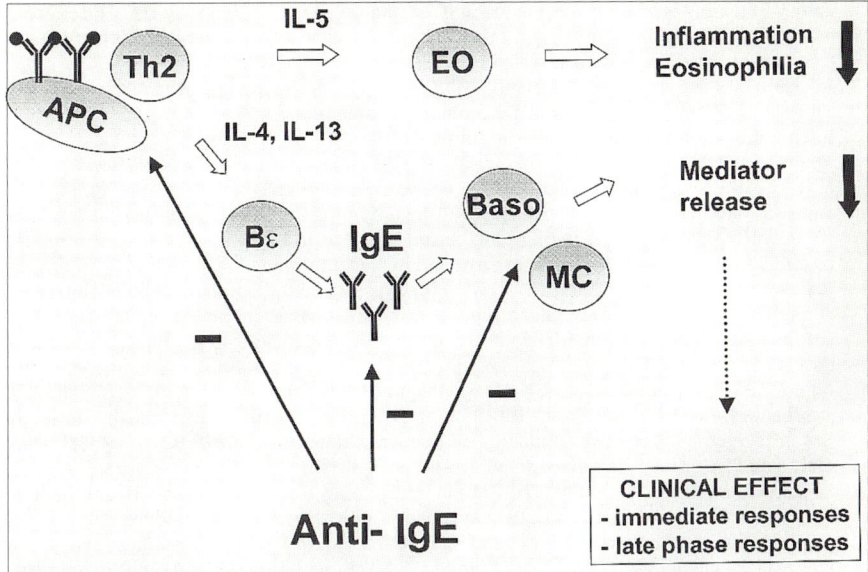

Fig. 2. Schematic representation of mechanisms of anti-IgE treatment

In addition, because IgE-mediated side effects may occur after specific allergy vaccination, anti-IgE in combination with specific allergy vaccination may enhance the safety profile and efficacy of allergy vaccination with allergenic extracts.

References

1. Presta L, Shields R, O'Connell L, Lahr S, Porter J, Gorman C, Jardieu,P. The binding site on human immunoglobulin E for its high affinity receptor. J.Biol.Chem. 1994 269:26368–26373
2. Chang TW, Davis FM, Sun NC, Sun CRY, MacGlashan DW, and Hamilton RG. Monoclonal antibodies specific for human IgE-producing B cells: a potential therapeutic for IgE mediated allergic disease. BioTechnology 1990, 8:122–126
3. Corne J, Djukanovic R, Thomas L, Warner J, Botta L, Grandordy B, Gygax D, Heusser C, Patalano F, Richardson W, Kilchherr E, Staehelin T, Davis F, Gordon W, Sun L, Liou R, Wang G, Chang TW, Holgate S.. The effect of intravenous administration of a chimeric anti-IgE antibody on serum IgE levels in atopic subjects: Efficacy, safety and pharmacokinetics. J.Clin.Invest. 1997 99:879–887
4. Casale TB, Bernstein L, Busse WW, LaForce CF, Tinkelman DG, Stoltz RR, Dockhorn RJ, Reimann J, Su JQ, Fick RB, Adelman DC. Use of an anti-IgE monoclonal antibody in ragweed-induced allergic rhinitis. J.Allergy Clin.Immunol. 1997. 100:110–121.
5. Fahy JV, Cockroft DW, Boulet LP, Wong HH, Deschenes F, Davis EE, Ruppel J, Su JQ, Adelman DC. Effect of aerosolized anti-IgE (E25) on airway responses to inhaled allergen in asthmatic subjects. Am.J.Resp.Crit. Care Med. 1999 160:1023–1027
6. MacGlashan DW Jr, Bochner BS, Adelman DC, Jardieu PM, Togias A, McKenzie-White J, Sterbinsky SA, Hamilton RG, Lichtenstein LM. Down-regulation of FcεRI expression on human basophils during in vivo treatment of atopic patients with anti-IgE antibody. J Immunol 1997;158:1438–1445

7. Fahy JV, Fleming HE,Wong HH, Liu JT, Su JQ, Reimann J, Fick RB, Boushey HA. The effect of an anti-IgE monoclonal antibody on the early- and late-phase responses to allergen inhalation in asthmatic subjects. Am.J.Respir. Crit.Care Med. 1997. 155:1828–1834.
8. Adelroth E, Rak S, Haahtela T, Aasand G, Rosenhall L, Zetterstrom O, Byrne A, Champain K, Thirlwell J, Cioppa GD, Sandstrom T. Recombinant humanized mAb-E25, an anti-IgE mAb, in birch pollen induced seasonal allergic rhinitis. J.Allergy Clin.Immunol. 2000;106:253–259.
9. Milgrom H, Fick RB Jr, Su JQ, Reimann JD, Bush RK, Watrous ML, Metzger WJ. Treatment of allergic asthma with monoclonal anti-IgE antibody. N Engl J Med 1999;341:1966–1973
10. Saini SS, MacGlashan DW Jr, Sterbinski SA, Togias A, Adelman DC, Lichtenstein LM, Bochner BS. Down-regulation of human basophil IgE and Fc?RI? surface densities and mediator release by anti-IgE-infusions is reversible in vitro and in vivo. J.Immunol. 1999; 162:5624–5630.
11. Racine-Poon A, Botta L, Chang TW, Davis FM, Gygax D, Liou RS, Rohane P, Staehelin T, van Steijn AMP, Frank W. Efficacy, pharmacodynamics, and pharmacokinetics of CGP 51901, and anti-immunoglobulin E chimeric monoclonal antibody, in patients with seasonal allergic rhinitis. Clin.Pharmacol. Ther. 1997 62:675–690.
12. Boulet LP, Chapman, KR, Cote J, Kalra S., Bhagat R, Swystun VA, Laviolette M, Cleland LD, Deschenes F, Su JQ, Devault A, Fick RB, Cockroft DW. Inhibitory effects of an anti-IgE antibody E25 on allergen-induced early asthmatic response. Am.J.Respir.Crit. Care Med. 1997 155:1835–1840.
13. Malveaux FJ, Conroy MC, Adkinson NF Jr, and Lichtenstein LM. J Clin Invest 1978;62:176.
14. Yamaguchi M, Lantz CS, Oettgen HC, Katona IM, Fleming T, Miyajima I, Kinet JP, and Galli SJ. IgE enhances mouse mast cell FcεRI expression in vitro and in vivo: evidence for a novel amplification mechanism in IgE-dependent reactions. J.Exp.Med. 1997 185:663–672
15. Lantz CS, Yamaguchi M, Oettgen HC, Katona IM, Miyajima I, Kinet JP, and Galli, SJ. IgE regulates mouse basophil FceRI expression in vivo. J.Immunol.1997 158:2517–2521.
16. Yamaguchi M, Sayama K, Yano K, Lantz CS, Noben-Trauth N, Ra C, Costa JJ, and Galli SJ. IgE enhances Fce receptor I expression and IgE dependent release of histamine and lipid mediators from human umbilical cord blood-derived mast cells: Synergistic effect of IL-4 and IgE on human mast cell Fce Receptor I expression and mediator release. J.Immunol. 1999 162:5455–5465
17. MacGlashan D, McKenzie-White J, Chichester K, Bochner BS, Davis FM, Schroeder JT, Lichtenstein LM. In vitro regulation of FcεRIα expression on human basophils by IgE antibody. Blood 1998; 91:1633–1643
18. Kinet JP. The high affinity IgE receptor (FcεRI): from physiology to pathology. Annu. Rev. Immunol. 1999. 17:931–972.
19. Toru H, Ra C, Nonoyama S, Suzuki K, Yata J, Nakahata T. Induction of the high affinity IgE receptor (Fc epsilon R I) on human mast cells by IL-4. Int. Immunol. 1996. 8:1367–1373
20. Nishiyama C, Toyokazu T, Okumura K, and Ra C. The transcription factors Elf-1 and GATA-1 bind to cell-specific enhancer elements of human high-affinity IgE receptor alpha-chain gene. J.Immunol. 1999.163:623–630.
21. Bieber T, De la Salle H, Wollenberg A, Hakimi J, Chizzonite R, Ring J, et al. Human epidermal Langerhans cells express the high affinity receptor for immunoglobulim E (Fc epsilon RI). 1992 J.Exp.Med. 175:1285–1290
22. Maurer, D., E. Fiebiger, B. Reininger, B. Wolff-Winiski, M. H. Jouvin, O. Kilgus, J. P. Kinet, and G. Stingl. Expression of functional high affinity immunoglobulin E receptors (FcεRI) on monocytes of atopic individuals. 1994.J. Exp. Med. 179:745–750.
23. Maurer D, Fiebiger E, Ebner C, Reiniger B, Fischer GF, Wichlas S, Jouvin MH, Schmitt-Egenolf M, Kraft D, Kinet JP, and Stingl G. Peripheral blood dendritic cells express FceRI as a complex composed of FceRIa and FceRIg-chains and can use this receptor for IgE –mediated allergen presentation. J.Immunol. 1996 157:607–616.
24. Wollenberg A, Kraft S, Hanau D, and Bieber T. Immunomorphological and ultrastructural characterization of epidermal Langerhans cells and a novel, inflammatory dendritic cell (IDEC) population in lesional skin of atopic eczema. J Invest Dermatol. 1996 ;106:446–453.
25. Kraft S, Wessendorf JH, Hanau D, and Bieber T. Regulation of the high affinity receptor for IgE on human epidermal Langerhans cells. J Immunol. 1998;161:1000–1006.
26. Reischl IG, Corvaia N, Effenberger F, Wolff-Winiski B, Krömer E, and Mudde GC. Function and regulation of FcεRI expression on monocytes from non-atopic donors. Clin Exp Allergy. 1996;26:630–641.

27. Geiger E, Magerstaedt R, Wessendorf JH, Kraft S, Hanau D, and Bieber T. IL-4 induces the intracellular expression of the a chain of the high-affinity receptor for IgE in in vitro generated dendritic cells. J Allergy Clin Immunol. 2000;105:150–156.

28. Kisselgof AB, and Oettgen HC. The expression of murine B cell CD23, in vivo, is regulated by its ligand, IgE. Int. Immunol. 1998 10:1377–1384.

29. Haak-Frandscho M, Robbins K, Lyon R, Shields R, Hooley J, Schoenhoff M, and Jardieu P. Administration of an anti-IgE antibody inhibits CD23 expression and IgE production in vivo. Immunology. 1994: 82:306–313.

30. Wierenga, E. A., M. Snoek, C. J. de Groot, I. Chrétien, J. D. Bos, H. M. Jansen, and M. L. Kapsenberg. 1990. Evidence for compartmentalization of functional subsets of CD4+ T lymphocytes in atopic patients. J. Immunol. 144:4651.

31. Parronchi, P., D. Macchia, M. Piccinni, P. Biswas, C. Simonelli, E. Maggi, M. Ricci, A. A. Ansari, and S. Romagnani. 1991. Allergen- and bacterial antigen-specific T-cell clones established from atopic donors show a different profile of cytokine production. Proc. Natl. Acad. Sci. USA 88:4538.

32. Takigawa, M., T. Tamamori, D. Horiguchi, T. Sakamoto, M. Yamada, A. Yoshioka, K. Toda, S. Imamura, and J. Yodo. 1991. Fce receptor II/CD23-positive lymphocytes in atopic dermatitis. I. The proportion of FcεRII+ lymphocytes correlates with the extent of skin lesions. Clin. Exp. Immunol. 84:275–282.

33. Mudde, G. C., F. C. van Reijsen, G. J. Boland, G. C. de Gast, P. L. B. Bruijnzeel, and C. A. F. M. Bruijnzeel-Koomen. 1990. Allergen presentation by epidermal Langerhans' cells from patients with atopic dermatitis is mediated by IgE. Immunology 69:335–641

34. van der Heijden FL, van Neerven RJJ, van Katwijk M, Bos JD, Kapsenberg ML. Serum IgE-facilitated allergen presentation in allergic disease. J. Immunol. 1993; 150:3643–3650.

35. Maurer D, Ebner C, Reininger B, Fiebiger E, Kraft D, Kinet JP, Stingl G. The High Affinity IgE Receptor (FcεRI) Mediates IgE-Dependent Allergen Presentation. J. Immunol. 1995;154:6285–6290.

36. Langeveld-Wilschut EG, Bruijnzeel PL, Mudde GC, Versluis C, van Ieperen-vanDijk AG, Bihari IC, Knol EF, Thepen T, Bruijnzeel-Koomen CA, and van Reijsen FC. Clinical and immunologic variables in skin of patients with atopic eczema and either positive or negative atopy patch test reactions. J. Allergy Clin. Immunol. 2000; 105:1008–1016.

37. Haselden BM, Kay AB, Larche M. Immunoglobulin E-independent major histocompatibility complex-restricted T-cell peptide epitope-induced late asthmatic reactions. J. Exp. Med. 1999; 189:1885–1894.

38. Krinzman SJ, Desanctis GT, Cernadas M, Mark D, Wang YS, Listman J, Kobzik L, Donovan C, Nassr K, Katona I, Christiani DC, Perkins DL, and Finn PW. Inhibition of T-cell costimulation abrogates airway hyperresponsiveness in a murine model. J. Clin. Invest. 1996;98:2693–2699.

39. van Neerven RJJ, Wikborg T, Lund G, Jakobsen B, Brinch-Nielsen Å, Arnved J, Ipsen H. Blocking antibodies induced by specific allergy vaccination prevent the activation of CD4+ T cells by Inhibiting serum-IgE-facilitated allergen presentation. J. Immunol. 1999;163: 2944–2952.

40. R.J.J. van Neerven, C.P.A.A. van Roomen, W. Thomas, M. de Boer, E.F. Knol and F.M. Davis. Humanized anti-IgE mAb Hu-901 prevents the activation of allergen-specific T cells. Int. Arch. Allergy Immunol In press.

Subject Index

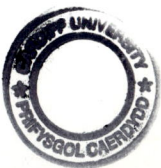

Printing (Computer to Film): Saladruck Berlin
Binding: Stürtz AG, Würzburg